PRINCIPLES AND PRACTICE OF BURN SURGERY

Juan P. Barret-Nerín, M.D.
*St. Andrew's Centre for Plastic Surgery and Burns,
Broomfield Hospital, Essex, United Kingdom*

David N. Herndon, M.D.
*Galveston Shriners Hospital, Texas
University of Texas Medical Branch, Houston, Texas*

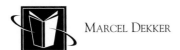 MARCEL DEKKER   NEW YORK

Library of Congress Cataloging-in-Publication Data
A catalog record for this book is available from the Library of Congress.

ISBN: 0-8247-5453-0

This book is printed on acid-free paper.

Headquarters
Marcel Dekker, 270 Madison Avenue, New York, NY 10016, U.S.A.
tel: 212-696-9000; fax: 212-685-4540

Distribution and Customer Service
Marcel Dekker, Cimarron Road, Monticello, New York 12701, U.S.A.
tel: 800-228-1160; fax: 845-796-1772

World Wide Web
http://www.dekker.com

The publisher offers discounts on this book when ordered in bulk quantities. For more information, write to Special Sales/Professional Marketing at the headquarters address above.

Current printing (last digit):

10 9 8 7 6 5 4 3 2 1

PRINTED IN THE UNITED STATES OF AMERICA

To my wife Esther, who is everything;
to my daughter Julia, who is even more;
and to my parents,
Juan Pedro (1933–2004) and Adelaida, who made me who I am.

Juan P. Barret

Preface

With an overall incidence of more than 800 cases per 1 million persons per year, only motor vehicle accidents cause more accidental deaths than burns. Advances in trauma and burn management over the past three decades have resulted in improved survival and reduced morbidity from major burns. Twenty-five years ago, the mortality rate of a 50% body surface area burn in a young adult was about 50%, despite treatment. Today, that same burn results in less than 10% mortality. Ten years ago, an 80 to 90% body surface area burn yielded 10% survival. Today, over 50% of these patients survive.

Nevertheless, although burn injuries are frequent in our society, many physicians feel uncomfortable managing patients with thermal injuries. Excellent textbooks about the pathophysiology of thermal injury and inhalation injury have recently been published. All new data produced by active research in the field of burn and trauma can be found in these books. Yet, the state-of-the-art techniques in the day-to-day care of burn patients—either as outpatients, in the operating room, or in the burn intensive care unit—have yet to be outlined in a single volume.

The current project includes all current techniques available today for the care of burn patients. Improved results in survival are due to advancements in resuscitation, operative techniques, infection control, and nutritional/metabolic support. All these improvements are included in the book, along with all the available techniques for burn shock treatment, hypermetabolic response support, new hemostatic and skin substitutes, and pain and psychology support and rehabilitation.

General surgeons, plastic surgeons, medical and surgical residents, emergency room physicians, senior students, and any kind of physician or burn team member involved in burn treatment in either community hospitals or burn centers would benefit from the present book, which not only outlines the basics of burn syndrome but also provides an overview of options for burn treatment. The book has been organized in a stepwise manner, with clear information as if the reader would be involved in weekly grand round, day-to-day work with the burn surgeon, anesthetist, or any other burn team member. We sincerely hope that it will serve its purpose of establishing the main principles of surgical treatment of burn injuries.

Juan P. Barret
David N. Herndon

Contents

Contributors

Juan P. Barret, MD, PhD Broomfield Hospital, Chelmsford, Essex, United Kingdom

Patricia Blakeney Shriners Burns Hospital, Galveston, Texas, U.S.A.

Peter Dziewulski Broomfield Hospital, Chelmsford, Essex, United Kingdom

Scott A. Farmer Shriners Burns Hospital, Galveston, Texas, U.S.A.

Lee D. Faucher University of Washington Burn Center, Seattle, Washington, U.S.A.

Tomás Gómez-Cía Hospital Universitario Virgen del Rocío, Seville, Spain

David M. Heimbach University of Washington Burn Center, Seattle, Washington, U.S.A.

David N. Herndon Shriners Hospital for Children and The University of the Texas Medical Branch, Galveston, Texas, U.S.A.

Jong O. Lee Shriners Hospital for Children and The University of the Texas Medical Branch, Galveston, Texas, U.S.A.

Walter J. Meyer III Shriners Burns Hospital, Galveston, Texas, U.S.A.

Ronald P. Mlcak   Shriners Hospitals for Children–Galveston and the University of Texas Medical Branch, Galveston, Texas, U.S.A.

Kevin D. Murphy   Shriners Hospital for Children and The University of the Texas Medical Branch, Galveston, Texas, U.S.A.

José I. Ortega-Martínez   Hospital Universitario Virgen del Rocío, Seville, Spain

Michael A. Serghiou   Shriners Burns Hospital, Galveston, Texas, U.S.A.

Edward R. Sherwood   Shriners Hospitals for Children–Galveston and the University of Texas Medical Branch, Galveston, Texas, U.S.A.

Steven E. Wolf   The University of Texas Medical Branch, Galveston, Texas, U.S.A.

Lee C. Woodson   Shriners Hospitals for Children–Galveston and the University of Texas Medical Branch, Galveston, Texas, U.S.A.

1

Initial Management and Resuscitation

Juan P. Barret
Broomfield Hospital, Chelmsford, Essex, United Kingdom

INTRODUCTION

Trauma can be defined as bodily injury severe enough to pose a threat to life, limbs, and tissues and organs, which requires the immediate intervention of specialized teams to provide adequate outcomes. Burn injury, unlike other traumas, can be quantified as to the exact percentage of body injured, and can be viewed as a paradigm of injury from which many lessons can be learned about critical illness involving multiple organ systems. Proper initial management is critical for the survival and good outcome of the victim of minor and major thermal trauma. However, even though burn injuries are frequent in our society, many surgeons feel uncomfortable in managing patients with major thermal trauma. Every year, 2.5 million Americans sustain a significant burn injury, 100,000 are hospitalized, and over 10,000 die. Only motor vehicle accidents cause more accidental deaths than burns. Advances in trauma and burn management over the past three decades have resulted in improved survival and reduced mortality from major burns. Twenty-five years ago, the mortality rate of a 50% body surface area (BSA) burn in a young adult was about 50%, despite treatment. Today, that same burn results in a lower than 10% mortality rate. Ten years ago, an 80–90% BSA burn yielded 10% survival. Today, over 50% of these patients are surviving. Improved results are due to advancements in resuscitation, surgical techniques, infection control, and nutritional/metabolic support.

1

The skin is the largest organ in the body, making up 15% of body weight, and covering approximately 1.7 m² in the average adult. The function of the skin is complex: it warms, it senses, and it protects. A burn injury implies damage or destruction of skin and/or its contents by thermal, chemical, electrical, or radiation energies or combinations thereof. Thermal injuries are by far the most common and frequently present with concomitant inhalation injuries. Of its two layers, only the epidermis is capable of true regeneration. When the skin is seriously damaged, this external barrier is violated and the internal milieu is altered.

Following a major burn injury, myriad physiological changes occur that together comprise the clinical scenario of the burn patient. These derangements include the following:

Fluid and electrolyte imbalance: The burn wound becomes rapidly edematous. In burns over 25% BSA, this edema develops in normal noninjured tissues. This results in systemic intravascular losses of water, sodium, albumin, and red blood cells. Unless intravascular volume is rapidly restored, shock develops.

Metabolic disturbances: This is evidenced by hypermetabolism and muscle catabolism. Unless early enteral nutrition and pharmacological intervention restore it, malnutrition and organ dysfunction develop.

Bacterial contamination of tissues.

Complications from vital organs.

The successful treatment of burn patients includes the intervention of a multidisciplinary burn team (Table 1). The purpose of the burn center and the burn team is to care for and treat persons with dangerous and potentially disabling burns from the time of the initial injury through rehabilitation. The philosophy of care is based on the concept that each patient is an individual with special needs. Each patient's care, from the day of admission, is designed to return him or her to society as a functional, adaptable, and integrated citizen.

INITIAL BURN MANAGEMENT

The general trauma guidelines apply to the initial burn assessment. A primary survey should be undertaken in the burn admission's room or in the Accidents and Emergency Department, followed by a secondary survey when resuscitation is underway.

The primary survey should focus on the following areas:

Airway (with C-spine control): Voice, air exchange, and patency should be noted.

Breathing: Check breath sounds, chest wall excursion, and neck veins.

Circulation: Mentation should be noted. Check skin color, pulse, blood pressure, neck veins, and any external bleeding.

TABLE 1 Members of the Burn Team

Burn surgeons (general and plastic surgeons)
Nurses
    Intensive care
    Acute and reconstructive wards
    Scrub and anesthesia nurses
Case managers (acute and reconstructive)
Anesthesiologists
Respiratory therapists
Rehabilitation therapists
Dietitians
Psychosocial experts
Social workers
Volunteers
Microbiologists
Research personnel
Quality control personnel
Support services

Neurological assessment: Check Glasgow coma score.
Expose the patient.

At this point a rough estimate of the extent of the injury should be made and resuscitation efforts focus on physiological derangements.

Initial resuscitation steps include the following:

1. Administer oxygen nasally or by mask. Intubate if patency of airway is at risk or massive edema is to be expected.
2. Insert at least two large peripheral intravenous (IV) catheters. Delays in resuscitation are costly. Therefore introduce IV catheter through burned or unburned skin.
3. Start Ringer's lactate at 1 L/h.
4. Insert nasogastric tube.
5. Insert urinary catheter.
6. Wrap patient in thermal blanket or place under thermal panel.
7. Splint deformed extremities.

The following are taken from the general Arrival Checklist at the University of Texas Medical Branch/Shriners Burns Hospital:

ABCs of Trauma:

Establish airway
Check breathing

Administer oxygen
Control external bleeding
Insert IVs, Foley catheter, nasogastric tube (NGT)
Initiate fluid resuscitation
Search for associated injuries

Patient Evaluation

AMPLE history (see below)
Immunization status
Check accompanying referral paperwork
Complete physical examination
Rule out occult injuries
Complete laboratory evaluation (see below)
Other x-ray exams if needed
Clean and gently debride wounds
Culture (blood, urine, wound, sputum)
Photographs
Burn diagrams: size and depth

Fluid Requirement Calculation

Measure height and weight
Determine total BSA and BSA burned
Resuscitation formula (see below)

Circulation Assessment

Escharotomies
Splint and elevate
Serial exams

Infection Prevention

Tetanus prophylaxis
Streptococcus prophylaxis 48 h (children only)
Major injuries: pre/perioperative systemic empirical antibiotics (based on
    local sensitivities)

Metabolic Support

Prevent hypothermia
Comfort measures: sedation, analgesics (see below)
Hormonal manipulation (see Chap. 13)

Burn Wound Treatment

Gentle debridement
Remove or aspirate blisters
Apply burn dressing (apply clear plastic film if patient is to be seen in the morning ward rounds)

Supportive Treatment

Ventilatory management
Physiotherapy
Psychosocial support

Surgical Wound Closure

Notify operating room and anesthesia service
Notify blood bank
Notify skin bank

INITIAL ASSESSMENT OF THE BURNED PATIENT

Treatment of the burn injury begins at the scene of the accident. The first priority is to stop the burning. The patient must be separated from the burning source. For thermal burns, immediate application of cold compresses can reduce the amount of damaged tissue. Prolonged cooling, however, can precipitate a dangerous hypothermia. For electrical burns, the source should be removed with a nonconducting object. In cases of chemical burns, the agent should be diluted with copious irrigation, not immersion. The initial physical examination of the burn victim should focus on assessing the airway, evaluating hemodynamic status, accurately determining burn size, and assessing burn wound depth. Immediate assessment of the airway is always the first priority. Massive airway edema can occur, leading to acute airway obstruction and death. If there is any question as to the adequacy of the airway, prompt endotracheal intubation is mandated. All burn victims should initially receive 100% oxygen by mask or tube to reduce the likelihood of problems from pulmonary dysfunction or carbon monoxide poisoning. The next step is to place two large-bore peripheral intravenous catheters, since delays in resuscitation carry a high mortality. Patients with burns of less than 15% (10% in children) BSA who are conscious and cooperative can often be resuscitated orally. The patient with more than 15% (10% in children) BSA burn requires IV access. Begin infusion of Ringer's lactate solution of about 1000 ml/h in adults, 400–500 ml/m^2 BSA/h in children, until more accurate assessments of burn size and fluid requirements can be made. An indwelling Foley catheter should be placed to monitor urinary output. A nasogastric tube is inserted for gastric decompression.

It is also imperative during the initial assessment to make a brief survey of associated injuries. A thorough secondary survey can be postponed, but life-threatening injuries such as cardiac tamponade, pneumothorax, hemothorax, external hemorrhage, and flail chest must be identified and treated promptly.

Patient evaluation should include what is termed an AMPLE history: allergies, medications, pre-existing diseases, last meal, and events of the injury, including time, location, and insults. In children the developmental status should be investigated and any suspicious injuries should raise the possibility of child abuse. A history of loss of consciousness should be sought. A complete physical examination should include a careful neurological examination, since evidence of cerebral anoxic injury can be subtle. While the initial resuscitation has been started, a thorough physical examination is performed. All systems should be examined, including genital and rectal examination. Associated injuries should be ruled out at this stage and treated accordingly. All extremities should be examined for pulses, especially in patients with circumferential burns. Evaluation of pulses can be assisted by use of a Doppler ultrasound flowmeter. If pulses are absent, and fluid resuscitation is adequate, the involved limb should undergo urgent escharotomy to release the constrictive eschar. It must be noted, however, that the most common cause of pulseless limbs is inadequate resuscitation. Therefore, the intravascular status of the patient must be assessed before proceeding with escharotomies.

Escharotmies can be performed at the bedside with IV sedation. It is preferable to use electrocautery to prevent excessive bleeding. Placement of escharotomies is shown in Figure 1. It is important to note that only the burned skin should be released. Incisions through the subcutaneous tissue do not increase the decompression and only add more scarring in the rehabilitation period. If excessive tension is noted after escharotomy, a formal fasciotomy should be considered. Linear scars should be avoided when crossing joints. Darts should be used in this anatomical location as well as in the neck. Patients with circumferential burns on the chest may also benefit from escharotomies to improve chest excursion and compliance.

The primary and secondary survey as well as the initial resuscitation should be performed under thermal panels or in a high-temperature environment. Burned patients can become rapidly hypothermic. Should this complication occur, it carries a high mortality. Thermal blankets and fluid warmers are good aids in fighting hypothermia. As a last resort, if all measures to prevent hypothermia fail or are not feasible, the patient should be urgently transferred to the operating room to continue resuscitation efforts where a well-controlled, high-temperature environ-

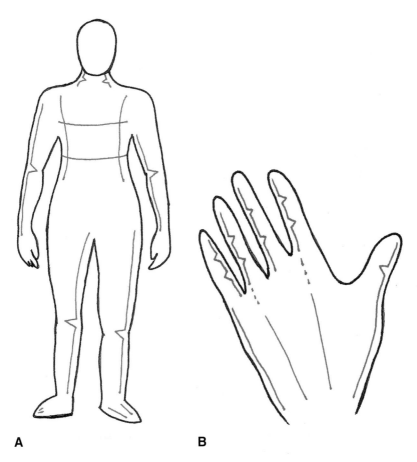

A   **B**

FIGURE 1 Suggested placement of escharotomies in the trunk and limbs (A) and on the hand (B). Note that darts should be included so that linear hypertrophic scar do not result.

TABLE 2 Primary Assessment

1. Administer 100% humidified oxygen.
2. Monitor respiratory status.
3. Endotracheal intubation if upper respiratory obstruction is likely.
4. Expose chest to assess ventilatory exchange (rule out circumferential burns).
5. Assess ventilatory exchange after establishing a clear airway.
6. Assess blood pressure and pulse
7. Accomplish cervical spine stabilization until the condition can be evaluated.
8. Identify life-threatening conditions (tension pneumothorax, open or flail chest, cardiac tamponade, acute hemorrhage, acute hypovolemic shock, etc.) and treat.

ment under thermal panels and fluid warmers is readily available. Primary and secondary assessments are summarized in Tables 2 and 3.

Burn Wound Assessment

After the patient's stabilization and initial resuscitation, physicians should focus on the burn wound. Burns are gently cleansed with warm saline and antiseptics, and the extent of the burn is assessed. Burn injury must be categorized as the exact percentage of BSA involved. The rule of nines is a very good approximation as an initial assessment (see Fig. 2). Another good rule of thumb is measuring the extent of the injury with the palm of the burn victim, which is estimated as 1% BSA. The area burned is transformed as the number of hand palms affected and then multiplied by 1%.

TABLE 3 Secondary Assessment

1. Initial trauma assessment and primary assessment completed.
2. Thorough head-to-toe evaluation.
3. Careful determination of trauma other than obvious burn wounds.
4. Use cervical collard, backboards, and splints before moving the patient.
5. Examine past medical history, medications, allergies, and mechanism of injury.
6. Establish intravenous access through large peripheral catheters (×2) and administer intravenous fluids through a warming system.
7. Protect wounds from the environment with application of clean dressings (topical antimicrobials not necessary).
8. Determine needs for transportation. Contact receiving facility for further instructions.

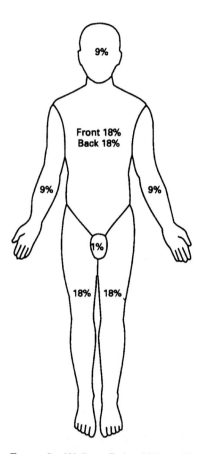

FIGURE 2 Wallace Rule of Nines. The extent of the injury can be estimated rapidly with this method. It may over- or underestimate the extent of the injury; therefore, a more accurate assessment is necessary on arrival at the admissions or emergency department, or burn center (see Fig. 3 for comparison).

The best way to measure the area burned accurately is the Lund and Browder Chart (see Fig. 3). In this method, the areas burned are plotted in the burn diagram, and every area burned is assigned an exact percentage. The Lund and Browder method takes into consideration the differences in anatomical location that exist in the pediatric population and therefore does not over or underestimate the burn size in patients of different ages. After the burn size is determined, the individual characteristics of the patient should be plotted in a standard nomogram to determine the body surface area and burned surface area of the patient (see Fig. 4). Measuring and weighing the patient in centimeters and kilograms provides the surface area of the patient in square meters. This measurement will help to calculate metabolic needs, blood loss, hemodynamic parameters, and skin substitutes.

At this point, the specific anatomical location of the burn should be noted as well as the depth of the burn per location. These measurements are to be noted also in the burn diagram, and will help in planning individual treatment for the patient. The eyes are explored with fluorescein and green lamp to rule out corneal damage; the oral cavity and perineum are explored to rule out any obvious internal damage.

Age	0–1	1–4	5–9	10–14	15
A – $\frac{1}{2}$ of head	$9\frac{1}{2}$%	$8\frac{1}{2}$%	$6\frac{1}{2}$%	$5\frac{1}{2}$%	$4\frac{1}{2}$%
B – $\frac{1}{2}$ of one thigh	$2\frac{3}{4}$%	$3\frac{1}{4}$%	4%	$4\frac{1}{4}$%	$4\frac{1}{2}$%
C – $\frac{1}{2}$ of one leg	$2\frac{1}{2}$%	$2\frac{1}{2}$%	$2\frac{3}{4}$%	3%	$3\frac{1}{4}$%

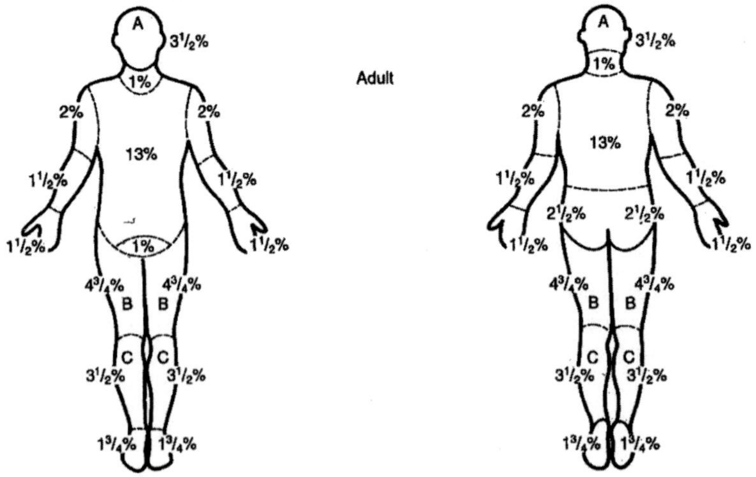

FIGURE 3 The Lund and Browder Chart is a good estimate of burn surface area (A).

BURN DIAGRAM   Shriners Burns Institute – Galveston Unit

Age:_____ Sex:_____ Date of admission_____

Type of burn: Flame ☐   Electrical ☐   Scald ☐   Chemical ☐   Inhalation injury ☐

Date of burn: _____

Date completed: _____

Completed by: _____

Date revised: _____

Revised by: _____

Approved by: _____

■ 3rd°

▨ 2nd°

Height (cm)_____
Weight (kg)_____
Body surface (m²)_____
Total burn (m²)_____
3° Burn (m²)_____

Associated injuries/comments:

_____
_____
_____

BURN ESTIMATE – AGE VS. AREA

Area	Birth–1 year	1–4 years	5–9 years	10–14 years	15 years	Adult	2°	3°	TBSA %
Head	19	17	13	11	9	7			
Neck	2	2	2	2	2	2			
Ant. trunk	13	13	13	13	13	13			
Post. trunk	13	13	13	13	13	13			
R. buttock	2.5	2.5	2.5	2.5	2.5	2.5			
L. buttock	2.5	2.5	2.5	2.5	2.5	2.5			
Genitalia	1	1	1	1	1	1			
R.U. arm	4	4	4	4	4	4			
L.U. arm	4	4	4	4	4	4			
R.L. arm	3	3	3	3	3	3			
L.L. arm	3	3	3	3	3	3			
R. hand	2.5	2.5	2.5	2.5	2.5	2.5			
L. hand	2.5	2.5	2.5	2.5	2.5	2.5			
R. thigh	5.5	6.5	8	8.5	9	9.5			
L. thigh	5.5	6.5	8	8.5	9	9.5			
R. leg	5	5	5.5	6	6.5	7			
L. leg	5	5	5.5	6	6.5	7			
R. foot	3.5	3.5	3.5	3.5	3.5	3.5			
L. foot	3.5	3.5	3.5	3.5	3.5	3.5			
						TOTAL			

B

FIGURE 3 (Cont.) It takes into account the differences in size of different anatomical locations to prevent any over- or underestimation of burn size. It is strongly advised to use the chart together with the rest of the initial assessment documentation (B).

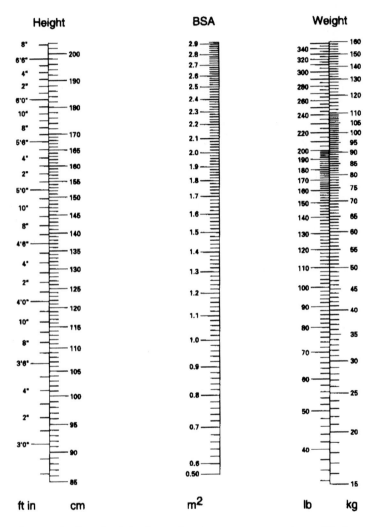

FIGURE 4 Standard body surface nomogram and modified nomogram for children (A).

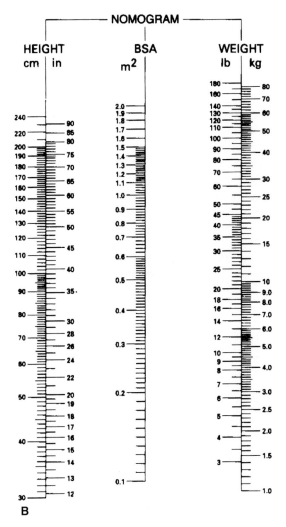

FIGURE 4 (**Cont.**) Modified nomogram for children. Weight and height are connected with a straight line, pointing to the body surface area in the center column (B).

In ventilated patients or patients with suspected smoke inhalation injury, direct bronchoscopy should be performed to determine the extent of the injury and start treatment if necessary. In nonintubated patients, a tube can be mounted on the bronchoscope to help nasotracheal intubation if this maneuver is deemed necessary (see Fig. 5). After direct bronchoscopic examination is completed, a definitive diagnosis is made based on clinical, laboratory, and bronchoscopic

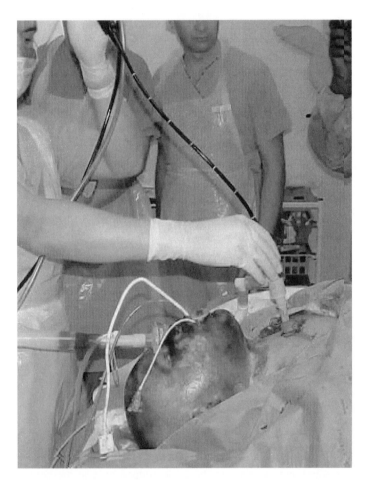

FIGURE 5   Direct bronchoscopy remains the gold standard diagnostic test for inhalation injury. It is readily available and allows diagnosis and therapeutic lavage of soot and damaged epithelium. If it is performed nasally in an orally intubated patient, an endotracheal tube can be mounted with the bronchoscope to convert it to nasotracheal intubation.

findings. Patients with inhalation injury are then started in the inhalation injury protocol (see below).

After definitive assessment in the burn center (see Table 4), a final diagnosis regarding the burn wounds (extent and depth), accompanying injuries, and smoke inhalation injury is reached. At this point burn wounds should be covered with a clean burn wound dressing. Compressive dressings should be avoided, because they can induce further hypoperfusion and conversion of partial-thickness wounds to full-thickness. Different dressings are available in the market. If the definitive treatment includes immediate burn wound excision, burns should be covered with Telfa clear (Kendall) or plastic film, while the patient is awaiting definitive surgery. Topical antimicrobials are not necessary if this treatment is chosen. When the treatment of choice of full-thickness burns is early burn wound excision in 72 h, after resuscitation is completed, burns can be treated either with 1% silver sulfadiazine (Flammazine, Silvadene) or cerium nitrate–silver sulfadiazine (Flammacerium) during the period between the accident and the definitive surgery. Partial-thickness burns are treated in a similar initial manner. Patients are covered with plastic film or Telfa clear until definitive assessment by a senior surgeon is performed. Small superficial burns are usually treated with Mepitel (Monlicke) or any other semiocclusive method. Large superficial burns are treated with Biobrane (Bertek Pharmaceuticals Inc) or TransCyte (Infromagen Inc) (see Table 5).

Determining burn depth requires experience. It is an important part of the burn assessment because the depth of the burn will determine the treatment option and the patient's outcome. It must be noted, however, that even in the hands of experienced burn surgeons clinical inspection alone can be misleading in more than 40% of patients, leading to an under-or overestimate of the depth of the burn wound. Laser Doppler scanning has emerged as a good tool in the diagnosis

TABLE 4 Definitive Assessment in the Burn Center

---

1. Primary assessment.
2. Secondary assessment.
3. Establish intravenous line and initiate resuscitation if not started.
4. Establish history of the injury and obtain AMPLE history.
5. Perform complete physical examination (with neurological and corneal examination).
6. Examine extremities and record circumferential burns and pulses.
7. Perform escharotomies if needed.
8. Evaluate wounds.
9. Evaluate airway and perform direct bronchoscopy if needed.
10. Estimate burn size and depth.
11. Conduct laboratory tests.

TABLE 5   Initial Burn Wound Treatment

Partial-Thickness Burns

Cover burns with Telfa-clear or plastic film until definitive diagnosis by experienced burn surgeon.

Minor burn: Mepitel or semiocclusive dressing (special locations: silver sulfadiazine)

Large burn: Synthetic artificial skin (Biobrane, TransCyte) or pig skin

Full-Thickness Burns

Immediate burn wound excision protocol (24 h): – Telfa clear or plastic film

Early burn wound excision protocol (72 h): silver sulfadiazine or cerium nitrate–silver sulfadiazine

Staged excision protocol (first week): cerium nitrate silver sulfadiazine

---

of burn depth. It provides good mapping of the depth of the wound, especially in those burns defined as of indeterminate depth (Fig. 6).

Burn wound have been classically categorized as first-, second-, and third-degree. First-degree burns are superficial and involve just the epidermis. Typified by sunburn, first-degree burns are inconsequential in subsequent burn management. They heal in 5–7 days. Oral intolerance and severe discomfort requiring hospitalization may accompany large first-degree burns. These burns have a red, hyperemic appearance of the surface, which, along with the hypersensibility and discomfort, is typical of these injuries (see Fig. 7).

Second-degree burns, also called partial-thickness burns, involve variable amounts of dermis (see Fig. 8). Second-degree burns are subdivided into superficial and deep second-degree wounds. In superficial second-degree burns, the epidermis and the superficial (papillary) dermis have been damaged. Blistering and extreme pain are typical. Sensation is preserved with different degrees of hyperesthesia. A moist, pink appearance that blanches with pressure, along with extreme pain and hyperesthesia, is common in these injuries. Regeneration occurs by proliferation of epithelial cells from hair follicles and sweat gland ducts. Healing is almost complete within 3 weeks, leaving no scarring if no complications occur. Surgery is seldom needed in this injury.

In deep second-degree burns, however, the epidermis, papillary dermis, and various depths of the reticular (deep) dermis have been damaged. Regeneration occurs much more slowly than in superficial burns. Complete healing take more than 3 weeks and scarring and infection are common. These injuries are best treated surgically, since excision of the dead tissue and skin grafting shorten hospital stay and improve outcomes. Deep second-degree burns tend to be hypoesthetic, presenting with less pain than superficial burns. They have a white–pink appearance and blistering does not normally occur, or is present many hours after the injury. A dry appearance is common.

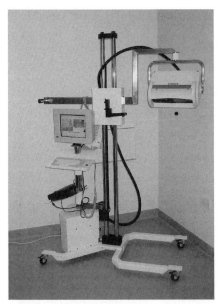

A

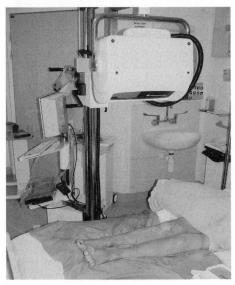

B

FIGURE 6 The laser Doppler scanner (A) is helpful for the diagnosis of burn wound depth. Its sensitivity and specificity are best between 48 and 72 h after the injury. It is placed over the area to be scanned (B), and in few seconds it produces a digitized image of the burn wound.

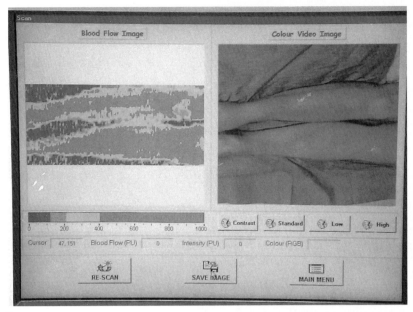

C

FIGURE 6 (Cont.)   Red areas are superficial burns with strong dermal vascularization. Blue areas are full-thickness burns (C). Air and normal skin show as blue areas.

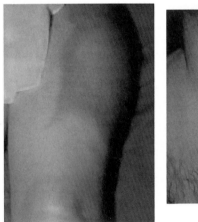 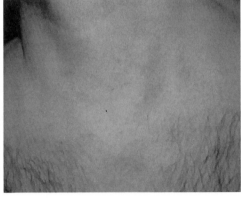

FIGURE 7   First-degree burns. Only the epidermis has been damaged. Typical appearance is that of a hyperemic area with severe discomfort and hyperestesia. Such burns do not blister, and they generally desquamate between 4 and 7 days after injury.

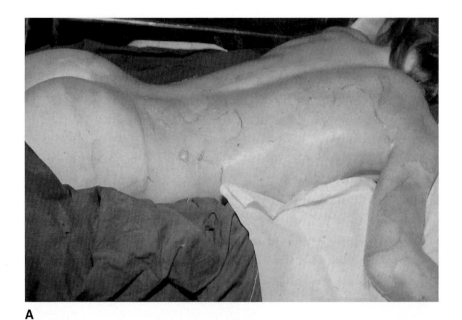

A

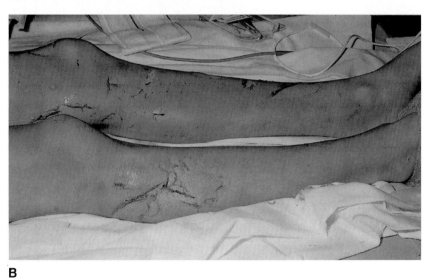

B

FIGURE 8 Second-degree burn injuries (or partial-thickness burns) present with different degrees of damage to the dermis. Pain is very intense (A, B). They usually blach with pressure and do not usually leave any permanent scarring.

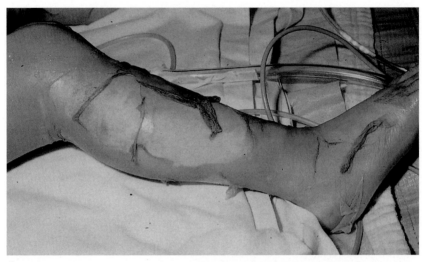

C

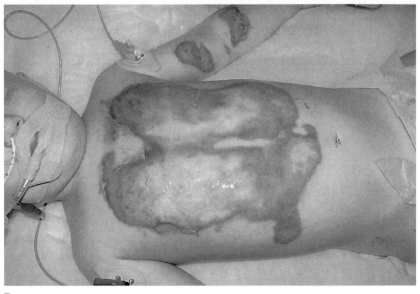

D

Figure 8 (Cont.)   Deep second-degree burns present with lesser degrees of pain and usually a prolonged healing time. Deep portions of the dermis have been damaged and they tend to leave permanent changes on the skin (C, D).

In contrast to the former injuries, third degree burns or full-thickness burns never heal spontaneously, and treatment involves excision of all injured tissue (Fig. 9). In these injuries, epidermis, dermis, and different depths of subcutaneous and deep tissues have been damaged. Pain involved is very low (usually with marginal partial-thickness burns) or absent. The potential for infection if left nonexcised is very high. A dry, white, or charred appearance is common. In infants and patients with immersion scalds, the burns may appear cherry red, and they may be misleading in nonexperienced hands.

Burns that affect deep structures, such as bones and internal organs, are categorized as fourth-degree burns. These injuries are typical of high-voltage electrical injuries and flammable agents, and have a high mortality rate. Some partial-thickness burns, however, present with a mixture of depths, with areas that are very difficult to categorize either as superficial or deep partial-thickness. They are usually termed indeterminate depth burns. Management of these injuries has been conservative treatment for 10–14 days followed by a second assessment and definitive diagnosis. Burns that then have the potential to heal in less than 3 weeks do not require skin grafting. In contrast, burns that will not heal at that point within 3 weeks are then operated on and skin grafted. We do know that burns that heal in less than 3 weeks do so without scarring or with minimal changes in pigmentation. With the aid of laser Doppler scanning, however, most of these burns can be categorized at 48 h after the injury as either superficial or deep, and definitive treatment can be begun without much delay.

After a definitive diagnosis has been made regarding size and depth, burns can be classified as minor, moderate, or major injuries (see Table 6). A major burn injury is defined as greater than 25% BSA involvement (15% in children) or more than 10% BSA full-thickness involvement. Major burns require aggressive resuscitation, hospitalization, and appropriate burn care. Additional criteria for major burns include deep burns of the hands, feet, eyes, ears, face, or perineum; inhalation injuries; associated medical conditions; extreme age; and electrical burns. All the former are formal criteria for transfer to a burn center. Moderate thermal burns of 15–25% BSA or 3–10% BSA full-thickness often require hospitalization to ensure optimal patient care. Other criteria for admission include concomitant trauma, significant pre-existing disease, and suspicion of child abuse. Minor burns can generally be treated on an outpatient basis.

LABORATORY AND COMPLEMENTARY TESTS

Routine admission laboratory evaluations should include the following:

Complete blood count
Coagulation tests, including D-dimmers and fibrinogen
Blood group type and screen

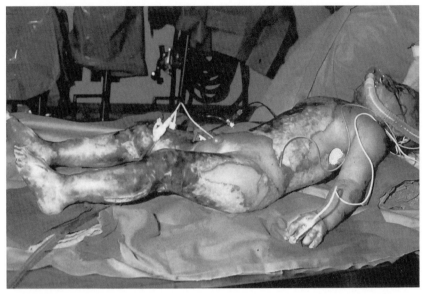

A

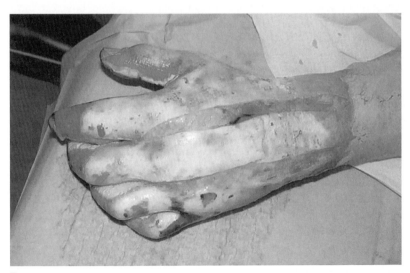

B

Figure 9 Third-degree burns present with complete destruction of the skin and different degrees of soft tissues (A). Their appearance ranges from white, non-blanching, and leathery (B) to nonblanching, red discoloration due to hemoglobin denaturation

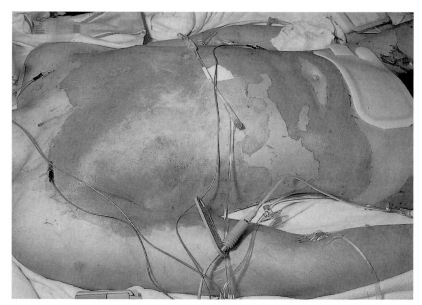

C

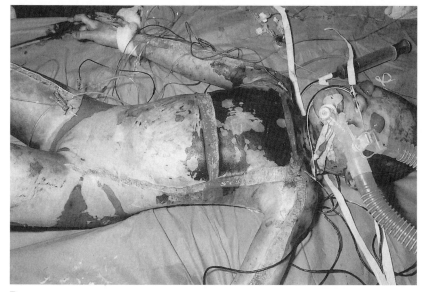

D

FIGURE 9 (Cont.) (C, D). A charred leathery dry eschar is typical of flame burns, more obvious in burns caused by ignited liquid flammables.

TABLE 6 Classification of Burn Injuries

Minor Burns
1. Less than 15% body surface area (less than 10% in children)
2. Less than 3% full-thickness
3. Not involving the head, feet, hands, or perineum

Moderate Burns
1. Burn area of 15–25% body surface area (10–15% in children)
2. Full-thickness burns involving 3–10% body surface area
3. Superficial partial-thickness burns of the head, hands, feet, or perineum
4. Suspected child abuse
5. Concomitant trauma
6. Significant pre-existing disease
7. Extreme age

Major Burns
1. Burn surface involvement of more than 25% body surface area (15% in children)
2. Full-thickness burns of more than 10% body surface area
3. Deep burns of the head, hands, feet, and perineum
4. Inhalation injury
5. Chemical burns
6. Electrical burns

>Serum electrolytes
>Glucose
>Blood urea nitrogen (BUN)
>Creatinine
>Total proteins, albumin, and globulins
>Calcium, phosphorus, and magnesium
>Osmolality
>Liver function test
>C-reactive protein
>Total CO_2
>Arterial blood gas, including lactate and Carboxyhemoglobin (HbCO)
>Urine analysis, including urine electrolytes
>Creatine phosphokinase (CPK), CPK-MB, and troponine in electrical injuries

These tests should be performed on admission, and every 8 h during the resuscitation phase. After the first 72 h they should done routinely as a daily basis, repeating the determination on an individual basis depending on the abnormalities encountered. When patients are admitted to the ward or transferred from the burns intensive care unit (BICU), lab tests are performed twice per week, unless the clinical condition dictates otherwise.

Other complementary tests include chest x-ray and other x-ray examinations performed on an individual basis. A 12 lead electrocardiogram should be obtained in all patients on admission and should repeated periodically in all electrical injuries.

Routine cultures are obtained on admission as part of the infection control protocol. They are then repeated twice per week unless dictated otherwise by the patient's clinical picture. Cultures should include blood, urine, sputum, throat, wound, and gastric/jejunal aspirates. Feces are sent for culture when available.

Ultrasonography, endoscopy, bronchoscopy, and other evaluations should be readily available on an individual patient basis.

FLUID RESUSCITATION

The most crucial aspect of early care of the burn patient is prompt initiation of volume replacement of large quantities of salt-containing fluids to maintain adequate perfusion of vital organs. Many formulas for burn resuscitation have proven clinically efficacious, and each differs in volume, sodium, and colloid content. The aim of any fluid resuscitation is to have a lucid, alert, and cooperative patient with good urine output.

Guidelines for correct resuscitation include the following:

Do not delay resuscitation.
Estimate burn size and calculate fluid requirements.
Fluid formulas are only a guideline; monitor urine output and tailor intravenous fluids to the response of the patient.
Monitor peripheral pulses, blood pressure, respiration rate, heart rate, urine output, oxygen saturation, and temperature (core/peripheral).
Monitor central venous pressure and/or cardiac output and hemodynamic parameters in severe burns or patients at risk for complications.
Achieve a urine output of 0.5 ml/kg/h in adults and 1 ml/kg/h in children, *no more, no less*
Elevate the head, limbs, and genitalia; elevate all that can be elevated.
Maintain the core temperature of the patient over 37°C.
Start enteral feeding on admission.
The aim is to obtain an awake, alert, conscious, and cooperative patient.
Do not obtain a replica of the Michelin Man; prevent edema.

The recommended resuscitation formulas for adults and children are the modified Parkland formula for adults and the Galveston formula for children. In each, half of the volume is administered in the first 8 h and the rest in the second 16 h.

Adult burn patients are resuscitated with the modified Parkland formula. It calls for the infusion of 3 ml/kg/% burn in the first 24 h postburn of Ringer's lactate solution. In the subsequent 24 h, transcutaneous evaporative losses from burn wounds are replaced at 1 ml/kg/% burn daily. The rate is adjusted hourly to ensure a urinary output of 0.5 ml/h.

Resuscitation of burned children differs in two aspects. First, the Parkland formula commonly underestimates fluid requirements in a burned child and may not provide even the usual daily maintenance requirements. There is great variability between body surface area and weight in a growing child. More accurate estimation of resuscitation requirements in burned children can be based on BSA determined from nomograms of height and weight (Fig. 4). For children, recommended initial resuscitation is 5000 ml/m^2 BSA burned/day plus 2000 ml/m^2 BSA total/day of Ringer's lactate. Again, one-half is given over the first 8 h and the rest in the next 16 h during the first 24 h postburn. Due to small glycogen stores, infants require glucose since they are prone to hypoglycemia in the initial resuscitation period; therefore, the basal maintenance fluid administration is given as 5% glucose-containing solutions. In the subsequent 24 h fluid requirements are 3750 ml/m^2 BSA burned/day plus 1500 ml/m^2 BSA total/day. Care should be taken to avoid rapid shifts in serum sodium concentration, which may cause cerebral edema and neuroconvulsive activity. The rate is adjusted to ensure a urinary output of 1 ml/kg/h (Table 7). Patients in air-fluidized (Clinitron) beds should receive 1000 ml/m^2 BSA/24 h extra fluids to replace the evaporative fluid loss produced by the bed.

Enteral feeding is usually started on admission and gradually increased until the maximum full rate is achieved. As the enteral feeding volume is increased and absorbed by the patient, intravenous fluid are diminished at the same rate, so that the total amount of resuscitation needs are met as a mixture of IV fluids and enteral feeding. By 48 h, most of the fluid replacement should be provided via the enteral route.

All resuscitation formulas are meant to serve as guides only. The response to fluid administration and physiological tolerance of the patient is most important.

TABLE 7   Resuscitation Formulas for Pediatric and Adult Patients

---

Pediatric Patients
First 24 h:
5000 ml/m^2 BSA burned/day + 2000 ml/m^2 BSA total/day of Ringer's lactate (give half in first 8 h and the second half in the following 16 h)
Subsequent 24 h:
3750 ml/m^2 BSA burned/day + 1500 ml/m^2 BSA total/day (to maintain urine output of 1ml/kg/h)
Adult Patients
First 24 h: 3 ml/kg/% BSA burned of Ringer's lactate (give half in first 8 h and the second half in the following 16 h)
Subsequent 24 h: 1 ml/kg/% burn daily (to maintain urine output of 0.5 ml/kg/h)

Additional fluids are commonly needed in patients with inhalation injuries, electrical burns, associated trauma, and delayed resuscitation. Fluid resuscitation should be started according to the fluid resuscitation formula. Fluid administration needs then to be tailored to the response of the patient based on urine output in a stable, lucid cooperative patient. The ideal is to reach the smallest fluid administration rate that provides an adequate urine output. The appropriate resuscitation regimen administers the minimal amount of fluid necessary for maintenance of vital organ perfusion. Inadequate resuscitation can cause further insult to pulmonary, renal, and mesenteric vascular beds. Fluid overload can produce undersized pulmonary or cerebral edema. It will also increase wound edema and thereby dermal ischemia, producing increased depth and extent of cutaneous damage.

Fluid requirements in patients with electrical injuries are often greater than those in patients with thermal injury. The main threat in the initial period is the development of acute tubular necrosis and acute renal insufficiency related to the precipitation of myoglobulin and other cellular products. A common finding in patients with electrical injuries is myoglobinuria, manifested as highly concentrated and pigmented urine. The goal under these circumstances is to maintain a urine output of 1–2 ml/kg/h until the urine clears. In nonresponding patients, alkalization of the urine and the use of osmotic agents may prevent death.

The use of colloid solutions for acute burn resuscitation remains debated. Development of hypoproteinemia in the early resuscitation period increases edema in nonburned tissues. In the absence of inhalation injury, however, lung water content does not increase. Early infusion of colloid solutions may decrease overall fluid requirements in the initial resuscitation period and reduce nonburn edema. However, injudicious use of colloid infusion may cause iatrogenic pulmonary edema, increasing pulmonary complications and mortality. The current recommendation is to add 25% albumin solution to maintain serum albumin > 2.5 g/100 ml after the first 8 h. In selected cases, it can be supplemented in the first 8 h postburn. Albumin solution 5% should be used instead of 25% solution in unstable patients with hypovolemia.

Fluid resuscitation should be monitored using clinical parameters. The best single indicator is urine output. Hypotension is a late finding in burn shock; therefore, pulse rate is much more sensitive than blood pressure. Normal sensorium, core temperature, and adequate peripheral capillary refill are additional clinical indicators of adequate organ perfusion. Fluid shifts are rapid during the acute resuscitation period (24–72 h), and serial determinations of hematocrit, serum electrolytes, osmolality, calcium, glucose, and albumin can help to direct appropriate fluid replacement.

Although overresuscitation is usually easy to detect, based on increasing edema and high urine output; underresuscitation may be much more difficult to diagnose and categorize. Persistent metabolic acidosis on measurement

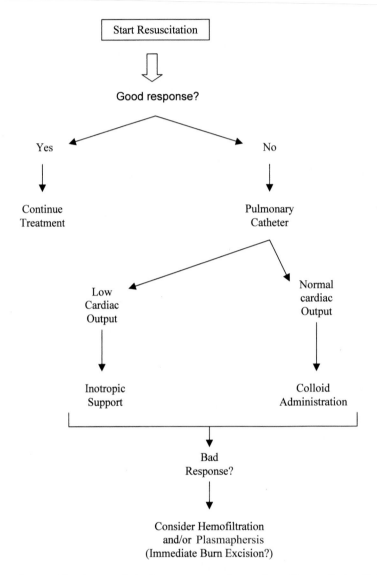

FIGURE 10 Approach to the nonresponding patient. Resuscitation fluids must be reviewed and corrected (including fluid boluses) before any other further action is taken.

of arterial blood gases may be indicative of continuing hypoperfusion from hypovolemia. As a general rule, patients who have a bad response to the standard Parkland formula and fluid boluses, and present with a continuous high base excess with increased lactate levels, are monitored with a pulmonary artery catheter. Patients with a low cardiac output despite correct resuscitation are candidates for inotropic support. On the other hand, if cardiac output is normal, patients are candidates for colloid administration. If patients do not respond to any of the resuscitation measures, continuous hemofiltration or plasmapheresis should be attempted (see Fig. 10).

MONITORING AND PATIENT CONTROL

Patients with major burns should receive full monitoring, including:

Continuous electrocardiograph monitoring
Continuous respiratory rate monitoring
Pulse oximetry
Central venous pressure
Arterial line
Foley catheter and urine output
Temperature probes
Capnometry (ventilated patients)
Pulmonary artery catheter (unstable severe burn patients)
Esophageal Doppler monitoring (alternative to Swan-Ganz catheters)
Doppler monitor for compartment syndromes

Central lines and arterial lines do carry some morbidity in burned patients. Judicious use of these otherwise helpful monitoring devices is advised. Monitoring of central venous pressure is indicated in patients with massive burns, those refractory to normal resuscitation maneuvers, elderly patients, and patients with significant pre-existing diseases. In general, a stable patient with burns under 40% BSA without significant pre-existing diseases can be managed without central line catheters. Control of blood pressure, pulse rate, pulse oximetry, respiratory rate, temperature, weight, and urine output should suffice in most of the patients. Blood pressure is often monitored using arterial lines. In most cases, however, indirect measure of blood pressure along with the physiological parameters mentioned earlier and the valuable addition of pulse oximetry are more than enough to monitor the patient. Arterial lines should be reserved for use in unstable patients, those with inhalation injury, unstable patients receiving ventilatory support, and patients who will need repeated blood gas analysis. Catheter-related sepsis has plagued burn patients for decades. With the advent of modern indwelling catheters, and strong policies for periodical line change, the incidence of catheter-related sepsis has declined dramatically. The usual recommendation is to change all lines every 7 days. Nevertheless, increasing evidence suggests that lines do not need to be changed unless they become infected. The question arises in the burn patient of differentiating between acute systemic inflammatory response syndrome and sepsis. Every burn center should make an effort to determine which protocol serves the best interest of patients in terms of infection control. General intensive care unit (ICU) guidelines regarding line protocols should be used. Care of the line should include daily inspection of entry point and daily dressing with dry compresses. Occlusive dressings and antibiotic creams are not effective to control infection, and there are reports that they may even increase the risk of infection.

After initial management in the admission room, patients are then transferred to their room. A controlled environment should be provided, with a high temperature (24–28°C) and at least 50% humidity. Patients are covered and placed under thermal panels. These panels provide a central area just over the patient with a high temperature (ideally 36°C) whereas in the rest of the room the environmental conditions, although still warm, are cool enough to allow reasonable comfort for health personnel (Figs. 11, 12). Head, limbs, and genitalia are to be elevated, and the patient should be positioned comfortably (see Chap. 14). Stable

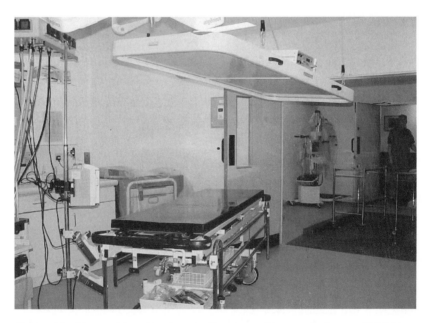

FIGURE 11 Thermal panels or heat radiators provide a central area of high temperature over the patient, allowing a lower temperature in the rest of the environment for staff and visitor comfort.

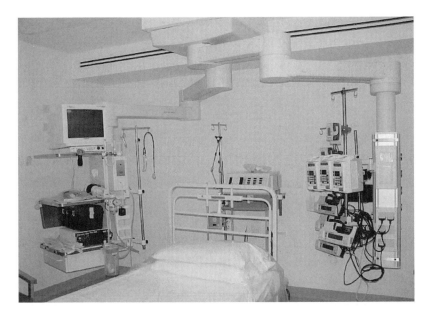

FIGURE 12 Burn ICU beds should be spacious and should have independent thermostats to permit changes in room environmental conditions according to patient needs.

patients should be encouraged to walk and mobilize as soon as possible, and early physiotherapy should be started. Patients should never be at bed rest unless absolutely necessary. Patients must be comfortable and pain free (see section below, Pain Control section), and patients and families should be trained in wound care and rehabilitation.

All patients need to be closely monitored by burn physicians. A formal morning round should be established, with review of all systems and wounds when deemed necessary. All altered parameters need to be corrected. We highly recommend performing an informal evening round to check the daily progress of the patient, and what corrections have been undertaken. At that time, it is useful to decide which patients need to have their wounds inspected the next morning. These multidisciplinary visits are completed with a biweekly multidisciplinary meeting at which the discharge planning for patients is discussed in full.

BIBLIOGRAPHY

1. Total Burn Care. Second Edition. Herndon David N, Ed. London. United Kingdom: WB Saunders, 2002.
2. Color Atlas of Burn Care. Barret Juan P, Herndon David N, Eds. London. United Kingdom: WB Saunders, 2002.

3. Burn Care. Wolf Steven E, Herndon David N, Eds. Austin. Texas: Landes Bioscience, 1999.
4. Surgical Management and Hypermetabolic Modulation of Pediatric Burns. Barret Juan P, Ed. Groningen. the Netherlands: University of Groningen, 2002.
5. Thermal InjuryRamzy Peter I, Barret Juan P, Herndon David N. Crit Care Clin 1999; 15(2).
6. Quantitative Microbiology: Its Role in the Surgical Armamentarium. Florida: CRC Press, 1991.
7. Principles and Practice of Burn Management. Settle John AD, Ed. Edinburgh. United Kingdom: Churchill Livingstone, 1996.

2

General Treatment of Burned Patients

Juan P. Barret
Broomfield Hospital, Chelmsford, Essex, United Kingdom

Advances in trauma and critical care have resulted in important improvements in burn management, improved survival, and reduced morbidity from major burns. Myriad physiological changes occur following thermal trauma, including fluid and electrolyte imbalances (systemic losses and shifts of water, sodium, albumin, and blood cells), metabolic disturbances (hypermetabolism, catabolism, and malnutrition), bacterial contamination of tissues and infection, complications in vital organs, and respiratory complication with or without the presence of inhalation injury.

Emergency treatment focuses on stabilization of patients, treatment of associated injuries, fluid resuscitation, initial respiratory support, and emergency treatment of the burn wound. Soon after stabilization and resuscitation, a formal discharge plan (treatment plan, rehabilitation plan, and social support) is established. Focus of burn treatment is then shifted to the definitive burn wound treatment and to the general support of the patient, which include:

Nutritional support
General patient support
Support of the hypermetabolic response
Treatment of inhalation injury
Pain management and psychosocial support

Infection control and treatment of critical conditions
Rehabilitation

The general treatment of burn patients is outlined in the following sections. For more specific issues, such as rehabilitation, psychosocial support, and support of the hypermetabolic response, the reader is referred to the relevant chapters in this book.

NUTRITIONAL SUPPORT

The hypermetabolic response to burns is the greatest of any other trauma or infection. A major burn injury provokes a complex disruption of hormonal homeostasis that induces an increased resting metabolic rate and oxygen consumption, increased nitrogen loss, increased lipolysis, increased glucose flow, and loss of body mass. To meet postburn energy demands, all main metabolic pathways are utilized. Carbohydrate stores are small; therefore, carbohydrate intermediate metabolites, which are also essential for fat catabolism, are obtained from skeletal muscle breakdown, thus increasing muscle catabolism. Prolonged inflammation, pain or anxiety, environmental cooling, and sepsis can further exaggerate this postburn hypermetabolic response.

One of the main principles underlying successful management of the postburn hypermetabolic response is providing adequate nutritional support. In general, patients affected with more than 25% body surface area (BSA) burned and those patients with malnutrition or who cannot cope with their metabolic demands as a result of concomitant injuries or diseases should receive nutritional support.

The nutritional formula of choice is enteral nutrition. Total parenteral nutrition should be abandoned and reserved for patients who cannot tolerate the enteral route. It carries a high mortality in burn patients.

A nasogastric tube should suffice in most patients. Placement of nasoduodenal or jejunal tubes is tedious and often not successful, and their advantages are dubious. They should be reserved for use in ventilated patients who are at risk for nosocomial pneumonia. When a nasoduodenal tube is used, it should be combined with a nasogastric tube. Ten percent of the enteral feeding is then infused via the nasogastric tube, and the rest via the nasoduodenal tube. In either tube-feeding regimen, the gastric residuals should be checked regularly. Once the residual has been checked, it is then infused back to the stomach to avoid electrolytic imbalances and alkalosis. If these residuals are more than a 2 h tube feeding infusion rate, the feeding should be stopped and the cause investigated. The most common cause of enteral feeding intolerance is tube malposition, although important causes of intolerance that all physicians should bear in mind are sepsis and multiple organ failure. The enteral feeding should be started on admission and continued until the wounds are 90% healed and the patient can maintain an oral intake of his or her caloric demand.

Enteral feeding is started on admission and, if absorbed, it is increased until full strength is obtained, ideally in the first 24 h. The hourly absorbed nutrition is subtracted from the total resuscitation hourly fluids the patient is receiving, in order to avoid overloading. When patients are scheduled for surgery, nutrition is stopped 2–4 h before surgery, and the stomach is aspirated prior to the induction of anesthesia. In ventilated patients, enteral nutrition is not stopped but is continued during surgery.

Caloric requirements in burn patients should be ideally calculated by means of indirect calorimetric measurement. This is an easy noninvasive bedside method. After measurement of the composition of expired gases, the calorimeter calculates the respiratory quotient and caloric requirement by means of standard equations. When indirect calorimetry is not available, calorie requirements are measured calculated on linear regression analysis of intake vs. weight loss. Patients should be assessed for nutritional status on admission, and reassessed on a daily basis. Patients should be weighed regularly to document their well being. Inadequate intake necessitates an alteration of the regimen. It is also important to determine whether the regimen is well tolerated. Initial nutritional assessment is depicted in Table 1. Patients should be investigated with a complete nutritional panel on admission and then once a week. This includes:

> Total lymphocyte count, white blood cells, hemoglobin and hematocrit, and mean corpuscular volume

TABLE 1 Initial Nutritional Assessment

Determine the caloric and protein needs of patients immediately upon admission
Assessment by physician and dietician
Assess:
– Personal background
– Chronic conditions
– Hypermetabolic conditions
– Physical conditions that may interfere with food intake
– Predisposing factors
– Recent weight loss or gain
– Food preference and allergies
– Weight and height for age and gender
– Total lymphocyte count
– White blood cells
– Hemoglobin and hematocrit
– Mean corpuscular volume
Perform indirect calorimetry if available
Calculate daily calorie and protein needs

Albumin, prealbumin, magnesium, phosphate, ionized calcium, copper, zinc, protoporphyrin/heme

24 h total urea nitrogen

Measurement of these variables, together with indirect calorimetry and the weight gain/loss of the patient will give a good estimate of his or her nutritional status.

Burn patients who can eat normally receive a high-protein, high-calorie diet. Liquids should be supplemented in the form of high-calorie fluids, such as milk or commercial milkshakes. Patients with burns over 25% BSA burned cannot cope with the caloric demands that trauma imposes on them, so that in all of them enteral supplementation is indicated.

Different enteral formulas are available. The most popular ones (Curreri and Harris Benedict for adults, and Galveston formula for children) are summarized in Table 2. Some of them (Curreri) may overestimate calorie requirements, whereas others (Harris-Benedict) may underestimate these needs. Therefore, they should be used as initial estimates, with patients needs titrated to their hypermetabolic response as measured by indirect calorimetry. It must be noted, however, that human hypermetabolic response reaches a maximum of about 200% of basal requirements. Above that, human physiology cannot increase the rate at which the fuels are utilized to transform them into energy and proteins. It means that supplementing above the 200% resting energy expenditure (REE) does not increase the absorption of nutrients. There is general agreement that this increase to 200% REE reaches the maximum with burn at or over 50% BSA.

The composition of the nutritional component is also important. Caloric replacement should be based on nonprotein calories only. Approximately 50%

TABLE 2 Nutritional Formulas

Nutritional formulas for pediatric burn patients
0–12 months: 2100 kcal/m^2 surface area + 1000 kcal/m^2 surface area burned
1–11 years: 1800 kcal/m^2 surface area + 1300 kcal/m^2 surface area burned
> 12 years: 1500 kcal/m^2 surface area + 1500 kcal/m^2 surface area burned
Nutritional formulas for adult burn patients
Curreri: 16–59 years: 25 kcal/kg + 40 kcal for each percentage of burn area
       60 years and more: 20 kcal/kg + 65 kcal for each percentage of burn area
Harris-Benedict: Basal energy expenditure (BEE) in kcal/day (at rest):
       Males: BEE = 66 + 13.7 (kg) + 5 (cm) − 6.8 (years)
       Females: BEE = 655 + 9.6 (kg) + 1.8 (cm) − 4.7 (years)
       Activity/injury factor:
       Bed rest 1.2, ambulatory 1.3, minor surgery 1.2, trauma 1.35, sepsis 1.6, severe burn 2.1
       Calculated caloric requirements
       = BEE × activity/injury factor

---

of the calories should be supplied as carbohydrates, 20% as proteins, and approximately 30% of the calories should be supplied as fat. Protein needs are 4.4 g/kg in infants (less than 6 months), 4.0 g/kg in small children (6–24 months), and a calorie to nitrogen ratio of 120:1 (kcal/N) in the rest of patients. For a balanced daily diet, administration of vitamins C, A, and E, B complex, zinc, iron, folate, and trace minerals is essential.

When the patient's wounds are virtually covered, the diet should transition from one in which the majority of the nutrition is supplied via tube feedings to a total oral diet. The transition should be slow and may take several days. The following steps should be followed:

1. Reduce tube feedings to a rate that with the oral intake equals 100% of reassessed goal.
2. As oral intake increases, provide only nocturnal tube feedings to equal 100% of goal.
3. When oral intake is at least 50% of goal, begin 3 day trial of oral diet with tube feedings held.
4. If goal is not being met at the end of the trial, re-evaluate feeding methods and, if necessary, resume tube feedings.
5. During all of the above steps, specific fluid orders with guidelines as to amounts and contents should be written

PATIENT SUPPORT

Hypoproteinemia and Anemia

Hypoproteinemia due to malnutrition, continuing serum protein losses, and post-burn sepsis and hepatic dysfunction will persist until wound closure is achieved. Intravascular proteins can be replaced by processed albumin (generally preferred), or fresh frozen plasma if a significant coagulopathy is also present. The efficacy of colloids is the subject of debate; therefore every effort should be made to correct hypoproteinemia with early enteral nutrition. Colloids should be reserved for patients with severely low protein levels and those with significant clinical effects of such hypoproteinemia.

Anemia is very common among burn patients. The initial thermal injury is accompanied by direct destruction of red cells. Other cells are not initially destroyed, but they are structurally damaged and the half-life of the red cell pool is significantly decreased. Repeated trips to the operating room makes this anemia even more profound, as a joint effect of hemorrhage and blood replacement, which decreases again the half-life of red cells. Initial blood loss can be corrected with incremental transfusions of 10–15 ml blood/kg/day. Operating blood loss should be replaced with 0.5–1 ml/cm^2 excised.

Environmental Control

Control of the surrounding environment is a well-recognized part of appropriate burn care. Burn patients lose some of their thermoregulatory abilities and are prone to hypothermia. An ambient room temperature of 28–33°C keeps the patient more comfortable and reduces his or her heat losses from evaporation. As mentioned before, the use of thermal panels in the patient's room helps to maintain the environment in close vicinity to the patient at a high temperature while the rest of the room is kept at a lower temperature (although still 24–26°C), which is much more comfortable for health personnel. Natural light and large windows help patients to maintain their well being. Strong noises should be avoided; and the area needs to be kept pleasant, clean, and relaxing. Play specialists and teachers for children; and occupational therapists, music therapy, and social activities for both children and adults facilitate the recovery of burned patients (Fig. 1).

Stress Ulcer Prophylaxis

The acid pH of the stomach plays an important role in infection control in the human body. This acid serves as a topical treatment for all foods that enter the digestive tube. This acid pH can be problematic when different problems collide in the same clinical situation. Tissue hypoperfusion (frequently measured by

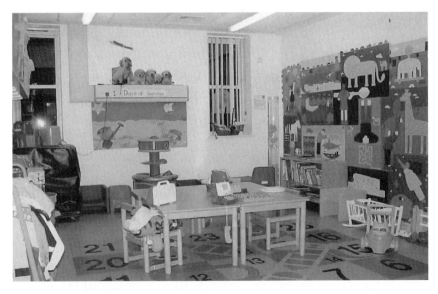

FIGURE 1   Control of the surrounding environmental is a well-recognized part of appropriate burn care that facilitates recovery.

gastric tonometry) and the depletion of reduction agents and free radical scavengers promote a progressive damage of gastric mucosa. This erodes and progresses to small ulcers by the action of gastric acid and digestive enzymes. Maintaining good patient support and preventing sepsis and multiple organ dysfunction is extremely important to prevent stress ulcers.

The best prophylaxis for stress ulcers is enteral nutrition. Burn patients need something in their stomachs at all times to prevent ulceration. Enteral feeding maintains gastric and intestinal mucosal integrity. It maintains organ perfusion and serves as a scavenger for gastric acid. Patients who are not receiving any enteral nutrition at any given time should receive sucralfate, which coats the gastric mucosa and prevents ulceration. H2 blockers and antacids should be reserved for patients whose condition cannot be managed properly with enteral nutrition and sucralfate. Changing the gastric pH encourages bacterial overgrowth and leads to a higher incidence of pneumonia. Acid kills bacteria, which is the most important action of acid in our stomachs.

Deep Venous Thrombosis Prophylaxis

Burn patients should be encouraged to be mobile except in the immediate postoperative period or if they are attached to a ventilator. Even ventilated patients, should be exercising. The rest of the patients should be up with their limbs sufficiently wrapped to prevent edema and graft loss. Early mobilization and ambulation are the best prophylaxis for deep venous thrombosis (DVT). Patients who are not able to exercise and ambulate should be started on subcutaneous low-molecular-weight heparin. Pneumatic boots with intermittent compression should be used during surgery to prevent the development of DVT during surgery. Patients in the intensive care unit (ICU) should be closely monitored for signs and symptoms of DVT and pulmonary embolism, and proper treatment begun as soon as the diagnosis is made.

TREATMENT OF INHALATION INJURY

Inhalation injury is evident in over 30% of hospitalized burn patients and in 20–84% of burn-related deaths. Heat can result in damage and edema to the upper airway, but uncommonly produces injury below the vocal cords except with steam burns. Acute asphyxia can occur due to environmental oxygen consumption or by reduction of oxygen transportation by carbon monoxide or cyanides. The majority of tissue damage attributed to inhalation injury is mediated by a chemical injury from incomplete combustion products carried by smoke, including aldehydes, oxides, sulfur, nitrogen compounds, and hydrochloric gases. This chemical damage to the lower airways and parenchyma is propagated by neutrophils. Lung vascular permeability is increased, promoting pulmonary edema. Desquamation of small airways along with inflammation produces airway casts, leading to areas of atelectatic lung alternating with emphysematous regions, acute pulmonary insufficiency, and bronchopneumonia.

Diagnosis of inhalation injury should be suspected in patients with facial burns, singed nasal hair, cough, carbonaceous sputum, or evidence of upper airway edema, including hoarseness, stridor, or wheezing. It should be considered in any patient with a history of burn in a closed space, loss of consciousness, or altered mental status. Arterial blood gases and carboxyhemoglobin content should be determined, but it may be misleading if initially normal. Diagnosis of inhalation injury is best confirmed by results of fiberoptic bronchoscopy. Chest x-ray is an insensitive initial test.

Treatment of inhalation injury should begin at the scene of the accident with immediate administration of 100% oxygen. Carbon monoxide poisoning produces asphyxia by binding competitively to hemoglobin and reducing oxygen-carrying capacity. Hemoglobin has a 210-times greater affinity for carbon monoxide than oxygen. On room air, carboxyhemoglobin (CO-Hgb) has a half-life of about 4 h in the bloodstream. The half-life of CO-Hgb is reduced to 20 min when the subject is breathing 100% oxygen. If oxygen supplementation is started promptly, anoxic cerebral injuries are reduced. Levels of CO-Hgb greater than 15% are clinically significant, and levels above 40% can produce coma.

Great debate still exists regarding intubation in patients with suspected inhalation injury. Maintenance of the airway is critical. If early evidence of upper airway edema is present, then early intubation is mandatory since airway edema increases over 12–18 h. Prophylactic intubation without a good indication should not be done, because intubation may otherwise increase pulmonary complications in burn patients. Early extubation should be performed in all patients (within 48–72 h), as soon as an air leak is detected around the tube cuff. Other patients who benefit from early intubation and extubation (after 48–72 h) are those with severe life-threatening burns. Controlling the upper airway by means of early intubation makes resuscitation much easier. The patients, however, should be extubated when resuscitation is over, in order to prevent the development of airway complications and acute respiratory distress syndrome (ARDS).

All patients with positive findings at bronchoscopy or with a suggestive history should be placed in an inhalation injury protocol. The nebulization of various substances and different respiratory therapy maneuvers have proved beneficial in the prevention of progression to tracheobronchitis, pulmonary edema, ARDS, and bronchopneumonia. The protocol is universal, and can be applied to patients with any sort of burn. It is summarized in Table 3.

Although the inhalation injury protocol is very effective in preventing the development of ARDS, some patients with inhalation injury do develop the whole picture of ARDS. Patients often have severe systemic inflammatory response syndrome (SIRS), and receive substantial second-hit insults from surgically induced bacteremia, sepsis, and repetitive hypovolemia. The strategy for managing

TABLE 3 Inhalation Injury Protocol

1. Titrate high-flow humidified oxygen to maintain arterial oxygen saturation > 90%
2. Cough, deep breathing exercises every 2 h
3. Turn patient from one side to the other every 2 h
4. Chest physiology and physiotherapy every 4 h
5. Nebulize 3 ml N-acetylcysteine 20% solution every 4 h for 7 days
6. Nebulize 500 units of heparin with 3 ml normal saline every 4 h for 7 days
7. Nebulize bronchodilators every 4 h for 7 days
8. Nasotracheal suctioning as needed
9. Early ambulation
10. Sputum cultures Monday, Wednesday, and Friday
11. Pulmonary function studies before discharge and at scheduled outpatients visits
12. Patient/parent education regarding injury process

respiratory distress syndrome is outlined in Table 4. In general, aggressive bronchial toilet with direct bronchoscopy and lavage to remove bronchial casts is one of the pillars of such strategy. In addition, tailoring ventilatory support to the individual needs helps to prevent barotrauma and other complications. When patients can no longer maintain their normal gas exchange, ventilatory support is necessary. Many different ventilatory modes are available, including high-frequency percussive ventilation. In general, the physician should choose a ventilator mode shown to be capable of supporting gas exchange in that particular circumstance. Acceptable oxygen saturation should be targeted, but normal levels should be not pursued. Oxygen saturation >90% should suffice in most of the

TABLE 4 Strategy for Managing Respiratory Distress Syndrome

1. Humidified gas for spontaneous or artificial ventilation.
2. Artificial airway for bronchial toilet if secretions are unmanageable.
3. Increase functional residual capacity (using positive end-respiratory pressure) to reduce toxic fractional inspired oxygen.
4. Add mechanical ventilation if work of breathing is excessive.
5. Adjust tidal volume and positive end-expiratory pressure according to arterial oxygen tension, fractional inspired oxygen, and peak inspiratory pressure.
6. Avoid neuromuscular blockers if possible.
7. Consider specialized measures (extracorporeal membrane oxygenation, permissive hypercapnia, high-frequency percussive ventilation) to improve gas exchange and oxygen delivery while reducing pulmonary trauma

TABLE 5 American College of Chest Physicians Consensus Conference on
Mechanical Ventilation

– The clinician should choose a ventilator mode shown to be capable of supporting
oxygenation/ventilation in patients with adult respiratory distress syndrome and
that the clinician has experience in using.
– An acceptable oxygen saturation should be targeted.
– When plateau pressure equals or exceeds 35 cmH$_2$O, the tidal volume should be
decreased (to as low as 5 ml/kg, and lower if necessary); in conditions where
chest wall compliance is low, plateau pressure somewhat greater than 35 cm
H$_2$O may be acceptable.
– To limit plateau pressures, permissive hypercapnia should be considered, unless
other contraindications exist that demand a more normal carbon dioxide tension
(P_{co_2}) and pH.
– Positive end-expiratory pressure (PEEP) is useful in supporting oxygenation.
The level of PEEP required should be established by empirical trials and
re-evaluated on a regular basis.
– Large tidal volumes (12–15 ml/kg) may be needed to improve oxygenation. Peak
flow rates should be adjusted as needed to meet the patient's inspiratory
demands.
– Current opinion is that fractional inspired oxygen (FiO$_2$) should be kept as low as
possible. However, to maintain oxygenation at lower FiO$_2$ levels, higher alveolar
pressures may be needed. When both high alveolar pressures and FiO$_2$ levels
are required to maintain oxygenation, it is reasonable to accept an arterial
oxygen saturation slightly less than 90%
– When oxygenation is inadequate, sedation, paralysis, and position changes are
possible corrective measures. Other factors in oxygen delivery, such as cardiac
output and hemoglobin, should also be considered

Source: Adapted from Chest 1993; 104 : 1833–1859.

cases. More important is to maintain good tissue oxygenation and an acceptable
mixed venous oxygen tension. The rest of the recommendations of the American
College of Chest Physicians Consensus Conference also apply (Table 5). Burn
patients with ARDS are also surgical candidates. Respiratory distress should never
prevent patients from being treated surgically. Only patients who are too unstable
to be moved and could experience cardiac arrest in transfer to the operating room
have relative contraindications to surgery.

PAIN MANAGEMENT

Burns hurt, and so does burn treatment. Pain is the most immediate concern of
the burn patients. Suffering a combination of physical discomfort and mental
torment increases the postburn hypermetabolic stress response. Treatment for a
patient's suffering, however, involves more than control of pain. Emotional sup-

port is essential, and uninterrupted sleep is beneficial. Other problems burn patients often experience are anxiety, itching, and posttraumatic stress disorder.

There are two types of burn pain. The first type is background pain. Background pain is always present and its range of fluctuation is very small. The second type of pain is the excruciating, intolerable pain that occurs when something is done to the patient, such as procedural pain during dressing changes, line change, or physiotherapy. It is the worst pain a patient can encounter, and patients cannot make any comparison to other experiences in life. Pain control is one of the great challenges in the burn unit, and it is an unsolved problem. Anxiety, sleep disorders, and posttraumatic stress are problems often encountered along with pain. They need to be treated at the same time in order to obtain a perfect response. It must be remembered, however, that anxiety or other disorders are not treated with opioids, and pain should likewise not be treated with anxiolytics. Patient responses to pain stimulus vary significantly. The patient's pre-existing psychological make-up, ethnocultural background, the experience of the injury, and its meaning modulate the individual response to pain.

General recommendations for Pain control

1. If patient says he or she has pain, then he or she has pain.
2. Analgesics are most effective when given on a regular basis (not as needed or required).
3. Intramuscular injections are not usually appropriate because the patient fears the injection and intramuscular flow may be altered.
4. Bowel management begins with the narcotic pain management.
5. Pain management protocol should be initiated with the starting doses, which can be modified as the situation dictates.

Pain Assessment

The patient's pain can be assessed using the 10-point scale or the Faces scale (Fig. 2). In the 10-point scale, the sliding scale is moved until the patient feels

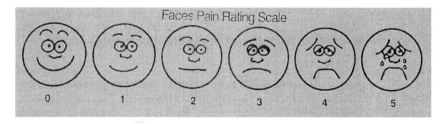

FIGURE 2 Faces pain rating scale. Patients point at the face that best describes the pain they are suffering. A laughing face means no pain at all; a sad, crying face describes intensive, non-bearable pain.

TABLE 6 The Observer Pain Scale

Score	Observation
1	Laughing, euphoria
2	Happy, contented, smiling, playing
3	Neutral (asleep or calm)
4	Mild–moderate pain: expresses, vocalizes pain, wrinkles brow, but can be distracted with toy or food or TV
5	Moderate–severe pain: expresses severe pain, crying inconsolably, screaming, hysteria, sobbing

that the number expressed matches the pain he or she is experiencing. A scale of 1 hurts just a little bit, whereas 10 is the worst experience a person can ever imagine. For children less than 3 years old, the Faces pain-rating scale is best used. The child points to the face that best describes the pain he or she is experiencing. A smiling face with a pain score of 0 is happy because it does not hurt at all. Face 5 is crying and sad because it hurts as much as you can imagine. For children who are preverbal or communicate nonverbally, the observer scale is used (see Table 6).

Both background and procedural pain occur in the emergency, acute, and rehabilitation phase. Therefore different methodologies should be applied depending on the patient's phase of the disease in order to obtain good pain control. In general, liberal use of opioids and benzodiazepines is advised. Unless patients have a pre-existing drug abuse problem, they will not become opioid dependent from its use during the acute phase of the burn.

General Issues

Burn patients should always receive baseline analgesia. Drugs need to be scheduled in order to maintain a basal level of painkillers that will make controlling the pain much easier. Therefore, do not order analgesics at the patient's request (PRN). The best practice in patients who are candidates for opioid analgesia is patient-controlled analgesia (PCA) pumps. They decrease patients' anxiety by putting them in control of the pain regimen. Furthermore, by calculating the PCA use, the analgesic needs for patients can be determined in an individual basis. Children of 8 years and older are candidates for PCA. Patients receiving opioids need to be started on a bowel regimen to prevent the development of constipation. In general, prune juice or lactulose will suffice in most. When patients get constipated, mineral oil should be started, followed by enemas if a good response is not obtained. The bowel regimen is represented in Table 7.

TABLE 7   Bowel Regimen

– Start with the following any time opiates are administered: prune juice or
  Lactulose
– Then add one of the following if the patient becomes constipated: mineral oil and
  Minienema if no bowel movement by noon; enema if no bowel movement after
  previous measures.

Pain vs. Anxiety

Anxiety can be very debilitating in the acute situation, and it often accompanies pain. It can be very diffcult to differentiate between them. It can not be overemphasized, however, that pain should not be treated with anxiolytics, and, likewise, anxiety is not treated with opiates. Pain must be always addressed first as well as acute stress disorder problems. When pain is under control, anxiety may disappear in some patients. Anxiety can be measured similarly to pain. Anxiety can be defined in a simplistic manner as fear. Often it is experienced as an anticipation of extreme pain. Patients learn quickly their routine in the burn unit and anticipate the pain with enormous amounts of stress and anxiety. The fear thermometer is a good way of measuring anxiety. A fear scale of 1 means no fear at all, a fear scale of 5 means very much fear. Patients point at the scale that best represents their fear at a specific time, and treatment is given accordingly. It is important to note that anxiolytics are also not to be given PRN. In order to achieve a good level of anxiolysis, patients need to receive a regular dose of drugs. Anxiolytics can be added to the procedural pain management regimen to decrease fear and add a certain degree of amnestic properties to the analgesia.

Pain Management Protocol

Background Pain Management

Start with one drug. Do not give drugs PRN. If pain is not controlled, give additional drugs on top of the previously administered drug. Consider posttraumatic stress disorder and anxiety if pain is not well controlled.

> For **ICU patients:**
>
> Morphine or fentanyl drips or morphine via PCA, and
> Midazolam or lorazepam for anxiety or agitation
> When patients are stable and in an subacute phase, change to slow-release
>   oral morphine
>
> For **patients** not in the ICU:
>
> Slow-release oral morphine or morphine via PCA, or
> Acetaminophen + codeine, or

Tramadol

Consider ibuprofen when anti-inflammatory action is also indicated (not in young children)

Sympathetic discharge symptoms such as sweating, palpitations, and abdominal pain can be blocked by clonidine. Hypotension may occur; thus monitoring is a must.

Procedural Pain Management

Many regimens may be useful. The following are some suggestions. Each must be tailored on an individual basis and per procedure. In general, a protocol including an anxiolytic and a hypnotic or analgesic should be used. Procedural pain management is indicated for all age groups and is administered in addition to background pain management.

For **ICU and non-ICU patients**, the general regimens available include: Morphine or fentanyl + lorazepam or midazolam; and Morphine + nitrous oxide. When the patient is undergoing major dressing change with debridement, regimens include ketamine (+ bezodiazepine in patients >16 years or >50 kg); and propofol.

It is important to mention that when patients receive procedural pain management regimens, they require full monitoring (pulse oxygen, electrocardiogram, blood pressure) monitoring of vital signs every 5 min. A physician or registered anesthesia nurse should be present. Procedural pain medication should be scheduled 30 min to 1 h pre-procedure rather than PRN. When hypnotic drugs are used, such as ketamine, propofol, or nitrous oxide, they should be administered and titrated to effect. Major dressing changes, debridement, line changes, and Biobrane application can be done using these regimens and full monitoring to avoid the need for multiples trips to the operating room.

Patients who need high dosages of morphine for pain control and escalating dosages of benzodiazepines may benefit from the addition to the pain regimen of gabapentin, clonidine, and methadone.

Management of Anxiety

As mentioned previously, burns hurt. This is well known, and, as such, people fear pain. Besides the fear that patients experience when they are confronted with multiple, repetitive, painful procedures, they may feel that they have lost control of life events. Both pain and loss of control are intensely anxiety-provoking situations. The anticipation of pain provokes a rise in the anxiety level, which is normally highest when health personnel enter the room. The loss of control maintains a background level of anxiety, which may increase in time as painful situations follow.

Fear and anxiety are best treated with the addition of anxiolytics. Before using them, however, pain management and acute stress disorder needs to be addressed first. The following agents are used:

1. Lorazepam: first choice in the acute phase
2. Diazepam: useful for rehabilitation therapy because it relaxes skeletal muscle
3. Midazolam: only when a short-acting agent is needed.

Patients who receive lorazepam for more than 15 days will need to have their dosage tapered. Diazepam has a longer half-life than lorazepam, and no taper in dosage is necessary.

Management of Acute Stress Disorder

A significant number of burn survivors will experience symptoms of posttraumatic stress disorder, including intrusive memories of the injury, during their acute recovery. If anxiety is associated with other symptoms of posttraumatic stress, such as hypervigilance or poor sleep, treatment should be considered. Symptoms commonly described include nightmares, flashbacks (re-experiencing the trauma while awake), difficulty falling sleep, difficulty staying asleep, hypervigilance, startle response, and dissociative feelings. Pharmacological management is usually the most helpful intervention in the acute phase. Treatment agents include imipramine and fluoxetine.

Management of Itch

Burn scars and wounds can produce severe itching that can become a very serious problem. Patients who experience severe itching excoriate grafts and produce open wounds on themselves. When pruritus is severe, they can not focus on anything else. Itching interferes with activity, and patients cannot concentrate.

The following protocol has proved beneficial in managing itching problems in burn patients. Each new step should be added to the previous treatment. Do not stop use of any of the drugs already being used, but add the new drug to provide an additive effect.

Topical treatments include moisturizing body shampoo and lotions to alleviate itching due to dry scaly skin, and adding Benadryl cream or astringent creams if this is not helpful.

Pharmacological management should start with diphenhydramine, which has sedative and antihistaminic properties. If this is not helpful, add hydroxyzine (the most effective antihistamine for chronic urticaria), and add cyproheptadine to the previous regimen in severe cases.

INFECTION CONTROL

Despite improvements in antimicrobial therapies and programs of early excision and grafting, sepsis continue to account for 50–60% of deaths in burn patients today. The burn wound is an ideal substrate for bacterial growth and provides a wide portal for microbial invasion. Microbial colonization of the open burn wounds, primarily from an endogenous source, is usually established by the end of the first week. Organisms isolated after the burn injury are predominantly gram positive. Seven days after the injury the burn wounds are colonized by the patient's endogenous flora, predominantly hospital-acquired gram-negative flora. Infection is promoted by loss of the epithelial barrier, by malnutrition induced by the hypermetabolic response to burn injury, and by a generalized postburn suppression of nearly all aspects of immune response. Postburn serum levels of immunoglobulins, fibronectin, and complement levels are reduced, as is the ability for opsonization. Chemotaxis, phagocytosis, and killing function of neutrophils, monocytes, and macrophages are impaired, and cellular immune response is impaired. This decrease in the immune response explains why bacteria that in normal hosts are not harmful present a high risk to burned patients. The avascular burn eschar is rapidly colonized despite the use of antimicrobial agents. If this bacterial density exceeds the immune defenses of the host, then invasive burn sepsis may ensue. When bacterial wound counts are $> 10^5$ micro-organisms per gram of tissue, risk of wound infection is great, skin graft survival is poor, and wound closure is delayed.

The goals of wound management are the prevention of desiccation of viable tissue and the control of bacteria. It is unrealistic to expect to keep a burn wound sterile. Bacterial counts less than 10^3 organisms per gram of tissue are not usually invasive and allow skin graft survival rates of more than 90%. The isolation of *Streptococcus* in the wound should be considered an exception to the former, since bacterial counts of less than 10^3 bacteria per gram of tissue can provoke invasive burn wound infection and should be treated.

Great debate still exists regarding the appropriate isolation regimen for burn patients. For decades, burned patients were treated in dedicated burn centers with strict isolation techniques. It is now common knowledge, however, that burned patients do become infected from endogenous gram-negative flora. Cross-contamination among patients is minimal; therefore, the standard practice of strict isolation is no longer needed. In general, barrier nursing and hand washing after every patient contact should suffice to control infection in the burn unit. More strict measures need to be implemented with the appearance of multiple resistant organisms.

Studies from several burn centers have laid to rest the idea that prophylactic antibiotics should be given to burn patients. This practice does not decrease the incidence of infection. It increases strains of multiple resistant organisms and challenges the posterior management of burn patients. It is advisable to administer antistreptococcal antibiotics in infants and small children for 24–48 h when surgery or application of synthetic dressing is considered. Children are often colonized by these organisms and are very sensitive to their growth. Perioperative systemic broad-spectrum antibiotics are advised when major surgery is performed. The manipulation of large burn wound surfaces produces a significant bacteremia and bacterial translocation in the digestive tract. It is advised to add this perioperative prophylaxis, which should be based on endogenous flora surveillance and include an antistaphylococcal agent in the acute period. Several studies have shown that burn patients experience sepsis 72 h after surgery if no antibiotics are used during major burn surgery. These agents should only be continued after surgery if evidence of sepsis is confirmed.

Bacterial surveillance through routine surface wound and sputum cultures is strongly advised. When patients become septic, cultures are helpful to direct antimicrobial therapy. Knowledge of local bacterial flora and local sensitivities patterns helps to rationalize antibiotic use, but they do not provide definitive data for the diagnosis of sepsis. Quantitative wound biopsies are a better determinant of significant pathogens than qualitative surface swabs. If bacterial counts are $>$ 10^5 (10^3 in *Streptococcus* isolates), wound infection should be suspected. Burn wound sepsis can however, only be determined by results of histopathological examination.

Diagnosis of sepsis in burn patients can be difficult to differentiate from the usual hyperdynamic, hyperthermic, hypermetabolic postburn state. Any significant burn will start an SIRS in patients (Table 8). Fever spikes are not always related to underlying infection, and blood cultures are commonly negative. Close monitoring and daily physical examination of burn patients are crucial for the prompt diagnosis of septic complications. In general, the most clinical subjective sign of infection is a sudden unexpected change in the patient's progress. The patient's hospital course is no longer smooth and going well. An increase in metabolic rate, feeding intolerance, change in mental orientation or gas exchange, increasing pain scores, or change in biochemistry will signal impending infections. Once this change has been detected, the cause should be investigated. Infection is the leading cause. The patient should be inspected thoroughly, all wounds exposed, and cultures and other relevant examinations performed. Local evidence of invasive wound infection includes the following:

Black or brown patches of wound discoloration
Rapid eschar separation
Conversion of wounds to full thickness
Spreading periwound erythema
Punctuate hemorrhagic subeschar lesions
Violaceous or black lesions in nonburned tissue (ecthyma gangrenosum)

TABLE 8 Definition of SIRS

Two or more of the following conditions must be present:
Body temperature $> 38\ °C$ or $< 36\ °C$
Heart rate > 90 beats/min
Respiratory rate > 20/min or $PaCO_2$ <32 mmHg
Leukocyte count $> 12,000/\mu l$, $< 4000/\ \mu l$, or 10% immature forms

The diagnosis of sepsis is made when at least five of the clinical criteria below are met, in addition to the documentation of a septic source such as:

> burn wound biopsy with $> 10^5$ organisms/g tissue and/or histological evidence of viable tissue invasion,
> positive blood culture,
> urinary tract infection with $> 10^5$ organisms/ml urine,
> pulmonary infection with positive bacteria and white cells on a class III or better sputum specimen

Clinical criteria for diagnosis of sepsis include the presence of at least five of the following:

1. Tachypnea (> 40 breaths/min in adults)
2. Prolonged paralytic ileus
3. Hyper- or hypothermia ($< 36.5°C$ or $> 38.5°C$)
4. Altered mental status
5. Thrombocytopenia ($<50,000$ platelets/mm^3)
6. Leukocytosis or leukopenia ($>15,000$ or <3500 cells/ mm^3)
7. Unexplained acidosis
8. Hyperglycemia

Other parameters often seen associated with sepsis are enteral feeding intolerance, hypernatremia, and coagulopathy. Cardinal signs of gram positive and gram-negative sepsis are summarized in Table 9.

In the absence of a confirmed organism or site, antibiotic selection should be based on routine surveillance cultures. Empirical antibiotic choice should also be based on sensitivities of the burn facility's endogenous organisms. Routine perioperative antibiotics should also take ward-endogenous organisms into account. Systemic empirical antibiotics should be continued until micro-organisms are identified; use of agents is changed based on microbiology results. Treatment is continued for at least 72 h after evidence of sepsis has resolved.

If the wounds appear clean and there is no suspicion of burn wound sepsis, other sources such as the lungs, urinary tract, and catheter should be suspected. Pneumonia or bronchopneumonia is the most frequent site of infection in burn patients after burn wounds.

Pneumonia

The diagnosis of pneumonia in severely burned patients is exceedingly problematic. Many of the usual signs and symptoms of pneumonia are unreliable in burn patients. Fever, leukocytosis, tachypnea, and tachycardia may all be present in the absence of infection. Sputum examination is often contaminated with oropharyngeal flora. A class III sputum sample should be obtained in order to make a

TABLE 9 Cardinal signs of gram-positive and gram-negative burn wound sepsis

Grain-positive sepsis
1. Burn wound biopsy with $> 10^5$ organisms/ g tissue and/ or histological evidence of viable tissue invasion
2. Symptoms develop gradually
3. Increased temperature to $> 40°C$ or higher
4. Leukocytosis $>20,000/\mu l$
5. Decreased hematocrit
6. Wound macerated in appearance with exudates
7. Anorexic and irrational
8. Decreased bowel sounds
9. Decreased blood pressure and urinary output

Gram-negative sepsis
1. Burn wound biopsy with $> 10^5$ organisms/ g tissue and/ or histological evidence of viable tissue invasion
2. Rapid onset (8–12 h)
3. Increased temperature 38–39°C (may be normal)
4. Normal or high white cell count
5. If not controlled, patient become hypothermic (34–35°C) plus leukopenia
6. Decreased bowel sounds
7. Decreased blood pressure and urinary output
8. Wounds develop focal gangrene
9. Satellite lesions away from burn wound
10. Mental obtundation

diagnosis. More invasive sampling techniques such as bronchoalveolar lavage have been advocated; however, these have been also shown to be less than ideal for establishing a diagnosis of pneumonia. Concomitant inhalation injury and changes in pulmonary vascular permeability result in diffuse nonspecific radiographic changes. Radiographic findings can only be helpful if they reveal lobar consolidation. Current parameters for diagnosis of pneumonia are summarized in Table 10. Pneumonia can result from descending infection of the tracheobronchial tree or from hematogenous dissemination of microbial pathogens. Inhalation injury is associated with descending infection. Patients with inhalation injury who sustain nosocomial pneumonia have concomitant atelectasis, ventilation–perfu-

TABLE 10 Diagnosis of Pneumonia

Systemic inflammatory response syndrome
Radiographic evidence of a new or progressive infiltrate
Class 3 sputum or better with presence of micro-organisms and white blood cells

sion mismatch, arterial hypoxia, and respiratory failure. Critically ill burned patients present with a high risk for respiratory infections. Besides the already mentioned inhalation injury, patients have consecutive septic showers, during subsequent trips for surgery, dressing changes, or septic episodes. Moreover, burn patients often have problems with deglutition that pose a risk of aspiration pneumonia. Sudden changes in the patient's hospital course and in his or her respiratory status should alert the physician to seek respiratory complications. Aggressive respiratory toilet and empirical systemic antibiotics should be started and ventilatory support reserved for cases of frank respiratory failure. Nosocomial pneumonia is generally a gram-negative infection and systemic antimicrobial therapy with multiple agents is generally required until the infection resolves clinically. Burn wound bacterial surveillance is of added value to direct empirical antibiotics, since organisms isolated in respiratory infections reflect burn wound flora in many instances. On the other hand, patients with ventilatory support present with a microbial spectrum that resembles the typical ventilatory-dependent patient pneumonia. Tracheobronchitis presents with a heavy gram-positive colonization, putting patients at risk for gram-positive pneumonia.

Urinary Tract Infections

Urinary tract infections can be classified into upper and lower urinary tract infection. True pyelonephritis is very rare in burn patients; however, lower urinary tract infection can occur as a result of a chronic indwelling Foley catheter. Urinary tract infections are diagnosed based on positive culture greater than 1×10^5 organisms cultured from a urine specimen. Urinalysis may reveal white cells and cellular debris associated with active infection. Positive urinary cultures are common during the course of sepsis, and they are also treated in the general context of that particular septic episode. It must be noted, however, that the association of clinical signs of sepsis with burn wound cultures or blood cultures with positive urinary cultures make the final diagnosis of sepsis. Isolation of *Candida sp.* in the urine does not make a definitive diagnosis of candidiasis. Other information about organ involvement, such as positive findings on funduscopic examination, is necessary to make this diagnosis. In general, isolated urinary tract infections are treated with appropriate systemic therapy with good urinary extraction. Gram-negative coverage should usually be provided. If there is suspicion of an ascending infection or sepsis, more aggressive treatment with prolonged systemic antimicrobials is warranted.

Catheter Related Infections

Central and arterial line placement, catheter care, and protocol have been discussed in Chapter 1. Catheter-related sepsis is associated with prolonged indwelling central and arterial catheters. Catheter sepsis may be primary, in which the catheter is the original focus of infection; or secondary, in which the catheter tip is seeded and serves as a nidus for continued shedding of micro-organisms into the bloodstream. Lines can be associated with the development of both gram-negative and gram-positive sepsis. Central and arterial lines represent an avascular foreign body and, as such, are prone to microbial seeding. Infectious complications associated with indwelling catheters represent a major problem. Burned patients appear to be especially susceptible to this complication, with rates quoted as high as 50%. There is a strong correlation between micro-organisms recovered from catheter tips and skin flora, and pathogens can be traced in up to 96% of cases to bacteria isolated in the burn wound. The former supports the idea that bacteria migrate down the catheter to the tip. Persistent positive blood cultures, redness and purulent discharge around catheter insertion, and persistent high fever without other signs or sites of sepsis should arise the suspicion of catheter-related sepsis. Contemporary cultures from the central line and peripheral blood semi-quantitative culture aid in the diagnosis, although many physicians choose to remove of the suspected infected line and catheter tip culture. Treatment involves removal of all infected lines and placement of new lines through new sites. Suppurative thrombophlebitis should be suspected in patients who do not recover from the septic episode and show persistent positive cultures despite appropriate treatment. Immediate operative excision of the affected vein to the port of entry into the central circulation and packing of subcutaneous tissue are essential for the treatment of this complication.

Other sources of septic complications in burned patients that need to be ruled out include the following:

Acalculous cholecystitis
Cholangitis
Regional enteritis
Necrotizing enterocolitis
Pancreatitis
Suppurative thrombophlebitis
Pelvic infections
Suppurative chondritis
Subacute bacterial endocarditis
Suppurative sinusitis

BIBLIOGRAPHY

1. Total Burn Care. Second Edition. Herndon David N, Ed. London. United Kingdom: WB Saunders, 2002.
2. Color Atlas of Burn Care. Barret Juan P, Herndon David N, Eds. London. United Kingdom: WB Saunders, 2002.

3. Burn Care. Wolf Steven E, Herndon David N, Eds. Austin. TX: Landes Bioscience, 1999.
4. Surgical Management and Hypermetabolic Modulation of Paediatric Burns. Barret Juan P, Ed. Groningen. The Netherlands: University of Groningen, 2002.
5. Thermal injuryRamzy Peter I, Barret Juan P, Herndon David N. Crit Care Clin 1999; 15(2).
6. Quantitative Microbiology: Its Role in the Surgical Armamentarium. Heggers JP, Robson MC. Eds. Boca Raton Florida: CRC Press, 1991.
7. Principles and Practice of Burn Management . Settle John AD, Ed. Edinburgh. United Kingdom: Churchill Livingstone, 1996.

3

Diagnosis and Treatment of Inhalation Injury

Lee C. Woodson, Ronald P. Mlcak, and Edward R. Sherwood
Shriners Hospital for Children and the University of Texas Medical Branch, Galveston, Texas, U.S.A.

INTRODUCTION

Inhalation injury is a nonspecific term describing the harmful effects of aspiration of any of a large number of materials that can damage the airways or pulmonary parenchyma. Inhalation injury is produced by either thermal or chemical irritation due to aspiration of smoke, burning embers, steam, or other irritant or cytotoxic materials in the form of fumes, mists, particulates, or gases. The damage can be the result of direct cytotoxic effects of the aspirated materials or secondary injury due to an inflammatory response. In addition to damage to the airways and pulmonary parenchyma, inhalation of toxic substances such as carbon monoxide or cyanide can produce harmful systemic effects.

Inhalation injury is very common in patients who sustain burns. Incidence of inhalation injury among patients with major burns is often estimated at 33%. Presence of inhalation injury by itself or in combination with cutaneous burns has great clinical significance. Inhalation injury can be lethal by itself and increases the mortality associated with cutaneous burns. It continues to be the main cause of death in over 50% of fire-related deaths in the United States. A variety of factors have led to a dramatic reduction in the mortality associated with cutaneous burns. Now most patients will survive burns of 80% or more if treated promptly and transferred to a burn center. With reduced mortality due to initial burn shock or later sepsis, the presence of an inhalation injury has become an even more important determinant of survival for fire-injured patients.

There are many clinical consequences of inhalation injury. For example, patients with combined smoke inhalation injury and cutaneous burns are more hemodynamically unstable than patients with burn injury alone. The volume of intravenous fluids required for resuscitation of patients with acute burns is increased as much as 50% when the patient has also sustained a smoke inhalation injury. Inhalation injury can lead to pneumonia and/or acute respiratory distress syndrome (ARDS), which are risk factors for multiorgan system dysfunction. In addition, thermal or chemical injuries to the larynx can lead to scars that impair voice quality or compromise airway protection and lead to chronic aspiration pneumonitis, while tracheal injuries can induce subglottic stenosis.

With establishment of specialized burn centers and general improvements in the care of burn patients, survival of patients with inhalation injury has also improved. This improvement has not come from the development of therapies that specifically alter pathophysiological effects of smoke inhalation. Treatment of inhalation injuries still depends on appropriate resuscitation, prevention of infection, grafting of burn wounds, and nonspecific respiratory support as needed. Although management of inhalation injuries remains largely supportive, early recognition and appropriate treatment can greatly reduce associated morbidity and mortality. Early prophylactic intubation can prevent asphyxiation due to airway obstruction from edema. Recognition and treatment of the systemic effects of inhaled toxins such as carbon monoxide or cyanide may prevent death or severe neurological deficit. Adequate fluid resuscitation for patients with cutaneous burns can limit the pulmonary damage due to inhalation injury. In addition, early airway management decisions in patients with laryngeal injuries can influence subsequent development of glottic and subglottic stenosis. There are many management decisions to make for patients presenting with risk factors for significant inhalation injury. An understanding of both the pathophysiology of inhalation injury and therapeutic options is necessary to minimize the harmful effects of these potentially devastating injuries.

Despite much work carried out to date, a number of controversies still remain regarding fundamental clinical issues in the treatment of patients with inhalation injury. Some uncertainty exists in the management of inhalation injuries due to the fact that the severity of the inhalation injury is difficult to quantitate early in the course. The appropriate technique for long-term airway management in patients with burn injuries remains controversial. The popularity of tracheostomy for early airway management in burn patients is increasing again. The decision to perform tracheostomy, however, should be made only when potential benefits outweigh the risks of the procedure.

PATHOPHYSIOLOGY

There are three forms of inhalation injury (Table 1). Inhalation of extremely hot materials can cause direct thermal injury. As explained in more detail below, however, in those who initially survive burn injuries, thermal damage to the airways is generally restricted to the upper airways. Another form of inhalation injury is damage by inhaled chemical irritants. Depending on the substances inhaled, chemical irritation can extend throughout the airways and can also include the pulmonary parenchyma. A third form of inhalation injury involves the systemic effects of inhaled toxins, most commonly carbon monoxide or cyanide. These three forms of injury can exist alone or in combination with each of the other two forms. Each form of injury requires specific diagnostic and therapeutic intervention.

Thermal Injury

Foley [1] described findings from 335 autopsies performed on patients who died from extensive burns. Thermal injury to intraoral, palatal, and laryngeal mucosal surfaces were not uncommon among those with inhalation injuries. The most common sites of laryngeal burns were the epiglottis and vocal folds where their edges are exposed. In contrast, burn injury to tissues below the glottis and upper trachea was not observed in any of their patients. Thermal injury below the glottis is limited by the very efficient heat-exchanging function of the upper airway. In the same way that the upper airways heat and humidify cool dry inspired air, the lower airways are also protected from extreme heat. An exception is exposure to steam, which has a much greater heat capacity than that of dry gases and can overwhelm protection by the upper airway mucosa. Inhalation of steam can produce thermal injury throughout the major bronchioles. An additional protective mechanism is reflex laryngeal closure in response to intense thermal or chemical irritation in conscious victims. Unconscious victims lack this protection and are more vulnerable to inhalation injury. Thermal injury to the lower airways and pulmonary parenchyma implies exposure to very intense heat and is usually rapidly fatal.

When inhaled materials are hot enough, mucosal injury is immediate. Areas of blistering, ulceration, hemorrhage and rapidly developing edema can be observed soon after injury. The pharyngeal mucosa offers little resistance to edema

TABLE 1   Three forms of inhalation injury

Thermal Injury (usually before vocal cords)
Chemical irritation
Systemic toxicity

formation, which can be massive, especially during resuscitation with large amounts of crystalloid fluids.

Heat denatures tissue proteins that activate complement and initiate a cascade of inflammatory mediator release and activation. Most of the variables of the Starling equation are altered in favor of increased transvascular fluid flux. Capillary permeability is greatly increased (reduced reflection coefficient), microvascular hydrostatic pressure is increased, interstitial hydrostatic pressure decreases, and there is an increase in interstitial oncotic pressure. As plasma proteins are lost at the burn injury sites and resuscitation progresses, with large volumes of crystalloid plasma colloid oncotic pressure decreases dramatically. Lymphatic drainage is soon overwhelmed and interstitial volume increases (edema formation). In the extremities this edema from burns can increase interstitial pressures sufficiently to impair tissue perfusion. In a similar manner, burns to the head and neck can cause impaired ventilation when the airways are obstructed by mucosal edema or by extrinsic compression from tense circumferential edema of the neck, especially in young children.

Chemical Irritation

As a rule, except in the case of steam or when effects of heat are immediately lethal, the injury to the airways and pulmonary parenchyma caused by chemical irritants is much more damaging than the effects of heat. Toxic gases in the smoke are inhaled as well as carbon particles coated with other irritants deposited in the airways as soot. Water in secretions of the mucosa dissolves these materials, resulting in concentrated solutions of caustic materials bathing the sensitive airway mucosa.

The acute response to inhalation of chemical irritants involves injury to the respiratory epithelium followed by hyperemia, edema, inflammatory infiltrate, and formation of a protein-rich exudate. Much of the descriptive work regarding pathophysiological changes after inhalation injury has come from experimental animals. Early effects of smoke injury include separation of ciliated respiratory epithelial cells from the basement membrane and increased mucosal blood flow. Damage to the epithelium allows formation of exudate from the exposed interstitium and impairs mucociliary clearance. The hyperemic response results from increased bronchial blood flow, which facilitates edema formation and brings inflammatory cells to the injury site. Chemical irritants also induce bronchoconstriction and mucus secretion.

Much of the pathology associated with smoke inhalation injury is a result of the inflammatory response to the initial chemical irritation. It has been stated that understanding the inflammatory response to smoke inhalation depends more on understanding inflammation than on understanding a specific kind of smoke or the specific histopathological damage that smoke might initially evoke. The inflammatory response to smoke injury is very similar to the injury produced by acid aspiration.

The combination of disrupted epithelium, impaired mucociliary clearance, and bronchorrhea results in accumulation within the airways of necrotic debris, mucus and other secretions, and a protein-rich exudate. Fibrin is formed within this mixture and the combination creates a thick coagulum that forms casts adherent to the injured surface of the airways (Fig. 1). Together the effects of airway edema, bronchoconstriction, retained debris, and casts cause obstruction of airways. This results in areas of atelectasis and sequestration of materials that provide medium for growth of bacteria. Impaired function of alveolar macrophages also allows bacteria to proliferate. Further tissue damage results from recruitment and activation of neutrophils that produce extracellular proteases and oxygen radicals.

Pulmonary gas exchange is impaired by widespread ventilation perfusion mismatch and shunt. Bronchospasm and impaired hypoxic pulmonary vasoconstriction contribute to the mismatch of ventilation and perfusion. Shunt results from patchy areas of airway obstruction, atelectasis, alveolar flooding, and consol-

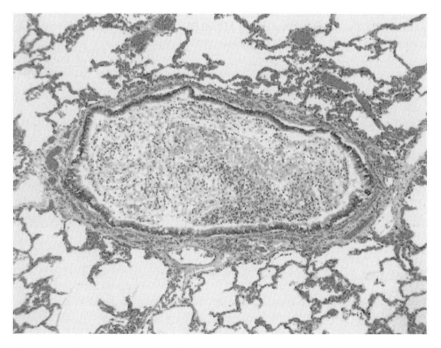

FIGURE 1 Bronchiole cast. Small airways may be completely obstructed by casts formed from inspissated secretions, fibrin, sloughed mucosa, and, as in this image, inflammatory cell infiltrate.

idation. Work of breathing is greatly increased by decreased compliance and increased respiratory rate.

Systemic Toxicity

Carbon monoxide (CO) and cyanide (CN) are clinically the two most important toxic components of smoke. Along with asphyxiation, CO accounts for most fatalities at the fire scene. Any patient with significant risk factors for smoke inhalation (e.g., exposure in a closed space, carbonaceous sputum, singed facial hair, or facial burns) should be evaluated for exposure to these toxins. CO has 200 times the affinity of hemoglobin for oxygen. CO decreases oxygen-carrying capacity by displacing oxygen from its binding sites on hemoglobin. CO further decreases oxygen delivery by preventing release of oxygen from oxyhemoglobin (shift of the oxyhemoglobin dissociation curve to the left). At some point this decrease in oxygen delivery limits cellular metabolism, leading to hypoxic insult, anaerobic metabolism and metabolic acidosis. Signs of CO toxicity include headache, mental status changes, dyspnea, nausea, weakness, and tachycardia. These are all nonspecific signs and may be masked by other effects of the burn or inhalation injuries. Patients with CO toxicity have a normal PaO_2 and oxygen saturation measured by routine pulse oximetry. They are not cyanotic. The definitive diagnosis is measurement of carboxyhemoglobin levels by co-oximetry.

CN is another common component of smoke and results from burning of certain plastic materials. CO and CN may be synergistic so that in combination sublethal concentrations of each may be much more dangerous than subtoxic levels of either alone. Some authors have suggested that the incidence of CN toxicity is underestimated. CN produces tissue hypoxia by inactivating cytochrome oxidase and blocking cellular oxygen utilization. Anaerobic metabolism results despite normal O_2 content and leads to a high anion gap metabolic acidosis. As with CO, the clinical signs of cyanide toxicity are nonspecific: headache, mental status changes, nausea, lethargy, and weakness. CN toxicity may be associated with an odor of bitter almonds. It should be suspected when high anion gap metabolic acidosis persists despite oxygen therapy and adequate circulatory resuscitation.

DIAGNOSIS

Early identification of an inhalation injury is important for optimal care of the fire-injured patient. Initially after injuries, breathing and pulmonary gas exchange may not be significantly impaired but knowledge of an inhalation injury at this time can influence a number of management decisions including airway management, fluid resuscitation, and diagnosis of systemic toxicity from inhaled substances.

History

Definitive diagnosis of inhalation injury will ultimately depend on endoscopic observations of damaged airway mucosa or development of respiratory failure. Timely management, however, begins with a heightened suspicion based on clinical evaluation. Information from a history and physical examination can be used to identify many patients with inhalation injury.

A number of historical features identify victims at increased risk for inhalation injury (Table 2). One of the most important is a history of smoke exposure in an enclosed space, which prevents dilution of the smoke and impairs the victim's ability to escape. Some forms of physical or mental impairment likewise prevent avoidance behavior and increase the risk of smoke inhalation. Physical impairment might be due to traumatic injury, while mental impairment could include extremes of age or depressed consciousness due to hypoxia or intoxication (substance abuse or toxic smoke components). Information regarding duration should be sought: prolonged exposure implies higher risk.

The nature of exposure is also an important determinant of injury. Flash or explosive fires can result in thermal injury to both the upper and lower airways. The trachea may be burned if the upper airway heat exchange capacity is overwhelmed and hot gases are forced through the glottis before laryngeal closure is possible. As mentioned earlier, inhalation of steam can cause thermal injuries distal to the larynx. Aspirated or swallowed hot liquids may also cause pharyngeal and laryngeal burns. Exposure to caustic fumes may cause serious injury to the airways and lung parenchyma. If the composition of inhaled fumes is known, the harmful effects of the chemical irritants can be predicted from knowledge of the chemicals' solubility. Effects of water-soluble irritants are generally seen in the airways because they dissolve in and are sequestered in airway secretions more proximately. Less soluble irritants are carried more distally and may cause delayed pulmonary edema from parenchymal injury.

TABLE 2 Features of patient history associated with increased risk of inhalation injury

Smoke exposure in an enclosed space
Prolonged exposure to smoke
Physical or mental impairment
Fire conditions and fuel
   Explosions
   Steam
   Caustic Fumes
Pre-existing pulmonary disease
Aspirated or swallowed hot liquid

It is important to obtain a history of pre-existing medical conditions. The impact of an inhalation injury depends in part on the patient's physiological reserve, which may be limited by the presence of pre-existing disease.

Physical Examination

Physical examination also reveals clues to underlying inhalation injury. Injuries of a critical nature are generally picked up during the initial trauma survey (advanced trauma life support protocol). Respiratory distress from airway obstruction or impaired pulmonary gas exchange usually presents with obvious signs and symptoms. Other patients with serious inhalation injury may present without respiratory distress and the insidious nature of the progressive respiratory failure may make inhalation injury less obvious initially. Physical examination can identify individuals at increased risk (Table 3).

Soot covering the face is clear evidence of exposure to smoke but not necessarily inhalation injury. Carbonaceous sputum is stronger evidence of smoke inhalation but may also be a false-positive indicator. Coughing up cabonaceous secretions can occur when soot deposits are restricted to the nasal passages. Carbonized nasal secretions may be aspirated and appear in tracheal aspirates. In addition, smoke inhalation and smoke inhalation injury are not always synonymous. Damage to the tissues in the airways or lung parenchyma does not always occur when smoke is inhaled. Inhalation injury will depend on the amount of exposure, the heat and composition of the smoke, and probably the individual susceptibility of the victim.

Cutaneous burns over the face and singed facial or nasal hair are evidence of exposure to intense heat near the airways. It also means that the victim was unable to escape exposure or injury, since the face is generally protected from

TABLE 3   Physical examination
findings associated with
inhalation injury

Respiratory distress
Soot over face or in sputum
Burns over face or neck
Singed facial or nasal hair
Oropharyngeal burns
Tachypnea
Hoarseness
Strider
Drooling
Signs of airway obstruction

---

heat by vigorous avoidance behavior. Patients with facial burns should be observed closely for signs and symptoms of upper airway obstruction by edema. These patients should also have their oropharynx examined for mucosal burns.

Respiratory impairment may present subtly as tachypnea. The patient may also show preference for the upright position for breathing. Hypoxia can cause altered mental status, confusion, or a decreased level of consciousness. These findings are also consistent with systemic CO or CN toxicity.

The thorax should be examined for burn injury. Extensive full-thickness burns to the chest, especially circumferential injuries, may result in a restrictive ventilatory defect. More superficial thoracic burns can cause a similar defect as thoracic compliance is decreased slowly by edema that develops during resuscitation with fluids.

Dyspnea, hoarseness, and coughing are often present initially in burn patients but often resolve spontaneously. Stridor should be differentiated from hoarseness as a more ominous sign. High-pitched inspiratory noise over the upper airway is characteristic of critical narrowing of the airway. In the context of fluid resuscitation for burn injuries, this can be rapidly progressive and demands immediate evaluation and probably intervention as well. Other signs of airway obstruction include use of accessory respiratory muscles, sternal and suprasternal retractions, and paradoxical thoracoabdominal movement.

Evaluation of the impact of an inhalation injury must take into account the presence of associated injuries. The combination of full-thickness burns with inhalation injury requires a larger volume of fluid for resuscitation than for the burns alone. Underresuscitation as well as overresuscitation of cutaneous burns can exacerbate the effects of an inhalation injury. The ability of a patient to compensate for an inhalation injury is diminished by injuries that make breathing difficult (e.g., fractured ribs or pneumothorax).

None of the above observations from the history and physical examination can be considered 100% sensitive and specific for inhalation injury. The value of these clinical indicators increases when multiple risk factors coexist. It has been stated that the diagnosis of inhalation injury becomes easier with the passage of time. However, morbidity is minimized by early diagnosis and treatment of inhalation injury.

Diagnostic Studies

History and physical examination will identify patients at risk for inhalation injury as well as those who urgently need intubation and mechanical ventilation. For patients at risk for injury but not currently experiencing respiratory failure, additional information is necessary. Diagnostic studies can provide objective information about extent of injury and physiological status (Table 4). This information

TABLE 4   Diagnostic studies for
evaluation of inhalation injury

Pulse oximetry
Arterial blood gas analysis
Chest radiograph
Fiberoptic bronchoscopy
Pulmonary function tests
Radionuclide ventilation–perfusion scans

---

can be critical for timely decisions. Serial measurements may be necessary for
some studies because the pathophysiological changes develop with time.

Pulse Oximetry

Pulse oximetry provides a sensitive and continuous means of assessing oxygenation. The continuous tone produced by the instrument allows practitioners to
monitor oxygenation constantly while concentrating on other aspects of patient
care. A change in tone is readily recognized by experienced clinicians despite
other distracting noises or activities. The plethysmograph function of the pulse
oximeter can be used to help assess peripheral perfusion in extremities that may
be compromised by tense edema or vascular injury. Pulse oximeter function
requires adequate peripheral flow and pulse. Loss of pulse oximeter signal in a
finger or toe may indicate deterioration in perfusion.

   Monitoring with pulse oximetry also has limitations. Since function requires
an extremity with a pulse, it may be difficult to find a suitable site for the probe
in some patients. Ear or lip probes may be suitable in some patients. In addition,
standard pulse oximeters cannot identify carboxyhemoglobin. This means that
patients with tissue hypoxia due to carbon monoxide toxicity cannot be diagnosed
using pulse oximetry.

Arterial Blood Gas Analysis

Arterial blood gas analysis provides a definitive measure of pulmonary gas exchange. Initial measurement of PaO_2 is an insensitive marker for inhalation injury
because there is usually some delay in development of gas exchange impairment
after smoke inhalation. Although this method is an insensitive prognostic marker,
early hypoxia is an ominous sign of severe injury. Analysis of arterial blood gases
provides useful information in patients with inhalation injury, especially in the
presence of cutaneous burns. Even if results are normal, early blood gas analysis
provides a baseline for comparison with later measurements as pulmonary function deteriorates. When interpreted in the context of the concentration of inspired
oxygen, the PaO_2 can allow estimation of physiological shunt. Serial measurements show disease progression or resolution and, along with $PaCO_2$, are used
to determine decisions about therapeutic support.

Early measurement of carboxyhemoglobin can identify patients with carbon monoxide toxicity. Initial carboxyhemoglobin concentration greater than 10% has been found to correlate with smoke exposure. Normal carboxyhemoglobin levels range from 1–2% in urban nonsmokers to 5–6% in smokers. Levels above 15% are toxic and levels above 50% can be lethal.

High concentrations of CO have been associated with combined toxicity with CN. Persistent metabolic acidosis despite appropriate resuscitation and normal hemodynamic function suggests cyanide toxicity. CN can be measured: levels greater than 0.5 μg/ml are potentially toxic and levels above 3 μg/ml are lethal [2]. Unfortunately laboratory measurement is frequently unavailable in a timely manner. The diagnosis should be made clinically based on history (substantial smoke exposure, plastic or furniture fire), unexplained metabolic acidosis, and elevated venous oxygen level. To minimize toxicity treatment should begin before laboratory measurements are available.

Blood gas analysis can also be used to assess response to fluid resuscitation for burn injuries. Metabolic acidosis is consistent with inadequate tissue perfusion and may indicate the need for more aggressive resuscitation efforts. Inhalation injury can increase the fluid required for resuscitation by almost 50%. Adequate resuscitation is even more important in the presence of inhalation injury, since underresuscitation exacerbates the effects of inhalation injury.

Chest Radiograph

Even when ventilation–perfusion scans indicate an inhalation injury, initial chest x-ray studies are usually normal in patients with inhalation injury. There is usually a delay in the development of small airway obstruction and atelectasis that are responsible for the initial chest x-ray changes caused by smoke inhalation. Because of this, initial chest x-ray studies have a very low negative predictive value. Despite this, chest x-ray studies are indicated for all patients at risk for inhalation injury. Identification of underlying pulmonary disease or early changes due to inhalation injury can significantly influence the patient's course. A chest radiograph is also important to exclude other thoracic injuries associated with the accident.

Fiberoptic Bronchoscopy

Inhalation injury is manifest largely as injury to the mucosa of the airways. Endoscopy provides immediate direct observation of mucosa in the larger airways. Results of a bronchoscopic examination are immediate and definitive. Flexible fiberoptic bronchoscopy is generally considered safe and accurate for the diagnosis of inhalation injury. The procedure allows detailed examination of supraglottic structures and tracheobronchial passages. Diagnosis of subglottic inhalation injury (Table 5) is based on findings of soot deposits, inflammatory changes (hyperemia, edema, bronchorrhea, and excessive mucus secretion), and/

TABLE 5 Endoscopic findings
with inhalation injury

Erythema
Edema
Soot
Bronchorrhea
Mucosal disruption
  Blistering
  Sloughing
  Ulceration
Exudates
Hemorrhage

---

or disruption of mucosa (mucosal blistering, sloughing, ulceration, exudates, and hemorrhages). These alterations generally precede impaired oxygenation and respiratory failure. Although these changes provide reliable diagnosis of the presence of inhalation injury, bronchoscopic evaluation has not proved accurate in quantitating the degree of injury.

When indicated, serial examination can help to avoid unnecessary intubations and at the same time allow intubation before severe airway obstruction and emergent conditions occur. In this situation the flexible bronchoscope can also be used as a means safely to secure the airway in patients who might otherwise be difficult to intubate. Intubation while maintaining spontaneous ventilation is considered the safest way of securing a difficult airway. In adults this can be accomplished with topical local anesthesia (nasal local anesthetic gel and glottic and subglottic local anesthetic sprayed through the suction port of the bronchoscope) and sedation if required. Most pediatric patients will not cooperate with such procedures while awake. Ketamine (5–10 mg/kg intramuscularly or 1–2 mg/kg intravenously) provides excellent conditions for bronchoscopy. Unlike other sedatives, ketamine does not reduce pharyngeal motor tone and cause airway obstruction from collapse of pharyngeal soft tissues. With the patient under ketamine sedation, topical local anesthetic must be administered to the larynx prior to instrumentation with the bronchoscope. A drying agent such as glycopyrrolate 0.1–0.2 mg intravenously is useful to reduce secretions during ketamine sedation. Ketamine can also be used with uncooperative adults; however, they are more prone to dysphoric effects of ketamine and may require benzodiazepine treatment during recovery from sedation. Sedation with any agent should be avoided in patients in significant respiratory distress if it appears that intubation by direct laryngoscopy would be difficult and fiberoptic intubation is required. Sedation can reduce respiratory drive and lead to airway collapse, making it difficult or impossible to ventilate or intubate with the bronchoscope.

Pulmonary Function Tests

Pulmonary function tests (PFTs) are effort dependent and so are of limited value for patients who are unable to cooperate. In the early phase of burn injury many factors such as pain, anxiety, and analgesic medications can impair compliance with the examination. As a result, PFTs are more useful for long-term follow-up care of patients with inhalation injury. Early testing of pulmonary function can be useful, however, when results are within normal limits. The negative predictive value of PFTs has been found to be in the range of 94–100%. Normal PFTs can be used to rule out early airway obstruction. The ratio of forced expiratory volume in 1s to functional vital capacity (FEV$_1$/FVC) is sensitive to small airway obstruction. In patients who can comply with testing, the value will decrease with injury. Flow volume loops have also been found reliably to rule out upper airway obstruction by edema. Obstruction due to upper airway edema presents as a variable extrathoracic obstruction when flow volume loops are obtained. Inspiratory flows are selectively reduced while expiratory flows are unimpaired (Fig. 2).

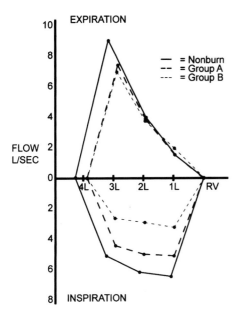

FIGURE 2 Flow–volume loops based on spirometry and forced vital capacity measurements in nonburn controls and in burn patients with inhalation injury. Group B had more airway inflammatory changes than group A. Note the selective reduction of inspiratory flow rates.

Radionuclide Scans

Xenon 133 ventilation–perfusion scans have been found useful in the early diagnosis of inhalation injury and this technique is included in most reviews of inhalation injury. The radionuclide is excreted by the lungs after intravenous injection. Small-airway obstruction delays clearance of the radionuclide from the airways. Interpretation of results can be complicated when patients have pre-existing lung disease. The examination also requires transportation of the patient to a facility remote from the burn ICU at a time when the patient's condition is relatively unstable. As a result, lung scans are not used extensively to diagnose inhalation injury.

TREATMENT

Treatment of inhalation injury is largely supportive in nature. There are few specific treatments available, with the exception of identified systemic toxins such as CO or CN. Initially an advanced trauma life support (ATLS) survey and an airway, breathing, circulation (ABC) approach to resuscitation are indicated. Inhalation injury is usually encountered in combination with cutaneous burns. Each injury must be treated in the context of the effects of the other. Inhalation injury increases the risk of acute respiratory distress syndrome (ARDS) and other pulmonary complications with severe cutaneous burns. Presence of inhalation injury also increases the volume of fluid required for resuscitation of the cutaneous burns. It is important to keep this in mind because underresuscitation will exacerbate the effects of inhalation injury.

All patients at risk for significant smoke exposure should have their carboxyhemoglobin level measured by co-oximetry. Standard therapy for CO toxicity has been 100% oxygen provided by tight-fitting mask or endotracheal tube. The half-life of carboxyhemoglobin is approximately 320 min for a person breathing room air and approximately 80 min when breathing 100% oxygen. Hyperbaric oxygen therapy further reduces the half-life and increases oxygen delivery by dissolved oxygen, but the relative risk–benefit relationships for this intervention are still controversial [3].

When CN toxicity is suspected treatment is begun empirically based on a clinical diagnosis. Treatment includes administration of sodium thiosulfate (150 mg/kg over 15 min) to convert cyanide to thiocyanate. In severe cases sodium nitrate (5 mg/kg slowly intravenously) can be given to convert hemoglobin to methemoglobin, which will convert cyanide to cyanmethemoglobin [3a].

Circumferential full-thickness burns can dramatically reduce chest wall compliance. The resulting restrictive respiratory defect can significantly impair ventilation. When this occurs escharotomies should be performed in the anterior axillary lines and these incisions should be connected by a transverse subcostal incision (Fig. 3). In some cases the relief provided by this intervention is sufficient to avoid tracheal intubation.

Morbidity and mortality due to pneumonia and other delayed complications are best minimized by prevention. Scrupulous attention to wound care, cleanliness, pulmonary toilet, vascular access sites, and monitoring for signs and symptoms of infection and extubation as soon as possible all help to prevent infection and allow early intervention when it does occur. Early excision and grafting reduce the time that wounds are open and minimize the risk of infection. When

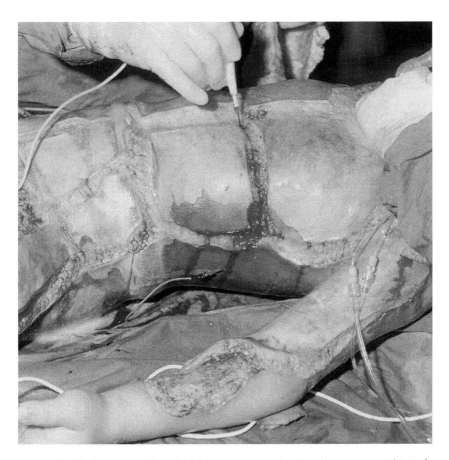

FIGURE 3 Escharotomy. Elevated tissue pressure due to edema can restrict perfusion in extremities and edema due to circumferential thoracic injuries can lead to a profound restrictive ventilatory deficit. Escharotomies can restore perfusion to extremities and may relieve restrictive ventilatory deficit enough to avoid intubation.

burn wounds are covered with autograft and are healing, systemic inflammatory activity abates, which speeds the resolution of residual inhalation injury.

Great improvements in survival from burn injuries have been made due to aggressive fluid resuscitation and coordination of multidisciplinary care in specialized burn centers. Seriously injured patients are best served by transfer to a tertiary center or burn center as soon as possible. Even with early transfer, during the first hours after injury there are important decisions and interventions necessary to minimize long-term sequelae.

Early prophylactic intubation

In patients with head and neck burns or inhalation injury, the most immediate danger during resuscitation is upper airway obstruction by edema. Burns to the face and neck can produce edema that progressively distorts anatomy and reduces range of motion, making direct laryngoscopy difficult or impossible. Acute lung injury due to smoke inhalation can also impair pulmonary gas exchange and lead to respiratory failure. Early prophylactic intubation is recommended when these complications threaten.

In some patients the need for immediate intubation of the trachea is obvious. Extensive and deep burns to the head and neck, hypoxia, depressed mental status, stridor or other overt signs of airway obstruction, and hemodynamic instability are among the list of strong indications for intubation (Table 6). Occasionally the signs and symptoms are more subtle or may be absent initially. With volume resuscitation, edema develops both in burned tissues and at sites distant from the injury. During resuscitation with large volumes of fluid, edema can cause airway obstruction rapidly in some patients. In these cases early prophylactic intubation can be life-saving.

Other patients may present with risk factors as well as signs and symptoms of inhalation injury and yet they may not benefit from intubation. In fact, most patients with inhalation injury do not require intubation and mechanical ventilation. Unnecessary intubation presents a number of serious risks to these patients

TABLE 6 Indications for Immediate Intubation in Patients at Risk for Inhalation Injury

---

Respiratory failure
Extensive full-thickness burns to head and neck
Stridor
Other overt signs and symptoms of airway obstruction
Endoscopic evidence of glottic closure by edema
Inability to protect airway
Hemodynamic instability

(Table 7). At a time when the burn patient is often at his or her most lucid, intubation precludes effective communication so that the history is limited, the patient's wishes cannot be expressed, and we cannot assess the patient's ability to comprehend information. It is often difficult to sedate the patient after intubation. Heavy sedation is often required and under these circumstances muscle relaxants are used in some institutions. Deep sedation and muscle relaxation increase the morbidity and mortality of unintended extubations, which have been found more frequent in this patient population. In addition, irritation to the larynx by an endotracheal tube is synergistic with inhalation injuries in producing laryngeal and tracheal injuries. Prophylactic intubation of all patients at risk will include many who would not benefit from intubation. These patients would be exposed to increased risk without benefit. As a result, it is important to exercise good clinical judgement in identifying patients for intubation. In order to make this distinction it is necessary to recognize which patients are at risk, understand the clinical course of inhalation injuries, utilize objective measurements of airway compromise (such as endoscopy), and follow the patient with close observation and serial re-evaluations when needed.

Several authors have concluded that clinical observations are not sufficiently sensitive or specific to identify reliably which patients will develop progressive edema and respiratory insufficiency due to the resultant obstruction. Clinical evaluation has been reported to either underestimate or overestimate the severity of inhalation injury and supraglottic edema [4,5]. As an example Muehlberger et al. [5] found that 6 of 11 patients in their series of patients with inhalation injury had traditional indications for intubation (Fig. 4), but upon fiberoptic endoscopy did not show significant obstruction to warrant intubation and were managed safely and effectively without and endotracheal tube.

An additional valuable observation of these studies is that when adequate resources are available, it is safe to observe without intubating select patients who are at risk for inhalation injury. Clinicians at the Baltimore Regional Burn

TABLE 7 Risks Associated With Unnecessary Intubations in Burn Patients

Intubation precludes effective communication with the patient.
Distorted anatomy and perceived urgency make traumatic or failed intubation more likely.
Endotracheal tubes are difficult to secure and incidence of self-extubation is high in acute burn patients.
Acute burn patients are often agitated after intubation and require heavy sedation, making unplanned extubation more dangerous.
Inhalation injury and mechanical trauma from the endotracheal tube are synergistic in producing laryngeal and tracheal injuries.

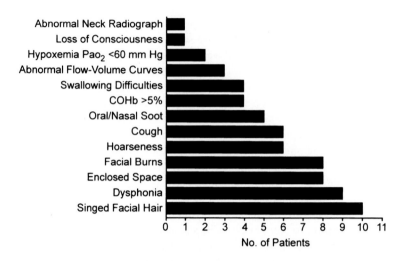

Figure 4   Frequency distribution of signs and systems of inhalation injury in 11 patients exposed to smoke and/or fire who presented without evidence of airway obstruction or respiratory distress. None of these patients required intubation despite the presence of multiple risk factors for inhalation injury.

Center [5] proposed an algorithm for airway management of burn patients at risk for airway compromise (Fig. 5). Initial ATLS survey can identify patients with impending respiratory failure or airway obstruction. These patients can be intubated before their airway status deteriorates further. Other patients at risk for inhalation injury but without obvious obstruction and distress initially can be evaluated endoscopically for direct evidence of airway obstruction.

When available, flexible fiberoptic endoscopy is very well tolerated by patients. Adults can be examined under topical local anesthesia and sedation as needed. Children in contrast, must be sedated for bronchoscopy. At our pediatric burn hospital, examinations are safely performed with patients under ketamine sedation and topical local anesthesia. Endoscopy allows direct and objective evaluation of the airway. If the airway appears patent with no significant obstruction the patient can be followed by close observation and, if necessary, serial examinations. If the glottic mucosa is pearly opalescent (edematous) and beginning to encroach on the glottic opening, intubation may be necessary. Presence of edema and inflammatory changes in the upper airway should be interpreted in the context of factors including but not limited to patients' pre-existing physical status, coexisting injuries, feasibility of rapid intubation, size and distribution of burns, and resuscitation requirements (volume and rate of infusion). During observation any significant clinical change, such as voice alteration, increased respiratory effort, or difficulty swallowing, warrants prompt re-evaluation.

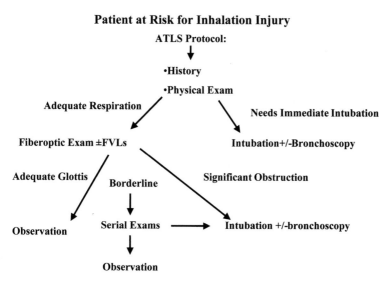

Patient at Risk for Inhalation Injury

FIGURE 5   Algorithm for airway management in patients at risk for inhalation injury.

Airway edema and occlusion can develop rapidly. Although there are risks associated with unnecessary intubations, in the absence of equipment or training for endoscopy or if close observation is not possible, empirical prophylactic intubation is the safest course of action if there is doubt about the status of the patient's upper airway. Special consideration must also be given to transportation of patients between institutions. This may involve a significant period of time (hours) in a setting of limited resources. When transferring the patient to a tertiary care or burn center airway management, decisions should be made in consultation with the accepting institution. Empirical prophylactic intubation may seem the safest choice. However, we have seen serious morbidity and even mortality due to airway complications in pediatric patients who had relatively trivial burns but were intubated for transport. Clearly defined indications for intubation should be identified prior to transport to justify the significant risks of intubation.

Inhalation Injuries to the Larynx and Tracheostomy

In addition to the more immediate airway concerns (obstruction and asphyxia) in the acute burn patient, management decisions must be made regarding more long-term consequences of thermal injuries to the larynx. Later sequelae include airway narrowing secondary to subglottic stenosis, compromise of laryngeal protection of lower airways and parenchyma from aspiration, and impaired voice quality. The arytenoids, true vocal cords, and the subglottic region are the areas most prone to long-term scarring.

Patients presenting with significant risk factors for inhalation injury should be examined endoscopically for evidence of laryngeal burns. Presence of significant thermal injury to the larynx makes it more prone to injury by an endotracheal tube. When possible, early extubation reduces the risk of exacerbating a laryngeal injury. When extubation is not possible tracheostomy is another option that may help to limit laryngeal injury.

Controversy exists regarding the use of tracheostomy in burn patients. The early popularity of tracheostomies for initial airway management in burn-injured patients gave way to reports of unacceptably high rates of complications. In the most often quoted study regarding the risks of tracheostomy in burn patients, Eckhauser et al. [6] reported much higher rates of pulmonary sepsis and mortality in burn patients with tracheostomies than in intubated patients without tracheostomy. Moreover, a 100% correlation was found between cultures of the burn wound and cultures of the endotracheal aspirate. Presence of a tracheostomy stoma, especially through a burn injury, was assumed to facilitate contamination of the respiratory tract with microorganisms from the burn wound. Tracheostomies were considered an increased risk in burn patients and a more conservative approach was recommended, with tracheostomies reserved for specific indications rather than for so-called prophylactic airway control [6,7].

More recently many clinicians have published comparisons of clinical outcomes for burn patients managed with translaryngeal endotracheal tubes and tracheostomy tubes. These studies indicate that the risk of pneumonia for patients with tracheostomies is the same as the risk for patients with translaryngeal endotracheal tubes [8,9]. The earlier study by Eckhauser et al. [6] has been criticized because of inadequate controls and other methodological deficiencies [7,10]. The general consensus now is that with current methods of supportive care, the risk of pneumonia appears similar in patients with tracheostomies and those with translaryngeal endotracheal tubes.

Tracheostomy offers several advantages over a translaryngeal endotracheal tube in certain patients. For those requiring prolonged mechanical ventilation, the tracheostomy tube has been reported to reduce dead space, improve compliance, lower peak inspiratory pressures, and facilitate airway suctioning. Tracheostomy also offers protection from laryngeal and tracheal injury. Prolonged translaryngeal intubation is associated with laryngeal injury. Tracheostomy is especially beneficial for patients who have sustained inhalation injury to the larynx. Mechanical irritation to the larynx by an endotracheal tube exacerbates inhalation injury to the larynx caused by heat or chemical irritants.

Several recent studies have described very low rates of morbidity associated with tracheostomy in small study groups of burn patients, especially young patients [11]. Some of these authors have recommended earlier and more aggressive use of tracheostomy in burn patients. A conservative reluctance to use tracheostomy in burn patients is now frequently replaced with a broader application of this technique, often in patients with normal airways and without need for long-term mechanical ventilation. Reluctance to perform tracheostomy in burn patients may increase risk of laryngeal injury in these patients, especially in those who have also sustained an inhalation injury to the larynx. At the same time, burn patients may experience an increased risk of morbidity when tracheostomy is performed in patients who will not benefit from the procedure (risk without benefit).

Many patients who have sustained major burn injury require intubation and mechanical ventilation soon after their injury. For most of these patients, intubation is only required for a short duration, often only until upper airway obstruction due to edema resolves. Even when inhalation injury is diagnosed endoscopically and pulmonary gas exchange is impaired, intubation and mechanical ventilation are not necessary unless there is profound respiratory failure. Under theses circumstances, tracheostomy offers little advantage over a translaryngeal endotracheal tube. In fact, in some burn patients initial management with tracheostomy presents an additional serious risk. A specific concern about the use of tracheostomy in burn patients is that, soon after burn, pronounced edema from cutaneous neck burns may cause dislodgment of the tracheostomy tube. Under these circumstances, loss of the airway may be life-threatening. Even in the presence of facial burns, an oral endotracheal tube may be more secure than a tracheostomy when thermal injury to the neck results in extensive edema.

One factor contributing to the controversy regarding the timing of conversion from translaryngeal intubation to tracheostomy in patients with inhalation injury is that it is very difficult to evaluate accurately the severity of an inhalation injury. This makes it difficult to predict which patients will require prolonged ventilation. Sellers et al. [10] have approached this problem using logistic regression to identify factors that correlated with prolonged ventilator dependence. The factors that they identified (percentage of body surface area with full-thickness burns, age, presence of inhalation injury, and worst PO_2/FiO_2 on postburn day 3) were used to develop an equation to predict the probability of prolonged ventilator dependence. Although this equation was found to be sensitive and specific for what they considered for prolonged ventilator dependence, many institutions will not perform tracheostomy at 2 weeks if there is no laryngeal injury and pulmonary function is improving. The reason to convert from translaryngeal intubation is to prevent mucosal disruption and subsequent scarring. The time required for mucosal disruption by an endotracheal tube will vary depending on presence of laryngeal inhalation injury, patient movement (e.g., swallowing, vocalization, and head movement), and systemic inflammatory processes. In the absence of laryngeal injury, conversion to tracheostomy can be delayed if there are indications that separation from mechanical ventilatory support may soon be possible.

Tracheostomy clearly offers advantages over translaryngeal intubation in certain patients in whom earlier conversion to tracheostomy reduces morbidity

[8]. However, tracheostomy does not offer advantages in all burn patients. Tracheostomy is an invasive procedure with a low but finite incidence of complications that can be very serious or lethal. The risk of subglottic stenosis in patients without laryngeal inhalation injury and who do not require prolonged ventilation should be higher after tracheostomy than after several atraumatic intubations for serial debridement and grafting procedures.

At present there are no unequivocal indications for timing the decision to convert to tracheostomy. It remains a judgment. The judgment applied by each center is most strongly influenced by local experience that will vary from center to center for many reasons. Because of this, all controversy will not likely be resolved any time soon. However, certain principles should be agreed upon.

In burn patients the increased risk of morbidity with tracheostomies is acceptable when the procedure also provides a significant advantage. However, when a patient has a normal airway without laryngeal injury and prolonged mechanical ventilation is not needed, tracheostomy does not offer benefit other than convenience during serial anesthetic administration for wound debridement and grafting. The decision to perform tracheostomy in burn patients should be individualized and based on specific indications. To reduce morbidity, the decision should be made as early as possible but not before a true indication is identified. Laryngeal injuries such as burns can be diagnosed immediately by endoscopy and tracheostomy can limit further injury. In this case tracheostomy should not be delayed. It is helpful to consult otolaryngologists as soon as a laryngeal injury is diagnosed. In the absence of upper airway injury, translaryngeal intubation can be continued without increased morbidity until it is clear that prolonged mechanical ventilation is needed.

Respiratory Care

The multitude of respiratory complications caused by smoke inhalation imposes heavy demands on the respiratory care practitioners who play a central role in its clinical management. Demands may include intubation and resuscitation of victims in emergency departments, assistance with bronchoscopy, performance of pulmonary function tests, monitoring blood gas analysis, pulmonary hygiene, chest physiotherapy, and management of mechanical ventilation. Effective respiratory care of patients with inhalation injury requires an organized, protocol-driven approach to therapy. This topic has been reviewed recently [12].

Bronchial Hygiene Therapy

Bronchial hygiene therapy techniques are an essential component of respiratory management of patients with inhalation injury. Therapeutic coughing, chest physiotherapy, early ambulation, airway suctioning, therapeutic bronchoscopy and use of pharmacological agents all may be effective in the mobilization and removal of retained secretions and fibrin casts. Retained secretions may result in life-threatening airway obstruction; they may also cause atelectasis, ventilation–perfusion mismatch, and ultimately contribute to the development of pneumonia, which will increase burn mortality.

Tracheobronchial suctioning and lavage are imperative for the removal of secretions and casts that cannot be cleared by the patient because of incapacitated mucociliary apparatus or ineffective cough. Scheduled, routine suctioning should be performed in all affected patients to aid in secretion removal. When secretions or casts become thick and adherent to the airways, bronchial lavage should be used as an adjunct to routine suctioning. Care must be taken not to use excessive lavage fluid because it may wash out surfactant. Nasotracheal suctioning may be performed in nonintubated patients as a mechanism to stimulate coughing and clear debris. Hazards that may occur with nasotracheal suctioning include mucosal irritation and bleeding, hypoxemia, vagal stimulation with bradycardia, and death.

Chest physiotherapy, postural drainage with elevation of the head of the bed, and routine repositioning of the patient every 2 h may be effective for secretion removal. Unfortunately, these techniques are frequently of limited use in burn patients because of concerns regarding the fragility of fresh skin grafts and donor sites.

Early after-injury out-of-bed activities including standing, sitting in a chair, and walking have been used as a means of expanding the lungs while gentle vibrations are performed to the affected area. Patients with inhalation injury are routinely moved out of bed to sit in a chair to help improve lung function. Parents of pediatric patients are encouraged to hold and rock their children as a means of therapy and to increase patient comfort.

When all other techniques fail to remove secretions, fiberoptic bronchoscopy has proven effective. Inspissated secretions and fibrin casts may prove resistant to all simpler methods of removal from the tracheobronchial tree. Fiberoptic bronchoscopy allows visualization of the airway and enables meticulous pulmonary toilet for clearance of retained secretions.

Pharmacological Treatment

Chemical tracheobronchitis resulting from inhalation can produce bronchospasm. Therefore the use of bronchodilators can be extremely useful in the pharmacological treatment of inhalation injury. This is especially true for patients with pre-existing reactive airway disease. Aerosolized sympathomimetics are effective in two ways: they result in bronchial muscle relaxation and they stimulate mucociliary clearance.

Aerosolized racemic epinephrine may be used as a vasoconstrictor. The vasoconstrictive action of racemic epinephrine is useful in reducing mucosal and submucosal vascular congestion and edema, especially in the upper airways. A secondary bronchodilator action serves to reduce potential spasm of the smooth muscles of the terminal bronchioles. Racemic epinephrine has also been used for the treatment of postextubation stridor. In our institution racemic epinephrine is used routinely after extubation in pediatric patients. Smaller pediatric patients are more sensitive to the effects of subglottic edema on airway narrowing.

Prospective clinical trials of corticosteroids have not shown a benefit for patients with inhalation injury. Despite the prominent role of inflammation in the pathophysiology of inhalation injury, not only did steroids fail to reduce morbidity or mortality they may also be associated with a higher rate of infections.

N-Acetylcysteine is a powerful mucolytic agent used in respiratory care. Its thiol group makes it a strong reducing agent capable of rupturing the disulfide bonds that stabilize the molecular mucoprotein network of mucus. Agents that break down these disulfide bonds produce the most effective mucolysis. Nebulized sympathomimetic bronchodilators are given along with N-acetylcysteine to counteract bronchial hyperreactivity.

A major problem for patients with smoke inhalation injury is the formation of fibrin casts in the small airways. These casts are composed of sloughed mucosa and other cellular debris and secretions held together by a tenacious fibrin clot formed from the protein-rich exudate that develops in the airways after inhalation injury. Fibrin casts block the airways and prevent ventilation of areas distal to the cast. This results in atelectasis, pulmonary shunt, and hypoxia. In addition, when mechanical ventilation is used with higher pressures and volumes to compensate for respiratory failure, normal areas of pulmonary parenchyma are injured and the acute lung injury is exacerbated. Distal to airways obstructed by casts, retained materials provide an excellent medium for microbial growth and greatly increase the risk of pneumonia.

Nebulized N-acetylcysteine and heparin administered to reduce formation of fibrin casts are the only specific agents with evidence of clinical efficacy for patients with inhalation injury. Desai et al. [13] treated pediatric patients with smoke inhalation injury using alternating doses of nebulized heparin (5,000–10,000u) and the mucolytic agent acetylcysteine (3 ml 20% solution). In a retrospective review of medical records of pediatric patients with inhalation injury, the authors observed a significant decrease in reintubation rates, incidence of atelectasis, and mortality in patients treated with nebulized heparin and N-acetylcysteine.

Effective respiratory care requires coordination of a variety of treatment modalities. The goals of this regimen is to maintain adequate ventilation and oxygenation, facilitate clearance of secretions and material from the airways, prevent atelectasis, and monitor function. Successful management requires a well-organized and protocol-driven approach. The inhalation injury pharmacological treatment protocol used at Shriners Burns Hospital–Galveston is described in Table 8.

TABLE 8   Shriners Burns Hospital-Galveston Inhalation injury treatment protocol

1. Titrate high-flow humidified oxygen to maintain SaO2 > 92%.
2. Cough, deep breathing exercises every 2 h.
3. Turn patient side to side every 2 h.
4. Chest physiotherapy every 4 h.
5. Nebulize 3 cc N-acetylcysteine 20% solution every 4 h for 7 days.
6. Alternate nebulizing 5000 units heparin with 3 cc normal saline every 4 h for 7 days.
7. Nasotracheal suctioning and lavage as needed.
8. Early ambulation.
9. Sputum cultures Monday, Wednesday, and Friday.
10. Pulmonary function studies prior to discharge and at outpatient visits.
11. Patient/parent education regarding disease process.

Mechanical Ventilation

Despite all conservative efforts to support unassisted ventilation, patients with moderate or severe inhalation injury may develop respiratory failure and require mechanical ventilation. Patients with severe inhalation injury are at a substantial risk for iatrogenic, ventilator-induced lung damage. Airway resistance is increased secondary to edema and cast formation; thus, higher airway pressures are required to provide sufficient flow to maintain minute ventilation. The optimal treatment of any disease reverses the pathophysiologic process without causing further injury. When inhalation injury is severe enough to require mechanical ventilation, such an outcome is not achieved. Conventional mechanical ventilation does not reverse the pathological process, is not characterized by improved clearance of secretions, and may actually compound the existing injury.

Over the past 30 years, and especially over the past decade, new ventilator techniques have become available that present alternatives for the treatment of patients with inhalation injury. Unfortunately, although the number of options available to the clinician has appeared to increase exponentially, well-controlled prospective trials defining the specific role for each of the modes of ventilation and comparing them to other modes of ventilation have not been performed.

The American College of Chest Physicians consensus conference on mechanical ventilation provided general guidelines that are applicable to inhalation injury patients. A summary of these guidelines is presented in Table 9.

A recent randomized study by the Acute Respiratory Distress Syndrome Network of the National Heart, Lung, and Blood Institute compared outcomes using large (12 ml/kg) tidal volume with airway pressure of 50 cmH_2O or less with outcomes with small (6 ml/kg) tidal volumes and pressure of 30 cmH_2O or less. The volume-assist-control mode was used for ventilation. The study was

TABLE 9 Recommendations from the American College of Chest Physicians
Consensus Conference on Mechanical Ventilationl

The clinician should choose a ventilator mode that he or she is familiar with and
    that has been shown capable of supporting oxygenation and ventilation.
A lower limit of acceptable oxygenation should be identified.
A plateau pressure greater than 35 cmH_2O is of concern; however, when chest wall
    compliance is reduced, greater pressures may be acceptable.
In order to limit airway pressure, PCO_2 should be permitted to rise (permissive
    hypercapnia) when tolerated.
PEEP is useful in supporting oxygenation and may help reduce lung damage. The
    optimal PEEP level should be chosen after empirical trials and re-evaluated
    regularly.
Large tidal volumes (12–15 ml/kg) with PEEP may be needed to improve
    oxygenation if the use of protective ventilatory strategies is ineffective

stopped early because of higher mortality in the group with higher tidal volumes
and pressures. It is now generally agreed that ventilation should be initiated with
tidal volumes of 6–8 ml/kg body weight. When acute increases in PCO_2 and
decreases in PO_2 occur, obstruction by fibrin casts should be considered, this
should be treated initially with aggressive pulmonary toilet. If this is unsuccessful,
physicians should consider changing to volume ventilation with higher tidal volumes as needed to provide oxygenation and ventilation.

Multiple studies have demonstrated that large portions of the lungs of patients ventilated for treatment of respiratory failure are consolidated and cannot
be ventilated. Under these circumstances, high airway pressures associated with
delivery of standard tidal volumes can cause pneumothorax. Overdistention of
patent alveoli also extends the lung injury by inducing interstitial edema, hemorrhage, and hyaline membrane formation in previously noninjured lung tissues.
Deliberate hypoventilation has been practiced in an attempt to reduce these
changes by lowering airway pressures associated with higher rates of ventilation
required to maintain a normal PCO_2. Hypercarbia and resultant respiratory acidosis are accepted as a tradeoff for lowered risk of ventilator-induced lung injury.
Hypercarbia has been well tolerated when the pH is maintained at 7.2 or higher.

High-frequency percussive ventilation (HFPV) has also been used following inhalation injury. This mode facilitates oxygenation at lower inspired oxygen
concentrations and adequate ventilation at lower peak and mean airway pressures.
In addition, a few reports have indicated increased secretion clearance with some
forms of high-frequency ventilation. The terms high-frequency flow interruption
and high-frequency percussive ventilation have been used to describe a technique
in which ventilation is accomplished by a positive-phase percussion delivered at
the proximal airway. In clinical trials, high-frequency percussive ventilation was

found to permit adequate ventilation and oxygenation in a small cohort of patients for whom conventional ventilatory support following inhalation injury had failed. A clinical trial has been published by Cioffi and colleagues in which a substantial decrease in inhalation injury-associated morbidity and mortality was noted [13a].

LATE COMPLICATIONS

With serious inhalation injuries, persistent systemic inflammation and prolonged ventilation at high pressures are associated with a variety of complications later in the patient's hospital course. High airway pressures and mechanical irritation from the endotracheal tube, tracheostomy tube, and a tracheal cuff combine to injure the airway further. Tubes and cuffs erode mucosa, exposing cartilage, and lead to laryngomalacia or tracheomalacia. Healing of denuded areas involves scar formation that can result in stenosis that impairs laryngeal motion and subglottic narrowing. High airway pressure impairs mucosal perfusion. This mucosal ischemia prevents healing, resulting in persistent inflammation and infection. Tissue responses vary with patient age. Children have a tendency to formation of granulation tissue and stenosis while older patients are more likely to experience necrosis and fistula formation.

Nearly all survivors of severe inhalation injury requiring prolonged ventilation, especially at higher airway pressures, retain some degree of respiratory dysfunction. Respiratory dysfunction can involve either upper airway or pulmonary parenchyma. Laryngeal injury can result in impaired vocal cord function, causing problems with phonation or lead to chronic aspiration. Pulmonary parenchymal pathological conditions include pulmonary fibrosis, reduced pulmonary capillary volume, bronchilolitis obliterans, chronic bronchitis, and bronchiectasis. These conditions can lead to a variety of associated pulmonary function problems including reactive airway disease, altered compliance, increased dead space and closing volume, and limitation of diffusion. Additional mechanical deficiencies also may impair pulmonary function. Prolonged ventilation and immobilization can cause atrophy and weakness of respiratory muscles. Thoracic burn scars (especially when circumferential) may contribute to a restrictive respiratory defect. Spinal deformities due to burn scar contractures can also cause a severe restrictive respiratory defect.

Long-term follow-up of pulmonary function among survivors of ARDS has revealed a large degree of heterogeneity. Function may be near normal in those who were young and did not smoke at the time of injury. However, respiratory function may be significantly impaired in older patients and in those who had additional comorbidities at the time of injury [14]. The most common abnormalities seen have been reduced diffusing capacity and easy fatigability. The observation that poor exercise tolerance did not correlate with the decrease in diffusion capacity suggests that the early fatigue seen in these patients is unrelated to pulmonary pathology [14]. Mlcak et al. [15] reported increased physiological dead space/tidal volume ratio during exercise in children 2 years after injury. This same group studied burned children out to 8 years and observed residual pulmonary pathology even at rest [16]. These changes included altered lung mechanics, gas exchange, decreased chest wall compliance due to scarring, and respiratory muscle weakness. Following severe thermal and inhalation injury, it is likely that these patients may never regain normal lung function.

SUMMARY

Inhalation injury either alone or in combination with cutaneous burns is associated with serious risk of morbidity and mortality. Early diagnosis and treatment are important because inhalation injury can lead to asphyxiation due to airway obstruction from edema, it increases volume requirements for fluid resuscitation in patients with cutaneous burns, and specific therapy may be needed for systemic toxins.

Overall mortality associated with burns has decreased dramatically and this includes patients with both burns and inhalation injury. Improved outcome is the result of many changes but includes aggressive fluid resuscitation, early excision, improvements in general care, along with the availability of specialized burn centers. These changes in care speed wound healing and reduce the incidence of serious infection and sepsis. These improvements also affect the course of inhalation injury by reducing systemic inflammation and pneumonia.

Beyond these improvements, the treatment of inhalation is largely supportive and nonspecific. Meticulous attention to details of bronchial hygiene can help prevent retention of secretions, airway obstruction, atelectasis, and pneumonia. Careful management of mechanical ventilation is needed to minimize ventilator-induced injury.

There are also specific therapeutic interventions for inhalation injury. Early prophylactic intubation can prevent lethal airway obstruction, but this decision must be weighed against the risks of unnecessary intubations. Hyperbaric oxygen therapy or pharmacological treatment of cyanide toxicity can prevent death or permanent neurological deficit. Nebulized heparin and a mucolytic agent can reduce cast formation, which leads to airway obstruction, atelectasis, hypoxia, and pneumonia. Later decisions include whether and when to convert from a translaryngeal endotracheal tube to a tracheostomy.

Patients at risk for inhalation injury can be identified by information obtained from their medical history and physical examination. Mucosal injury can be identified by endoscopic examination. At present it is not possible to predict which patients will experience progressive respiratory failure as a result of inhalation injury. Effective management requires continuous close observation and co-ordination of the efforts of all the burn care team.

REFERENCES

1. Foley FD. The burn autopsy: fatal complications of burns. Am J Clin Pathol 1969; 52(1):1–13.
2. Bakerman's ABC's of Interpretive Laboratory Data. 3rd Ed. Myrtle Beach. SC: Interpretive Laboratory Data, Inc., 1994.
3. Chou KJ, Fisher JL, Silver EJ. Characteristics and outcome of children with carbon monoxide poisoning with and without smoke exposure referred for hyperbaric oxygen therapy. Pediatr Emerg Care 2000; 16:151.
3a. Stoetting RK. Periphera Vasodilators. In: Pharmacology and Physiology in Anesthetic Practice. Philadelphia: J. B. Lippincott, 1991:327.
4. Haponik EF, Lykens MG. Acute upper airway obstruction in patients with burn. Crit Care Rep 1990; 2:28.
5. Muehlberger T, Kunar D, Munster A, Couch M. Efficacy of fiberoptic laryngoscopy in the diagnosis of inhalation injuries. Arch Otolaryngol Head Neck Surg 1998; 124: 1003–1007.
6. Eckhauser FE, Bollote J, Burke JF, Quinby WC. Tracheostomy complicating massive burn injury. A plea for conservatism. Am J Surg 1974; 127(4):418–423.
7. Hunt JL, Purdue GF, Gunning T. Is tracheostomy warranted in the burn patient? Indications and complications. J Burn Care Rehab 1986; 7:492.
8. Barret JP, Desai MH, Herndon DN. Effects of tracheostomies on infection and airway complications in pediatric burn patients. Burns 2000; 26:190.
9. Jones WG, Madden M, Finkelstein J, Yurt RW, Goodwin CW. Tracheostomies in burn patients. Ann Surg 1989; 209:471.
10. Sellers BJ, David BL, Larkin PW, Morris SE, Saffle JR. Early prediction of prolonged ventilator dependence in thermally injured patients. J Trauma 1997; 43:899.
11. Palmieri TL, Jackson W, Greenhalgh DG. Benefits of early tracheostomy in severely burned children. Crit Care Med 2002; 30:922.
12. Mlcak RP, Herndon DN. Respiratory care. In: Total Burn Care. 2nd Ed. Herndon DN, Ed. London: W.B. Saunders, 2001.
13. Desai MH, Mlcak RP, Richardson J, Nichols R, Herndon DN. Reduction in mortality in pediatric patients with inhalation injury with aerosolized heparin/acetylcystine therapy. J Burn Care Rehab 1998; 19:210–212.
13a. Cioffi WG, Rue LW, Graves TA, McManus WF, Mason AD, Pruitt BA. Prophylactic use of high-frequency percussive ventilation in patients with inhalation injury. Ann Surg 1991; 213:575–580.
14. Cooper AB, Ferguson ND, Hanly PJ, Meade MO, Kachura JR, Grantson JT, Slutsky AS, Stewart TE. Long-term follow-up of survivors of acute lung injury: Lack of effect of a ventilation strategy to prevent barotrauma. Crit Care Med 1999; 27(12): 2616–2621.
15. Mlcak RP, Desai MH, Robinson E, McCauley RL, Richardson J, Herndon DN. Increased physiological dead space/tidal volume ratio during exercise in burned children. Burns 1995; 21(5):337–339.

16. Mlcak RP, Desai MH, Robinson E, Nichols RJ. Lung function following thermal injury children—an 8-year follow up. Burns 1998; 24:213.

BIBLIOGRAPHY

1. Demling RH, Chen C. Pulmonary function in the burn patient. Semin Nephrol 1993; 13:371.
2. Fitzpatrick JC, Cioffi WG. Diagnosis and treatment of inhalation injury. In: Total Burn Care. 2nd Ed. Herndon DN, Ed. London: W.B. Saunders, 2001.
3. Practice Guidelines for Burn Care. J Burn Care Rehab Suppl 2001; 14S.
4. Haponik EF, Munster AM. Respiratory Injury. Smoke Inhalation and Burns. 1st Ed. New York. NY: McGraw-Hill, 1990.
5. Thompson JW. Inhalational and caustic injury to the larynx. In: The Larynx. Ossoff RH, Shapshay SM, Woodson GE, Nettercile JL, Eds. Lippincott Williams & Wilkins, 2003:421–430.
6. Traber DL, Herndon DN, Soejima K. The pathophysiology of inhalation injury. In: Total Burn Care. 2nd Ed. Herndon DN, Ed. London: W.B. Saunders, 2001.

4

Burn Wound Management and Preparation for Surgery

Juan P. Barret and Peter Dziewulski
Broomfield Hospital, Chelmsford, Essex, United Kingdom

After the size, site, and depth of the burn wound have been determined and all initial urgent measures are completed, a plan of treatment must be formulated for further management of the wound. Patients are transferred to their room where general treatment is continued and comfort measures, including warming and analgesia, are instituted. At this point, attention needs to be turned to the burn wound. A clear plan must be instituted, and repeated dressing changes to make management decisions should be avoided. Plastic wrap or Telfa clear dressings covered in warming blankets or any other material that keeps patients warm and comfortable should be used. This allows for easy inspection of the burn wound if a definitive plan of treatment is still to be outlined or a new or more senior burn surgeon needs to inspect the wound to make the final treatment plan. As soon as the initial management and resuscitation of burn patients is complete the determination of the wound treatment plan is the main focus during this phase of patient care.

It is essential to outline the surgical plan in order to institute the rationale of dressing changes and the choice of dressing materials. A proper diagnosis is necessary to start wound care. Depending on the size and depth of the burn wound, the approach to wound care and closure will differ, and so will the rationale for wound care and dressings.

The topical treatment applied to the burn wound will generally be based on two main criteria:

The depth of the burn wound
The type of surgical approach to the burn wound

Determination of burn depth crucial in formulating the treatment plan. Superficial burns require a well-developed wound care protocol. Wounds of this type heal without surgical intervention; therefore, the topical treatment and choice of dressings will have a direct impact on the patient's comfort and wound healing. The type of surgical intervention, especially the timing of excision and extent of the excision, will determine the type of wound care management patients require before and during burn wound closure.

BURN WOUND MANAGEMENT BASED ON THE DEPTH OF THE WOUND

Burn injuries damage different degrees of the epidermis, dermis, and soft tissues. Depending on the depth of the injury, wounds will present with different abilities for healing and re-epithelialization. Superficial wounds will present with good chances for complete wound healing within 3 weeks, whereas deep wounds have lost most or all possibilities for spontaneous wound healing. State-of-the-art wound care is therefore essential in superficial wounds to warrant and stimulate spontaneous wound healing. Surgery and operative wound closure will play a central role in the management of deep wounds.

In general, patients can be categorized to three broad groups depending on the type of injury sustained:

1. Superficial burn
2. Indeterminate-depth burn
3. Deep partial and full-thickness burn

Patients' local wound treatment and surgical plans are based essentially on the type of injury (see Table 1).

Superficial burns include all those injuries that have destroyed the epidermis and different degrees of the papillary dermis. They are represented by first-degree

TABLE 1 Management of the Burn Wound

Superficial partial-thickness burns: conservative treatment
Deep Partial and full-thickness burns: excision and autografting
Indeterminate-depth burns: Conservative treatment (10–14 days), followed by
   second inspection and definitive treatment (based on healing time)

(or epidermal burns) and superficial second-degree burns (or superficial partial thickness burns). Conservative management of these injuries is normally the rule. Indeterminate-depth burns include those injuries that can be classified neither as superficial nor as deep burns. Their potential for regeneration is also variable, and a period of conservative treatment followed by a second assessment and definitive treatment plan is usually required. Deep second-degree and third-degree burns represent deep partial and full-thickness burns. They do not represent any treatment problem, and surgery is normally the treatment of choice. Most or all dermal appendages have been destroyed, and regeneration proceeds slowly or never occurs. The debate continues as to the timing of surgery, especially for patients with massive injuries.

Superficial burns

A conservative approach is mandatory in this type of injury. Superficial burns heal by proliferation of skin appendages. When they heal in less than 3 weeks they leave minor skin changes or no scars at all. The period that these injuries require for complete healing is mandated by the speed of debridement of all devitalized tissues and the proliferation of basal cell epithelial cells. Treatment should be therefore directed to speed or promote debridement of all debris caused by burning and to provide a microenvironment that allows and promotes re-epithelialization. Many topical treatment regimens are available in the market for treatment of superficial burns. Many topical antimicrobial creams for the temporary skin substitutes are available. The application of topical creams for the treatment of partial-thickness burns has been and still is favored by many burn care physicians. This treatment protocol proved to be effective in the late 1960s and early 1970s and allowed for better control of burn wound sepsis. The application of topical creams requires frequent dressing changes and produces severe pain and anxiety. Patients refer to these as among the most painful and frightening experiences in their lives. Such treatment has been proved effective for the treatment of superficial burns, but its use presents with a series of drawbacks, including patient discomfort, difficulties in burn dressing, and delays in discharge from hospital. The former has stimulated the exploration of alternative treatments with temporary skin substitutes.

For many years, application of 1% silver sulfadiazine cream has been the standard choice. Its use, however, requires frequent dressing changes and a daily bath or shower that provokes pain and severe anxiety. Silver sulfadiazine works best when it is applied every 12 h, thus doubling pain discomfort and increasing nursing staff stress. The application of temporary skin substitutes is a good alternative to daily dressing changes, but their use requires a more sophisticated approach. They are also more expensive and their use must be rationalized to be able to extend the quality of care to all burn patients. The most commonly used temporary skin substitutes for the conservative treatment of superficial burns include Biobrane, TransCyte, and porcine xenografts. Their use and application are described in full in Chapter 7. Skin homografts are also a good alternative to temporary skin substitutes, but their particular characteristics and price mandates that their use be more restricted for patients with massive superficial burns.

Regardless of the dressing used on a superficial burn, it has to serve all the following purposes:

1.   Superficial burns need to be aggressively debrided prior to the application of the definitive dressing. In many circumstances it is best done under sedation or general anesthesia in patients with large superficial burns.
2.   The dressing has to provide a natural protection against infection. If subsequently infected, superficial burns may convert to full-thickness skin loss requiring formal excision and skin autografting, which leads to a worse cosmetic and functional outcome.
3.   The dressing has to provide comfort to patients and, ideally, should provide good analgesia.
4.   The dressing should permit patients' full range of motion and early rehabilitation.
5.   The dressing should be easy to care by patients and relatives.
6.   The dressing should permit early discharge of patients and subsequent control in the outpatient department.

The treatment of superficial burns is outlined in Chapter 7. However, the authors' choice of treatment for any significant superficial burn is temporary skin substitutes, which provide all former characteristics. Good quality of care can be achieved with conservative treatment with topical antimicrobial creams, but side effects and patient discomfort should preclude their use. Prospective studies have proved the superior outcome of superficial burns with the extensive use of temporary skin substitutes. Pain is absent or significantly reduced, patient discomfort is improved, and patients are discharged sooner from the hospital. Final outcome is similar with both treatments; therefore it is our criteria to treat any significant superficial burn with temporary skin substitutes.

Deep Partial and Full-thickness Burns

In deep partial and full-thickness burns a formal surgical approach should be followed. In deep partial-thickness burns most of the dermis has been destroyed. They usually heal after a prolonged period of time (more than 3 weeks) by proliferation of skin appendages that reside deep in dermis. After a variable time of bacterial and chemical debridement of the superficial dead tissue, epithelial cells migrate to the raw surface. The prolonged healing time and inflammation lead to scar formation and poor cosmetics and function, which provide the rationale for early excision of the dead tissue and skin autografting. The final outcome provided by skin autografts is regarded as far better than that of the natural healing process, which is usually complicated by hypertrophic scar formation, decreased function, prolonged rehabilitation, and poor cosmetic outcome.

Full-thickness burns present with a total loss of skin. Healing progresses by prolonged spontaneous debridement and eschar separation and the production of different amounts of granulation tissue. Small full-thickness skin losses may heal by contraction and re-epithelialization from the skin edges, whereas large full-thickness skin losses may progress to loss of limbs, granulation tissue formation, and septic complications. Those who survive the natural healing process are usually left with profound disabilities. Standard treatment of full-thickness burns includes formal early excision of all dead tissue and skin autografting. Deep injuries with bone, tendon, or other exposures of vital anatomical structures require flap coverage.

As mentioned before, treatment of choice for both deep partial-thickness and full-thickness burns includes excision and autografting. A temporary dressing needs to be applied while the patient is awaiting surgery. The application of 1% silver sulfadiazine or cerium nitrate–silver sulfadiazine provides good antimicrobial properties, although it may be not necessary if surgery is to be performed immediately. When burns are debrided and grafted immediately or few hours after the injury, a simple protective dressing may be applied to isolate the wound from the hostile environment. Topical antimicrobials are not necessary in these circumstances because wounds are sterile soon after burning. It is not until days after the injury that they are heavily colonized with pathogens. More insight into the treatment of these injuries in provided in Chapters 8 and 9.

Indeterminate-Depth Burns

Indeterminate-depth Burns fall between superficial and deep partial burns. In general, they present with a mixture of both injuries, such as burns with a so-called geographical appearance: presenting with patterns of superficial blanching areas together with whitish nonblanching areas, none of which is big enough to be diagnosed as true areas of deep partial thickness that could be treated surgically. In this case, sacrificing the mixture of superficial burns would worsen the final outcome, extending the area of grafting and scarring to areas of living tissue that would have healed otherwise without scars. These injuries have areas of superficial vital injuries that will heal with conservative treatment enclosed in regions of deep partial-thickness injuries. The treatment of the burns with early excision and grafting would sacrifice all these vital areas of skin. On the other hand, the appearance of the whole burn wound includes some deep injuries and wounds with doubtful vitality.

Treatment of these injuries calls for an initial conservative approach followed by a formal diagnosis and agreement. A diagram of all sites involved should be created. Burn wounds that heal in less than 3 weeks do so without scar formation; patients are therefore treated conservatively for 10–14 days. At that time, a new assessment is made and a decision is made as to whether the remaining will or will no heal within 3 weeks (counting day 0 as the day of the burn injury). If wounds appear to heal and complete wound closure is expected before day 21 postinjury, conservative treatment is continued. Wounds that will need more than 3 weeks to heal are treated then as deep partial-thickness wounds, excision and skin autografting are performed.

Conservative treatment that patients receive during the first 10 to 14 days is similar to that outlined for superficial wounds (see Chap. 7). Use of skin substitutes is also strongly advised, but they present with a higher tendency to collections and infection than do superficial wounds. Whichever treatment option is chosen, burn wounds need to be inspected periodically to detect any infectious complications. Systemic antibiotics and formal burn wound excision and autografting may be needed in the event of burn wound sepsis. Other than that, patients are reviewed but *no changes in the plan of management of burn wounds are made*. The initial decision must be maintained during the first 10–14 day period. Burn wounds are dynamic and change during that period. Changing the management decision half way through this time based on the wound appearance will inevitably lead to excision and autografting. This break in the practice will produce increased blood loss, sacrifice of living tissue, and grafting of burned areas that might have healed on their own (see Fig. 1).

Large life-threatening burns constitute an exception to this general management of indeterminate burns. Even though the vitality of these injuries is still in question and all the former considerations apply to these massive burns, these patients are candidates to early superficial excision or debridement and homografting. This aggressive surgical approach leads to an optimal survival rate and excellent outcome. These injuries carry a high likelihood of mortality. Removal of all devitalized tissues and wound closure with vital homografts, which close the wounds and provide growth factors, lessen this likelihood. Treatment does not differ from that of massive superficial burns, as described in Chapter 7.

BURN WOUND MANAGEMENT BASED ON THE SURGICAL APPROACH

Two basic general surgical approaches apply in burn surgery. How burn wounds are managed during the initial period, will significantly affect the way the wound is managed topically. Time delay between burn injury and surgery is the key element in the two main surgical approaches. They include:

1. Immediate burn wound excision
2. Early/serial burn wound excision

INDETERMINATE-DEPTH BURN WOUND

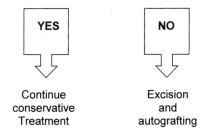

Conservative treatment for 10-14 days

**Second assessment at
10-14 days**

BURN WOUND TO HEAL IN THREE WEEKS?

YES   NO

Continue   Excision
conservative   and
Treatment   autografting

FIGURE 1   Protocol for treatment of indeterminate depth burn wounds. Once the master plan and management decision have been established, patients are treated conservatively for 10–14 days. At that time, a definitive plan is outlined.

These two main approaches differ in the timing of surgery, regardless of the type, diagnosis, and depth of the burn wound. The different philosophy in the surgical approaches resides in the general planning and the day surgery is started. The same burn wound may be treated successfully using either of the two ways, but differences in the postburn hypermetabolic and inflammatory response, blood loss, and possible sacrifice of viable tissue may result.

Immediate Burn Wound Excision

In this surgical approach all burn wounds are operated on within 24 h after the injury. Deep burns are excised and grafted, whereas superficial burns are treated with temporary skin substitutes. When this technique is utilized, topical management of the wound awaiting definitive surgical treatment includes the application of clean (nonsterile) plastic wrap or the application of petrolatum-based fine-mesh dressings. Telfa clear may serve the same purpose plastic wrap. It can also be applied nonsterile, but it can be purchased as long nonsterile rolls that can be easily autoclaved. Topical antimicrobials are not necessary. Burn wounds are sterile early after burning, and colonization has yet to begin by the time patients are sent to the operating room. Within 24 h after the burn injury, all wounds are surgically closed either with grafts or temporary skin substitutes; therefore the application of topical antimicrobials is not necessary. Less expensive materials should be always used, since temporary dressings applied after burn wound assessment are to be removed in few hours. The rationale for immediate burn wound excision includes the modulation of the hypermetabolic, catabolic, and inflammatory response of patients by immediate removal of dead tissue. More information regarding immediate burn wound excision is to be found in Chapters 9 and 10.

Early/Serial Burn Wound Excision

In early/serial burn wound excision, burns are excised within 72 h after the injury. Wounds are serially excised in sessions of up to 20–25% of the total body surface area involved in the injury. Patients return at intervals of 48 h to the operating room, with the aim of having the complete burn wound excised within 7–10 days after injury. Information on this approach is summarized in Chapter 10. Burn wounds that are not full thickness are dynamic during the first 48 h. Therefore, advocates for this technique prefer to delay surgery 48–72 h until resuscitation is complete and all burn wounds are stable to avoid the excision of potentially viable tissue. It is also accepted that a small delay in definitive treatment is not harmful in burn surgery, although increasing evidence in the trauma and burns literature claims otherwise.

Topical management of wounds is as follows:

1. Superficial and indeterminate wounds: The same approach outlined before and presented in Chapter 7 can be applied when using this approach. Superficial and indeterminate burn wounds can be treated with temporary skin substitutes after cleansing and superficial debridement.
2. Deep-partial and full-thickness burns: Burns of this nature should be treated with the application of topical antimicrobials until definitive surgical treatment is performed. One percent Silver sulfadiazine is the standard treatment in many burn centers, although cerium nitrate–silver sulfadiazine is a very good alternative. Definitive burn wound closure is achieved before colonization by multiply resistant gram-negative bacteria occurs, so no further antimicrobials are usually needed.

Burn wounds that are serially excised and covered with either autografts or skin substitutes will require the application of different ointments and topical solutions depending on the skin expansion and skin substitute used. The reader is referred to Chapter 10 for more information.

Another approach included in this less aggressive group of therapies is the conservative treatment of burns with cerium nitrate–silver sulfadiazine for a week followed by delayed serial burn wound excision. In this therapy, wounds are managed topically with daily application of cerium nitrate–silver sulfadiazine for a week. Patients then undergo surgery on limited areas of their body and return at weekly interval for further excision and autografting. The wounds that are left nonexcised after every operative session are treated with daily application of the same topical agent until complete wound closure has been achieved.

In any pragmatic approach, certain patients may not fit in the protocol. In these circumstances, an individual approach needs to be implemented to provide a good outcome. Good examples include the following:

> Non-life-threatening burns in patients with important associated medical conditions. Medical conditions need to be addressed first to decrease the morbidity and mortality of surgery
>
> Large superficial burns with small full-thickness patches are best treated as superficial burns and full-thickness areas addressed last when the rest of the burns are healed.
>
> Patients who experience extreme pain not controlled with analgesic regimens may benefit from early excision and grafting to decrease daily cleansing.
>
> Small deep–partial and full-thickness burns in patients who continue working and attending school are best treated conservatively and operated on as out patients procedures.
>
> Burns to the hands and feet benefit from an aggressive approach to permit the patient's early social and work reintegration

PREPARATION FOR SURGERY

Burn surgery requires commitment and cooperation from the whole burn team. Treatment of massive burns is an enterprise that matches the complexity of open-heart surgery or any other major surgical procedures based on the interaction of a multidisciplinary team. It should be only attempted in major tertiary hospital facilities where the whole spectrum of specialization is available. Even though burn wound excision and grafting may seem to the novice as a simple and easy surgical procedure, a profound understanding of the burn pathophysiology, dynamics of wounds, critical care, and wound healing is necessary to perform successful operations.

Preparation for surgery is based on three main principles:

1. Anesthetic evaluation
2. Preparation of patients
3. Preparation of the operating room.

Burn wound excision, either immediate/early or delayed should be considered an elective procedure and prepared and managed as such. Only emergency surgical airway access and escharotomy and fasciotomy should be undertaken without formal and proper evaluation. Experienced burn anesthetists and burn surgeons only should perform burn wound excision, since minor errors may lead result in the death of patients.

Anesthetic Evaluation

Destruction of skin by thermal injury disrupts the vital functions of the largest organ in the body and results in a systemic inflammatory response that alters function in virtually all organ systems. The metabolic rate and reserve of many organs are altered. All changes that occur during the resuscitation phase and postresuscitation phase should be noted and taken into account to provide safe anesthesia. Treatment of burn patients must compensate for loss of these functions, until the wounds are covered and healed. Preoperative evaluation of the burned patient is guided largely by knowledge of these pathophysiological changes. Good communication with the surgical team is essential in order to estimate the size and depth of the wound to be operated on. This will help in estimating the actual physiological insult to be expected during surgery. The trauma that surgery superimposes on the already increased metabolic rate of burn patients can result in it being impossible to ventilate patients during surgery. Accurate estimates of blood loss are crucial in planning the operative management of burn patients. Surgical blood loss depends on area to be excised (cm^2), time since injury, surgical plan, and presence of infection. Blood loss from skin graft donor sites will also vary depending on whether it is an initial or repeated harvest. Calculation of expected blood loss is calculated in Table 2. Special atten-

TABLE 2 Calculation of Expected Blood Loss

Time since burn injury	Predicted blood loss (cc/cm² burn area)
< 24 h	0.45
1–3 days	0.65
3–16 days	0.75
> 16 days	0.5–0.75
Infected wounds	1–1.25

tion must be paid to the airway and pulmonary function during preoperative evaluation. Anatomy can be distorted and range of mobility to allow enough exposure of the airway may be decreased. The level of respiratory support needs also to be assessed. The patient's hemodynamic status must be investigated to foresee any derangement that may occur during surgery and to establish the patient's inotropic support requirements. A thorough and systematic review of all systems should follow, noting all derangements, pre-existing conditions, and expected requirements during surgery and the immediate postoperative period. Any metabolic derangement should be corrected before the patient is taken to the operating room in order to avoid unexpected problems. The following is a summary of general preparation for surgery:

> Establish burn size, depth, and surgical plan.
> Communicate with surgical team.
> Establish expected physiological impact of surgery.
> Assess airway. Consider fiberoptic intubation.
> Assess level of respiratory support. Evaluate intraoperative requirements and make efforts to match requirements during surgery.
> Evaluate hemodynamic status and expected needs during surgery.
> Make a thorough and systematic evaluation of the patient. Detect any physiological derangements and pre-existing conditions and correct them before patient is taken to the operating room.
> Establish predicted blood loss and order blood products.
> Order coagulation products if needed.
> Make sufficient plans for patient transport, location of initial postoperative care, and fluid management, including enteral feeding regimen.
> Make adequate preparation in terms of monitors, vascular access, and availability of blood products, drugs, and any other medical equipment needed.
> Do not send for the patient until all equipment has been checked; all operating room settings are complete; operating room temperature is appropriate; and all drugs, fluids, and blood products are physically present in the room.

Success in major burn surgery requires anticipation of all possible problems. This can only be accomplished by profound knowledge of burn pathophysiology, state-of-the-art burn critical care, and good communication among burn team members.

Preparation of Patients

Patients and/or families should be informed of the impact of the injury and what is to be expected from the surgical procedure. Informed patients tend to present with lower levels of anxiety and their pain control is usually much better. Therefore, all efforts should be made to inform and calm patients during preparation for surgery. It is very important to inform patients and relatives in plain words about the extent of the injury and the implications this injury will pose in their hospital stay and future rehabilitation. An important dose of optimism, compassion, and support will be necessary to overcome problems during the acute phase. Patients and relatives need to be informed of all phases of treatment and the need for repeated surgical procedures. It is very important to explain that the patient will experience pain, stress, and anxiety during the acute and rehabilitation phase, and that the support of close family and relatives will be extremely important to overcome these problems. Rest and sleep are also extremely important, and their importance should also be emphasized.

Good pain control should be achieved and the type of postoperative analgesia discussed with the patient. All patients who are co-operative enough should be offered patient-controlled analgesia (PCA). If PCA pumps can be used, they provide good analgesia and also, which is more important, give patients control over pain and all painful procedures and situations they will have to face in the future.

Nonintubated patients should fast for at least 6 h. Enteral feeding and clear fluids can be continued until 2–3 h before surgery. The stomach is then to be aspirated via the nasogastric tube before induction of anesthesia. There is no need to stop enteral feeding in intubated patients. The stomach is also emptied at the beginning of surgery. Unless large residuals are present before surgery, the hourly amount of enteral feeding that patients receive is low enough to present only a minor risk of aspiration.

All metabolic and physiological derangements should be corrected, blood products ordered, and the patient prepared for surgery. In general, patients are treated as any other intensive care unit (ICU) patient. The particulars of the burn population must be taken into account when patients are prepared for surgery. Burn patients are more prone to metabolic and electrolyte imbalances and they must be closely monitored and all deviations corrected. Homografts, biological dressings, and skin substitutes should be also ordered.

Good vascular access is essential. Large infusion volumes are not uncommon during major burn surgery. Vascular access in major burn cases includes triple-lumen central venous lines, large-caliber peripheral access, and arterial lines. Trauma lines or Swann-Ganz introducers are very helpful to provide appropriate vascular access to allow the infusion of large volumes in short periods of time. Transfusion of large amounts of blood products, which have high viscosity characteristics, may be necessary during surgery. Therefore, trauma catheters or large peripheral catheters in low-pressure vascular beds can be considered for use during burn surgery. Lines should be placed before surgery, in order to expedite treatment.

Nursing staff should be informed of the surgical plan and the expected dressing and nursing requirements during and after surgery. Rehabilitation services are involved before surgery. All joints are well positioned and splints and physiotherapy requirements discussed. When intraoperative splinting is necessary, rehabilitation specialists should also be informed to make specific arrangements. Blood products, biological dressings, and skin substitutes including homografts are quantified using standard nomograms (see Chapt. 1, Fig. 4). The size of the burn to be excised is calculated by plotting height and weight onto the nomogram. Percentage of total surface area to be excised is then calculated. Predicted blood requirements are calculated per cm^2 (see Table 2), and the total amount of blood products ordered. The amount of skin homografts and skin substitutes are calculated based on the total surface area to be excised in cm^2.

Preparation of the Operating Room

Operating room staff has to be informed of any planned surgery as soon as possible in order to make all arrangements. As mentioned before, no random decisions should be made before or during surgery to avoid accidents. Operating nursing staff should be invited to make daily rounds with the rest of the team to get direct information about any surgery and major dressing changes to be performed in the operating room. Good communication is essential, and it is the responsibility of both the burn surgeon and the burn anesthetist to provide and allow the flow of information. A fixed and detailed plan of the surgical procedure must be outlined and passed on to the rest of the burn team and any other relevant personnel. To avoid contradictory and confusing information, the surgical plan should be only distributed when it is considered to be complete and final. If a change of plan or new information has to be distributed, it should be clearly stated that it is new information that invalidates the former plan. A new completed surgical plan should be provided that includes the new information. Amendments should be avoided.

The complete information that should be provided includes the following:

Size of the burn
Anatomical sites
Associated injuries and ventilatory requirements
Sequence of surgery
Position of patient
Change in position of patient during surgery
Blood requirements
Skin homograft and biological and skin substitute requirements
Equipment
Hemostatic agents and tourniquets
Postoperative requirements and type of bed
Postoperative positioning
Splint and rehabilitation requirements

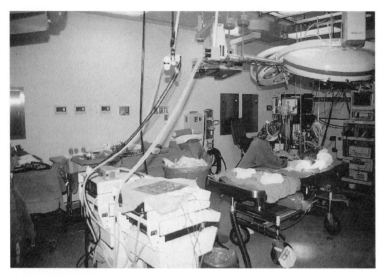

A

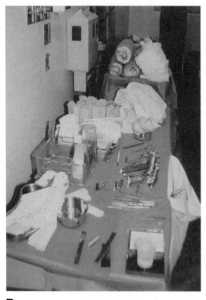

B

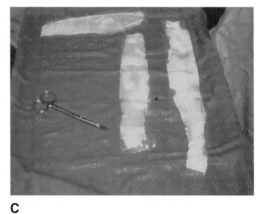

C

FIGURE 2   A. Typical operating room set-up. It is mandatory to have all equipment (B), blood products, and skin substitutes (C) ready before the patient is transferred to the operating room.

All blood products and skin substitutes must be physically present and all equipment and burn dressings ready (see Fig. 2). It cannot be overemphasized that it is imperative that surgery not begin until blood products are in the operating room. Blood loss is extensive during burn surgery, and the anesthetist should be always ahead of the surgeons. Even when blood transfusion is deemed not necessary, blood products should be readily available in the event of major unexpected blood loss.

Essential equipment includes the burn-operating table (Fig. 3). A modified autopsy table with hydraulic and a shower capabilities is very helpful. It permits full prepping of the patient and good access to both burn surgeons and burn anesthetist. The operating room should also be equipped with 4 ceiling hooks, two of them at shoulder level and two at hip level (Fig. 4). These are very helpful to elevate limbs, providing good access during excision and grafting. Operating rooms should have also a second operating table available for turning the patient when it is necessary to place patients in the prone position for harvesting donor sites from the back or to perform excision and grafting of burns on the back. The second operating table should be an ordinary table with hydraulic capabilities. This is normally used when minor burns are treated and full body prepping is not necessary. Arm tables and any other operating table accessories must be available to perform minor burn operations.

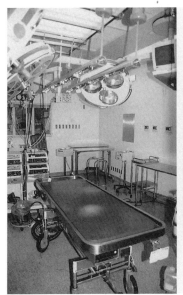 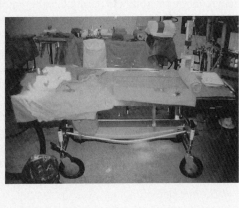

FIGURE 3 The burn operating table. It permits total body prepping and easy access for both surgeons and anesthetists.

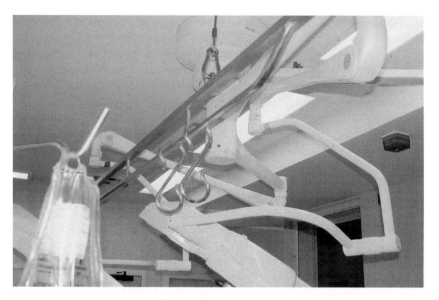

FIGURE 4   Ceiling hooks are very helpful to suspend limbs and provide good access for excision and grafting. It also avoids the need for assistants to hold limbs, so the operating team does not become exhausted.

The operating room should be as large as possible. The burns operating team is very numerous and the equipment required for major burn wound excision is extensive. Large and spacious rooms help to run the operation smoothly and allow circulating nurses and other assistants to perform their duties at easy and not interfering with the operating team. The room should also include individual thermostats to keep the room temperature at 32°C. The latent heat of evaporation of water is 31.5°C. Above this temperature, the energy source for evaporation will come from the environment rather than the patient. If the room temperature falls below 31.5°C (temperature corrected with room humidity), the caloric vector is reversed and energy radiates from the patient to the environment. In this situation, patients become hypothermic and their metabolic rate increases. In extreme circumstances, patients are at risk of death from hypothermia. Radiant heaters are also very helpful for perioperative thermoregulation (Fig. 5). They provide a warm microenvironment over the patient, whereas the room temperature can be kept at a more tolerable level for health workers. Other adjunctive measures include the use of thermal blankets, plastic sheeting over the head and face, and all intravenous fluids being given at 38°C through a warming coil. The operating room staff should be reminded to take fluids themselves every 30 min. The patient's core temperature needs to be controlled via an indwelling bladder cathe-

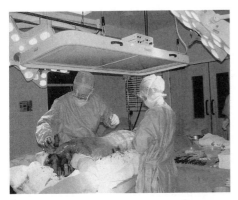
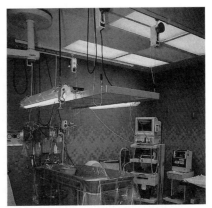

A

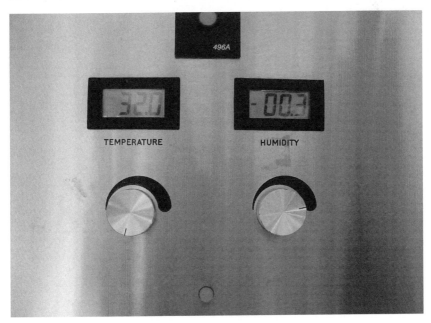

B

FIGURE 5   A. Thermal panels or radiators provide a warm microenvironment for burn patients. B. The operating room should also have independent thermostat to warm the room to 32°C.

ter or esophageal catheter. Two sets of lights are very important, although the gold standard is trauma resuscitation lighting.

Essential operating staff for burn surgery includes:

One scrub nurse per operating team
One scrub nurse for skin processing
One circulating nurse
Two anesthetists
Two surgeons per operating team

In summary, burn wound excision and closure require a profound understanding of burn pathophysiology and the outlining of protocols and master plans. Good communication among burn team members is essential to avoid accidents and unwanted outcomes. Complete preparation of patients, burn care providers, and operating room issues is mandatory, as well as the establishment of priorities for common goals.

BIBLIOGRAPHY

1. Barret JP. Surgical closure of the burn wound. In: Color Atlas of Burn Care Barret Juan P, Herndon David N, Eds. London: W.B. Saunders, 2001.
2. Heimbach DM, Engrav LE. Surgical Management of the Burn Wound. New York: Raven Press, 1984.
3. Wolf SE, Herndon DN. Burn Care Landes Bioscience. Austin. TX, 1999.
4. Klasen HJ. Preparation for surgery. In: Principles and Practice of Burns Management-Settle John AD, Ed. Edinburgh. UK: Churchill Livingstone, 1996.
5. Monafo WW, Bessey PQ. Wound care. In: Total Burn Care. Second Edition Herndon David N, Ed. London: WB Saunders, 2002.

5

Anesthesia for Acute Burn Injuries

Lee C. Woodson
Shriners Hospital for Children and the University of Texas Medical Branch, Galveston, Texas, U.S.A.

INTRODUCTION

Since the end of World War II there has been steady improvement in the clinical outcome for patients with serious burn injuries. Early and aggressive fluid resuscitation can usually prevent burn shock, except with the most extensive full-thickness burns and in patients with coexisting disease. This has dramatically increased initial survival from burn injuries. Early excision and grafting along with better antimicrobial therapy have reduced the incidence of sepsis. Refinements in nutritional support and general wound care have also facilitated wound healing. Improvements in clinical outcome have not been restricted to decreased mortality. In specialized burn centers, therapeutic interventions are influenced by rehabilitation issues from the time of admission. Better functional and cosmetic outcomes have resulted in improvements in quality of life for burn victims.

Modern burn care now depends on the coordinated effort of a multidisciplinary team. This approach is most effectively accomplished in specialized burn centers that bring together surgeons, intensive care specialists, nurse clinicians, nutritionists, rehabilitation therapists, pulmonary care therapists, and anesthesia providers. Anesthetic management is an important part of this multidisciplinary approach. Early excision and grafting of burn wounds limit systemic inflammatory activity, speed healing of injuries, and reduce sepsis. However, with this technique burn patients come to surgery so soon after injury that anesthetic care may include management of the initial resuscitation. Skills and experience of anesthesia providers also have value in burn intensive care units where airway management, vascular access, pulmonary care, fluid and electrolyte management, and pharmacological support of the circulation are central issues. Rational and effective anesthetic management of acute burn patients requires an understanding of the multidisciplinary approach so that perioperative care is compatible with the overall treatment goals for the patient. It is important to keep these goals in mind when making perioperative decisions so that overall care is not sacrificed for short-term benefit in the operating room. The anesthetist becomes one of the burn care team when the anesthetic care in the operating room is coordinated with the patient's care in the burn intensive care unit (ICU).

Major burn injuries result in pathophysiological changes in virtually all organ systems. As a result, the anesthetist is faced with multiple challenges in the care of severely burned patients (Table 1). The challenges are both technical (airway management and vascular access) and cognitive (e.g., systemic inflammatory response syndrome and multiorgan system dysfunction).

Challenges in the anesthetic management of burn patients do not end when the acute wounds are healed. With improved survival from burn injuries more

TABLE 1   Challenges in Management of the
Acute Burn Patient

– Airway compromise
– Pulmonary insufficiency
– Impaired Circulation due to:
　　Hypovolemia
　　Decrease myocardial contractility
　　Anemia
　　Compartment syndrome
– Difficult vascular assess due to:
　　Burn wounds at access site
　　Edema distorting/concealing landmarks
– Monitoring with cutaneous sensors difficult
　　Pulse oximetry, ECG difficult over burn wounds
　　ECG
– Rapid blood loss
– Altered drug response
– Renal insufficiency
– Infection/sepsis
– Impaired temperature regulation
– Associated injuries

---

patients will present for reconstructive correction of extensive deformities. Patients who have survived major burn injuries often require surgical reconstructive care for years after the initial injury in order to correct functional and cosmetic sequelae. These patients present their own unique challenges, both technical and otherwise. Airway management and vascular access can be very difficult in patients with extensive burn scar deformities. Altered response to anesthetic drugs and reduced pain tolerance are also central issues for these patients. This chapter, however, will focus on anesthetic management during the acute phase of burn injury.

PREOPERATIVE EVALUATION

Preoperative evaluation of acutely burned patients requires knowledge of the continuum of pathophysiological changes that occur in burn patients from the initial period after injury through the time that all wounds have healed. The dramatic changes that occur in virtually all organ systems directly affect anesthetic management. In addition to the routine features of the preoperative evaluation, evaluation of the acute burn patient requires special attention to airway management, pulmonary support, vascular access, adequacy of resuscitation, and associated injuries. Table 2 lists specific concerns that guide the preoperative evaluation.

The current standard of burn care calls for early excision and grafting of nonviable burn wounds. These wounds harbor pathogens and produce inflammatory mediators with systemic effects resulting in cardiopulmonary compromise. Early excision reduces systemic inflammation and risk of infection. After major burn injury, the systemic effects of inflammatory mediators on metabolism and cardiopulmonary function reduce physiological reserve and patients' tolerance to the stress of surgery deteriorates with time. Assuming that the patient has adequate

---

TABLE 2 Specific Concerns for Preoperative Evaluation

– Patient age
– Extent of injuries (% total body surface area)
– Burn depth and distribution (superficial or full-thickness)
– Mechanism of injury (flame, explosion, electrical, chemical, scald)
– Airway compromise
– Presence of inhalation injury
– Time elapsed since injury
– Adequacy of resuscitation
– Associated injuries
– Coexisting diseases
– Surgical plan

resuscitation, extensive surgery is best tolerated soon after the injury when the patient is most fit. Nevertheless, it must be recognized that resuscitation of burn injuries involves large fluid and electrolyte shifts and may be associated with hemodynamic instability and respiratory insufficiency. Effective anesthetic management of patients with extensive burn injuries requires an understanding of the pathophysiological changes that result from major burn and inhalation injuries. This is required in order to assess resuscitation accurately prior to surgery and to provide appropriate resuscitation intraoperatively. In fact, anesthesia for major burn surgery involves resuscitation from the initial injury and/or the effects of the burn wound excision.

Preoperative evaluation must be performed within the context of the planned surgical procedure, which will depend on the distribution and depth of burn wounds, time after injury, presence of infection, and existence of suitable donor sites for grafts. An anesthetic plan requires understanding of both the patient's physiological status and the surgeon's plan. The patient's physiological status is revealed by results of physical examination and review of the medical record. The medical record will provide information regarding previous medical history as well as a description of the injury and hospital course. When the burn wound has been previously excised, anesthetic records must be reviewed for information on how the patient tolerated previous operations. An understanding of the surgical plan requires close communication with the surgeons. Unlike many operations that follow a repeatable sequence (for example, appendectomy), no two burn wound excisions are the same. Each operation is guided by how much nonviable tissue is present and the condition of potential sites for split-thickness harvesting of skin for autografts. Often the surgical procedure depends on findings of close wound examination that can only be done in the operating room. The surgeons will nevertheless have some estimate of areas to be excised and donor sites to harvest. This information is necessary to estimate the amount of blood needed as well as what vascular catheters will be needed for replacement of volume and hemodynamic monitoring.

Evaluation of Cutaneous Burns

The skin has been described as the largest organ in the body. Thermal injury to the skin disrupts several vital protective and homeostatic functions (Table 3). Care of burn patients, either in the operating room or in the ICU must compensate for these functions until the wounds are healed.

The skin helps to maintain fluid and electrolyte balance by serving as a barrier to evaporation of water. Heat loss through evaporation and impairment of vasomotor regulation in burned skin diminish effective temperature regulation. Skin also protects from infection by providing a barrier to pathogens. Burned

TABLE 3 Functions of Skin

– Protective Barrier
   Immunological
   Fluid evaporation
   Thermal (insulation, sweat production, vasomotor
     thermoregulation)
– Sensory
– Metabolic (vitamin D synthesis and excretory
   function)
– Social (self-image, social image)

---

surfaces produce an exudate that is rich in protein. Loss of this protein along with diminished hepatic synthesis eventually reduces plasma protein concentration and contributes to accumulation of interstitial fluid (edema).

Morbidity and mortality due to burn injuries depend in large part on how much and how deeply the skin is burned. The extent of burn injury is expressed as the percent of total body surface area burned (TBSA). This area is then classified into the area burned superficially and the area burned through the full thickness of the skin. Partial-thickness burns will often heal but areas of full-thickness burn must be completely excised, sometimes down to fascia. Depth of excision is one of many factors that influence blood loss. Tangential excision is associated with more blood loss than occurs with excision down to fascia.

Volume resuscitation of burn-injured patients is guided by estimates of percentage TBSA burned. A quick estimate of percentage TBSA burned can be made with the so-called rule of nines (Fig. 1). More accurate estimates must take into account the changes in body proportion that occur with age (Fig. 2). In the early period after injury, the adequacy of resuscitation can be evaluated by comparing the volume of fluid administered with what the patient's predicted needs are based on common formulas.

A critical part of preoperative evaluation of patients for burn excision and grafting is an estimation of expected blood loss. Several key decisions in the anesthetic management plan depend on this information. Among other things, the expected blood loss determines what venous catheters will be needed and whether or not invasive monitors such as direct arterial pressure or central venous pressure will be required. Adequate blood should be typed and crossed and in the operating room prior to the start of surgery because blood loss can be very rapid during these procedures.

Surgical blood loss depends on the area to be excised (cm^2), time since injury, surgical plan (tangential vs. fascial excision), and the presence of infection

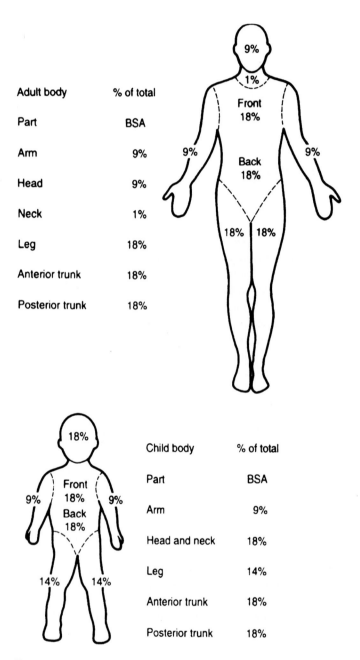

Adult body	% of total
Part	BSA
Arm	9%
Head	9%
Neck	1%
Leg	18%
Anterior trunk	18%
Posterior trunk	18%

Child body	% of total
Part	BSA
Arm	9%
Head and neck	18%
Leg	14%
Anterior trunk	18%
Posterior trunk	18%

FIGURE 1   A rough estimate of total body surface area burned can be made using the rule of nines.

OFFICIAL ASSESSMENT - 72 HOUR BURN DIAGRAM

Shriners Burns Institute
Galveston Unit

Age: ______________ Sex: ______________ Date of Admission ______________________

Type of Burn: Flame ☐ Electrical ☐ Scald ☐ Chemical ☐ Inhalation Injury ☐
Contact ☐

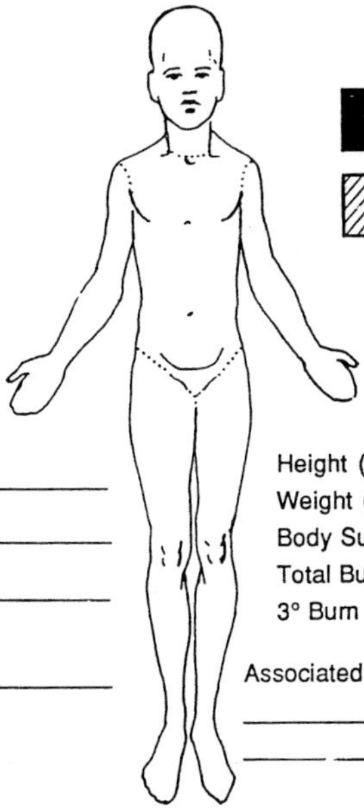

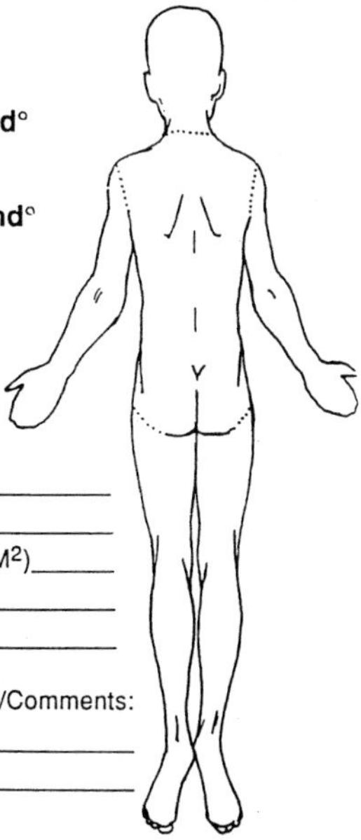

■ 3rd°

▨ 2nd°

Date of Burn: ______________________

Date Completed: ______________________

Completed By: ______________________

Attending Physician: ______________________

Height (cm) ____________

Weight (kg.) ____________

Body Surface (M^2) ________

Total Burn (M^2) ________

3° Burn (M^2) ________

Associated Injuries/Comments:

____

____

BURN ESTIMATE - AGE VS. AREA

	Area	Birth-1yr.	1-4 yrs.	5-9 yrs.	10-14 yrs.	15 yrs.	Adult	2°	3°	TBSA%
941.	Head	19	17	13	11	9	7			
941	Neck	2	2	2	2	2	2			
942	Ant.. Trunk	13	13	13	13	13	13			
942	Post. Trunk	13	13	13	13	13	13			
942	R. Buttock	2.5	2.5	2.5	2.5	2.5	2.5			
942	L. Buttock	2.5	2.5	2.5.	2:5	2.5	2.5			
942	Genitalia	1	1	1	1	1	1			
943	R.U. Arm	4	4	4	4	4	4			
943.	L.U. Arm	4	4	4	4	4	4			
943	R.L.Arm	3	3	3	3	3	3			
943	L.L. Arm	3	3	3	3	3	3			
944	R. Hand	2.5	2.5	2.5	2.5	2.5	2.5			
944	L. Hand	2.5	2.5	2.5	2.5	2.5	2.5			
945	R. Thigh	5.5	6.5	8	8.5	9	9.5			
5	L. Thigh	5.5	6.5	8	8.5	9	9.5			
,5	R. Leg	5	5	5.5	6	6.5	7			
945	L. Leg	5	5	5.5	6	6.5	7			
945	R. Foot	3.5	3.5	3.5	3.5	3.5	3.5			
'45	L. Foot	3.5	3.5	3.5	3.5	3.5	3.5			

Burn Assessment

Area Burned	TOTAL %	% 3°
Head & Neck		
Ant.Trunk		
Post. Trunk		
Right Arm		
Left Arm		
Right Leg		
Left Leg		
TOTAL		

FIGURE 2 An age-adjusted burn diagram can be used to estimate more accurately the total body surface area affected by burns.

TABLE 4 Expected Blood Loss During Burn Wound Excision

Days since surgical procedure	Predicted blood loss (ml/cm² burn area)
<24 h	0.45
1–3 days	0.65
2–16 days	0.75
>16 days	0.5–0.75
Infected wounds	1–1.25

Adapted from Desai et al., Ann Surg 1990.

(Table 4, Fig. 3). The area to be excised is estimated by multiplying the total body surface area (m^2) by the percentage TBSA burned. Blood loss expected per cm^2 can be estimated based on time since injury and presence or absence of wound infection. Table 5 gives an example calculation of estimated blood loss for a hypothetical case.

Effects on Circulation

Initially the most profound physiological effects of major burn injury are related to hemodynamic function and tissue perfusion. A state of burn shock develops from hypovolemia due to extravasation of intravascular fluid and often myocardial depression as well. Cardiac output is decreased, systemic vascular resistance is increased, and peripheral tissue perfusion is impaired. Hypovolemia results from increased capillary permeability and movement of protein-rich fluid from the vascular space to the interstitial space. Lymph flow is greatly increased but is overwhelmed and tissue edema results. Edema around burn-injured tissues can be massive. Permeability is also increased at sites distant from the burn injury.

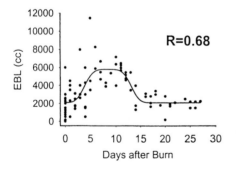

FIGURE 3 Blood loss during primary burn excision as a function of time. Correlation coefficient (R) of polynomial model equation was 0.68 (from Hart et al, 2001).

TABLE 5   Calculation of Estimated Blood Loss for
Hypothetical Burn Patient

Total body surface area $= 1.0m^2$
% Total body surface area burned 50%
2 weeks postinjury
Wounds infected
Estimate blood loss as 1 ml/cm^2 wound to be excised
$1m^2$TBSA $\times$ *50% TBSA burned* $= 0.5m^2$ burned area
$\times$ *10,000 cm^2/m^2* $= 5,000$ cm^2 burned area
$\times$ *1ml/cm^2* wound excised $= 5000$ ml expected blood loss

---

In addition to decreased cardiac output and vasoconstriction, tissue perfusion can be compromised by increased tissue pressure due to accumulation of edema fluid during the resuscitation. In the extremities this produces a compartment syndrome that must be relieved by escharotomy; otherwise necrosis will require amputation.

During the initial stage after injury, survival depends on timely and aggressive resuscitation to prevent or treat hypovolemia. Preoperative evaluation and preparation for surgery require accurate assessment of the effectiveness of the resuscitation.

Several resuscitation protocols have been described to guide the volume resuscitation of burn patients (Table 6). Buffered isotonic crystalloid solutions such as lactated Ringer's solution are preferred in most burn centers. At present there are no prospective data demonstrating improved clinical outcomes when colloids or hypertonic saline are used for resuscitation. Generalized increased endothelial permeability limits intravascular retention of colloids during the first 24 h after burns. As a result, colloids are usually restricted until the day after injury.

An exception is found in pediatric patients. Albumin is often added to the resuscitation fluids for children because of more rapid decrease in plasma albumin in these patients. The most widely recognized pediatric resuscitation protocols have been developed by Shriners Hospitals in Galveston and Cincinnati (Table 7). Both of these formulas include albumin during the first 24 h.

During preoperative evaluation resuscitation formulas can be used to help judge the adequacy of resuscitation. Comparing the volume predicted with the administered volume allows a quick and superficial estimate of the appropriateness of the amount of fluid administered. The history should also be reviewed for evidence of delay in starting resuscitation. This is a risk factor for increased morbidity and mortality in burn patients. Both over and underresuscitation can exacerbate the injury. Delay or underresuscitation, of course, can cause organ damage through ischemia. Overresuscitation can also cause problems such as

TABLE 6 Formulas for estimating adult fluid resuscitation needs

Formula	Crystalloid	Colloid
Crystalloid formulas		
Modified Brooke	Lactated Ringer's 2 mL/kg/% burn	
Parkland	Lactated Ringer's 2 mL/kg/% burn	
Colloid formulas		
Evans	Normal saline 1 mL/kg/% burn	1 mL/kg/% burn
Brooke	Lactated Ringer's 1.5 mL/kg/% burn	0.5 mL/kg
Slater	Lactated Ringer's 2L/24 h	FFP 75 mL/kg/24 h
Demling	Dextran 40 in saline 2 mL/kg/h	FFP 0.5–1 mL/kg/% burn
	Lactated Ringer's, maintain urine output	
Hypertonic formulas		
Hypertonic saline (Monafo)	250 mEq sodium/L (1–2 ml/kg/% burn)	
Modified Hypertonic (Warden)	Lactated Ringer's +50 mEq NaHCO$_3$ (4ml/kg/% burn/first 8h)	
	Lactated Ringer's (maintain urine output/second 8 h)	
	Lactated Ringer's + albumin (maintain urine output/third 8 h)	

pulmonary edema or compartment syndrome of either extremities or abdominal viscera. Pulmonary edema is unusual in burn patients unless intravascular filling pressure is increased above normal.

Certain features of the burn injury can increase fluid requirements beyond what the protocols predict. Smoke inhalation injury has been found to increase fluid requirements up to 50% above what would be estimated from accompanying cutaneous burns alone. This effect is more important with less extensive burns and the difference is less distinct with burns greater than 50% total body surface

TABLE 7 Formulas for Estimating Pediatric Fluid Resuscitation Needs

Formula	Volume	Timing	Composition
Cincinnati	4 ml/kg/% burn	1st 8 h	Lactated Ringer's + 50mEq NAHCO$_3$
	+ 1500 ml/m^2 burn		
		2nd 8 h	Lactated Ringer's
		3rd 8 h	Lactated Ringer's + 12.5 albumin
Galveston	+ 5000 ml/m^2 burn	1st 24 h	Ringer's Lactate
	+ 2000 ml/m^2 BSA		12.5 gm albumin

area. Extensive full-thickness burns also increase fluid requirements beyond the volumes estimated by formulas such as the Parkland formula.

Formulas and protocols for burn resuscitation are only rough guides and fluids must still be titrated according to the patient's response and physiological state. Resuscitation is an imprecise process: there is no single reliable end point to titrate to. Heart rate and mean arterial blood pressure along with a urine output of 0.5–1.0ml/kg/h continue to be favorite end points for resuscitation. However, numerous studies have shown that these indicators can be misleading. A state of what is termed compensated shock can persist for some time despite vital signs being within normal limits and an adequate urine output. Although these traditional guides are important targets during early resuscitation, other signs and physiological variables should be included in the assessment to avoid unrecognized underresuscitation. Base deficit is readily available from the arterial blood gas analysis and provides a sensitive marker for global hypoperfusion. Base deficit has been shown to correlate closely with blood lactate and provide a useful indicator of inadequate tissue oxygen delivery. Base deficit does not provide a convenient end point to titrate fluid administration to, but it does give an overall indication of the quality of the resuscitation. It must then be determined what needs to be changed in the resuscitation such as more volume, more oxygen-carrying capacity, or vasoactive infusions.

Physical examination also can be very helpful in evaluating resuscitation effectiveness. Warm extremities with easily palpable pulses and adequate capillary refill are present when resuscitation efforts are effective. Cool extremities with poor pulses and slow capillary refill indicate inadequate tissue perfusion.

If the patient survives the initial burn shock and is adequately resuscitated, a state of hyperdynamic circulation develops. Severe burn injuries produce a dramatic increase in metabolic rate. Oxygen consumption can be twice the normal rate. The increase in metabolic demand is associated with pronounced wasting of lean body mass. This response is the consequence of hormonal and inflammatory factors. From the second or third day postburn the cardiac output increases to meet increased metabolic demands and to compensate for decreased vascular resistance associated with the systemic inflammatory response (Fig. 4). Patients unable to compensate with an adequate increase in cardiac output have a higher mortality rate.

The hypermetabolic response to burns has profound effects on burn treatment. Inadequate nutritional support results in further stress and wasting, impaired wound healing, decreased immunity, and organ dysfunction. Interruption of nutritional support in the operative period along with stress of hypothermia and surgical trauma exacerbate this condition.

Airway and Pulmonary Function

In the preoperative evaluation of burn patients, the airway and pulmonary function are major specific concerns. Burn injuries and resultant head and neck edema can

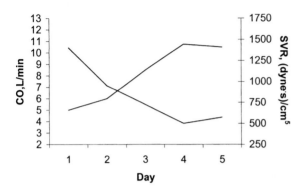

A hyperdynamic circulatory pattern develops during the first few days following extensive burn injuries. CO, cardiac output; SVR, systemic vascular resistance.

distort anatomy and reduce range of motion to the point that direct laryngoscopy is difficult or impossible. These changes may also compromise the patient's spontaneous ventilation and may make ventilation after induction of general anesthesia difficult or impossible. It is imperative that these conditions be identified early to allow adequate planning.

The history of injury and physical examination findings are important in identifying patients at risk for inhalation injury and airway compromise. Some patients who have sustained significant inhalation injury will present without signs or symptoms of airway obstruction or respiratory distress. As resuscitation progresses, edema fluid accumulates and inflammatory changes develop that may lead to an insidious and progressive respiratory embarrassment. Risk factors from the history and physical examination can identify patients who need closer and more objective examination.

When available, pulmonary function tests (PFT) with flow volume loops (FVL) can be used as a screen or triage tool to rule out progressive upper airway edema and obstruction. A normal FVL in these patients has been found to carry a greater than 98% negative predictive value for upper airway obstruction.

Flexible fiberoptic nasopharyngoscopy and bronchoscopy (FOB) provide direct objective evaluation of the major airways. Pharyngeal tissues offer little resistance to edema formation, when injured by heat, the swollen tissues can obliterate the airway. If tracheal intubation is not accomplished before this occurs, emergency tracheostomy may be the only way to secure the airway. More commonly thermal injury to the larynx results in boggy edema of the aryepiglottic folds and arytenoid eminences. This redundant tissue creates a dynamic obstruction to inspiratory flow by folding into the glottic inlet during inspiration. Early prophylactic intubation is indicated when upper airway edema threatens obstruction.

However, caution is advised because emergent intubation of acute burn patients is associated with serious morbidity and mortality, especially during transportation between institutions. These risks are justified when the patient will likely benefit from intubation. However, as a rule fewer than 50% of patients with inhalation injury require intubation and mechanical ventilation. Unfortunately, clinical evaluation is not sufficiently sensitive or selective to identify patients who will benefit from intubation. As mentioned above, FVLs or fiberoptic endoscopy provide reliable diagnostic information. Even in the presence of risk factors for inhalation injury, if there is no respiratory distress and objective information (e.g., fiberoptic endoscopy) indicates that airway obstruction is not present, it has been found safe to observe patients without intubation. Close observation is needed, however, and serial examinations are performed when conditions change. When resources do not allow endoscopy or close observation, a more conservative approach is required. This topic is discussed in more detail in Chapter 3.

In adults endoscopy can be performed with topical local anesthesia and sedation when appropriate and needed. In children, however, deep sedation is required. In our institution ketamine has been found to provide excellent conditions for FOB. Glycopyrrolate (0.1–0.2 mg intravenously) given at least 15 min before ketamine administration helps prevent problems with secretions. Ketamine (1–2 mg/kg) intravenously produces insensibility and profound analgesia. The primary advantage with ketamine is that respiratory drive and airway patency are not compromised. This is not the case with any of the other intravenous sedatives or analgesics used.

When the patient has already been intubated, a close examination is needed to ensure that the endotracheal tube is in proper position and that it is secured in a reliable fashion. It is important to know what the indications for intubation were: concern over airway edema, burn shock, inability to protect the airway from aspiration, respiratory failure, or other. It is also appropriate to determine if the initial indication has resolved. These questions must be answered in order to form a safe and effective plan for airway management, including during the postoperative period.

Airway edema can be evaluated by evacuating the endotracheal tube cuff to check for air leak between the endotracheal tube and the airway. If there is no leak, the endotracheal tube fits tightly in the airway. If it is removed, edematous tissue might collapse into the airway and block respiration. In this case the cuff should not be left inflated; this aggravates airway mucosal ischemia, which, after time, can lead to necrosis and eventual scar formation (stenosis). Direct laryngoscopy or fiberoptic endoscopy allows one to examine pharyngeal structures directly. When boggy edematous tissues fold around the endotracheal tube and no space can be viewed between the endotracheal tube and laryngeal structures, it is dangerous to remove the endotracheal tube. In this situation the airway should remain secured until the edema resolves (usually in 2–3 days). Fiberoptic endoscopy is a less stressful procedure and is better tolerated. When endoscopy reveals clear space around the larynx, and especially if laryngeal structures can be identified as well as space between the endotracheal tube and glottic rim, extubation or change of the endotracheal tube can be considered.

Effects on Renal Function

The kidneys are vulnerable to injury in patients with serious burn injury. Ischemic injury may occur during the resuscitation phase because of hypovolemia and burn shock, especially if there is a delay in resuscitation. Peripheral edema may be so severe that compartment syndrome develops in extremities. Rhabdomyolysis may result in release of myoglobin when perfusion is restored by escharotomy. Myoglobinemia is also associated with serious electrical burns. Myoglobin is toxic to kidneys and myoglobinuria should be treated with mannitol diuresis and alkalinization of the urine with bicarbonate. It is important to monitor urine color during resuscitation to check for development of myoglobinuria.

For patients who have survived the resuscitation phase with renal function intact, overwhelming infection and sepsis also pose a threat to the kidneys. In these cases every effort must be made to preserve renal perfusion and oxygen delivery. In the preoperative evaluation it is important to review laboratory values to check renal function.

PHARMACOLOGICAL CONSIDERATIONS

Physiological and metabolic changes resulting from large burn injuries and their medical treatment may dramatically alter patients' responses to drugs. Responses are altered by pharmacokinetic as well as pharmacodynamic determinants. These altered responses may have profound clinical relevance. At the very least, consideration of altered response may require deviation from usual dosages in order to avoid toxicity or decreased efficacy. At the other extreme, potentially lethal effects of succinylcholine contraindicate the use of this drug for a limited period following large burn injuries.

The complex nature of pathophysiological changes, interpatient variation in nature and extent of burns, as well as the dynamic nature of these changes during resuscitation and recovery make it difficult to formulate precise dosage guidelines for burn patients. With some agents (e.g., mivacurium), large changes in separate and distinct processes may negate each other, resulting in a drug response equivalent to that seen in nonburned patients. For other drugs, much higher dosages are required. Effective drug therapy in burn patients requires careful monitoring of effects and titration of dosage to the desired response.

The two phases of cardiovascular response to thermal injury affect pharmacokinetic parameters in different ways. During the resuscitation phase, loss of fluid from the vascular space causes decreased cardiac output and perfusion of tissues including kidney and liver where much drug elimination takes place. Decreased cardiac output will accelerate the rate of alveolar accumulation of inhalation agents and can result in exaggerated hypotension during induction of general anesthesia. Volume resuscitation during this phase dilutes plasma proteins and expands the extravascular space especially, but not exclusively, around the burn injury itself. These changes tend to increase sensitivity and prolong the action of many drugs during the first 1–2 days postinjury.

From 2 to 3 days after burn injury, a hypermetabolic and hyperdynamic circulatory phase is established that has different effects on pharmacokinetic variables and drug responses compared with the resuscitation phase. During this phase increased body temperature, oxygen consumption, and cardiac output are associated with increased perfusion of liver and kidney and increased activity of some drug-metabolizing enzymes. During this phase clearance of some drugs is increased to the point that increased dosages are required.

Plasma protein concentrations are greatly altered after large burns. This can affect drug response because many anesthetic drugs are highly protein-bound. For highly protein-bound drugs, drug action and elimination are often related to the unbound fraction of the drug available for receptor interaction, glomerular filtration, or enzymatic metabolism. There are two major drug-binding proteins in the plasma and they are affected in opposite ways by burn injury. Albumin binds mostly acidic and neutral drugs (e.g., diazepam or thiopental) and is decreased after burns. Plasma and total body albumin are greatly reduced after major burn injury because of losses in wound exudate and reduction in hepatic synthesis. Basic drugs ($pKa > 8$, e.g. propranolol, lidocaine, or imipramine) bind to alpha$_1$-acid glycoprotein. Alpha$_1$-acid glycoprotein is considered an acute-phase protein and its concentration may double after large burn injury. Since these important drug-binding proteins respond in opposite ways to burn injury, changes in drug binding, response, and clearance will depend on which protein binds the drug in question.

Clearance is the most important factor determining the maintenance dosage of drugs and can influence the response to drugs given by infusion or repeated bolus during anesthesia. Drug clearance is influenced by four factors: metabolism, protein binding, renal excretion, and novel excretion pathways (e.g., loss of drug in wound exudate). All of these factors are significantly altered in burns, often to the point that the dosage should be adjusted. The complexity of these changes make it difficult to describe specific guidelines for most drugs. The most important principle to remember is to monitor response and titrate the dosage of anesthetic drugs.

Altered response in burn patients is more easily predicted for muscle relaxants. This is fortunate because, in terms of anesthetic management, the most profound and clinically significant changes in drug response occur with this group of drugs. Large burns cause sensitization to succinylcholine and exaggeration of the hyperkalemic response to succinylcholine. In patients soon after burn injury, the hyperkalemic response to succinylcholine can be sufficient to cause cardiac arrest. It is not known for certain when this risk develops, but most agree that succinylcholine should not be used in burn patients after 48 h following injury. This problem is temporary and the length of time is also controversial. Succinylcholine probably should not be used until at least a year after wounds have healed.

In contrast to succinylcholine, most nondepolarizing muscle relaxants require larger and more frequent dosages to maintain muscle relaxation because of the marked resistance that occurs after burns. An exception is mivacurium. Standard dosages of mivacurium retain their efficacy in burn patients. Mivacurium is metabolized by plasma cholinesterase and this enzyme is decreased after burns. This is thought to increase the concentration of mivacurium at its site of action and delay its elimination, so that dosing need not be altered for burn patients.

MANAGEMENT OF ANESTHESIA

Monitors

The choice of hemodynamic monitors is a major concern in planning anesthetic management for burn patients. Since access may be limited and difficult in these patients, careful preoperative assessment is necessary for effective management.

As with any critically ill patient, the choice of monitors in burned patients depends on the extent of the patient's injury, physiological state, and planned surgery. An arterial catheter provides much information, including pulmonary and metabolic status as well as hemodynamic function. When blood loss is expected to be extensive and rapid, blood pressure may change more quickly than the interval between cycles of a noninvasive blood pressure monitor. In this case, an arterial catheter provides beat-to-beat monitoring capability. As explained below, direct arterial pressure monitoring also allows observation of wave form and respiratory variation in systolic blood pressure, which are very useful for titrating fluid administration for volume replacement during periods of rapid blood loss. An arterial catheter also allows arterial blood sampling for blood gas analysis. This helps with the assessment of tissue perfusion as well as pulmonary function.

In patients with large burn injuries, a central venous catheter serves several functions. Central venous pressure can be useful in titrating volume replacement. Although central venous pressure has been found to be a poor indicator of preload, it can quickly show if the filling pressure is low or very high. If the pressure is low, volume administration will probably be an effective intervention for hypotension, if the pressure is already high, a vasoactive infusion is more likely to help. Elevated central venous pressure in the presence of pulmonary capillary leak from inhalation injury or systemic inflammation is likely to cause pulmonary edema.

A pulmonary artery catheter is usually not helpful and may even be distracting during excision of a large burn. In some cases, however, measurement of cardiac output and pulmonary artery occlusion pressure may be of use when heavy inotropic support or high levels of positive end-expiratory pressure (PEEP) are needed.

Electrocardiographic electrodes and pulse oximeter probes may be difficult to maintain on burn patients. Burn wounds or antibiotic ointment prevent adherence of standard electrocardiographic gel electrodes. Metallic surgical staples and alligator clips are effective. Transmission pulse oximetry sites may be burned or included within the surgical field. Clips are available that attach to a lip or ear when these sites are not compromised. Some clinicians have modified standard pulse oximeter probes for application to the tongue. At times it may be necessary to draw back on the arterial catheter to examine the color of the arterial blood when acute changes occur and pulse oximetry is not reliable.

Urine output is the most useful perioperative monitor of renal function and in some circumstances it can also serve as an index of global perfusion. Chronic diuretic therapy can limit the usefulness of urine output as a monitor of perfusion. Another important use of monitoring urine output is to identify hemolytic transfusion reactions. During anesthesia and burn wound debridement, signs and symptoms of transfusion reaction are masked. Hemolysis, however, can be detected by observation of the urine color. Any burn patient expected to require transfusion while anesthetized should have a Foley catheter inserted for this purpose.

Vascular Access

If peripheral veins are available and central venous pressure is not needed, a peripheral vein catheter may be the most appropriate. These catheters should be sutured in place because full body preparation and movement of the patient during surgery often cause dislodgment of peripheral catheters taped in place.

As already mentioned, patients with extensive burns often lack peripheral venous access. A central venous catheter sutured in place provides secure venous access and is the preferable route of administration of vasoactive drugs. In the ICU a central venous catheter is helpful for blood sampling and as a secure route for prolonged antibiotic administration. If it is to be used for volume replacement during burn excision in the operating room, a central venous catheter should have a bore large enough to allow rapid infusion.

Central venous access can be made difficult in the resuscitation phase by edema that obscures landmarks and during the healing phase by scar formation that displaces and obscures landmarks. When burns are extensive, it may be necessary to insert lines through burned skin. When the burn is deep, it may be helpful to have the surgeon excise the area to facilitate insertion and to allow securing sutures to be placed in viable tissue. When a subclavian catheter is to be placed through edematous tissue, pitting edema can sometimes be displaced by firm continuous pressure applied to the site. This allows palpation of landmarks and passage of the needle beneath the clavicle without pointing the needle down toward the lung.

When vascular catheters have already been inserted, it is important to know how long they have been in place: most burn centers schedule regular line changes in order to reduce the risk of catheter-related infections and sepsis. At many centers central venous catheters are changed over a wire after 3 days and moved to a new site after 7 days. The risk of arterial catheter infection is less than with venous catheters. Also, the risk of mechanical complication is greater for arterial catheters. For this reason we do not change arterial catheters as often as venous catheters as long as the cutaneous site does not appear infected.

The operating room is an ideal location for line changes in these patients because sterility and patient positioning can be optimized here. Newly placed catheters from the ICU can be used in the operating room if they are an appropriate size for rapid volume infusion. The date and size of vascular catheters should be noted in order to plan line placement in the operating room.

Placement of arterial catheters also presents challenges in burn patients. In nonburned patients the radial artery is usually the preferred access site for direct measurement of arterial blood pressure. In patients with extensive burns, however, the radial artery is often not the best site. When the upper extremities are burned, the radial artery may not be accessible. In addition it is difficult to maintain radial artery catheters more than 48 h in burn patients because patients need to be moved frequently for wound care and examination. Radial artery catheters are especially difficult to maintain in small pediatric patients. Moreover, the pressures obtained from the radial artery often are significantly lower than observed with blood pressure cuff or femoral artery catheter.

Accessing the femoral artery is usually easier than the radial artery. Even in large burns the groin is frequently spared and the vessel is much larger. The risk of mechanical complication is higher when multiple attempts are needed (as may be the case during initial resuscitation) and when the ratio of arterial to catheter diameters is low (in smaller patients). In smaller patients (10–15 kg or less) a 2.5 Fr catheter is adequate for monitoring and is less likely to cause arterial thrombosis. The risk of mechanical complication from femoral arterial catheters is small even in pediatric patients. However, when this occurs it can be devastating as it may involve loss of limb. Placement of femoral arterial catheters in pediatric patients should be performed with great care and with an understanding of the risks. Benefits from the monitor should justify the risk or the monitor should not be used. The involved limb should be monitored closely for signs of impaired perfusion. Unilateral slowed capillary refill, loss of pulse, cool toes, and dusky appearance can be easily recognized. In most cases catheter-related vascular compromise resolves quickly after removal of the catheter. If not contraindicated, heparinization can prevent further thrombosis after a vascular injury.

Airway Management

Most patients with significant burns will receive continuous enteral feeding via a feeding tube placed in the duodenum. The hypermetabolic state following large burns requires aggressive nutritional support. It is impractical to fast these patients for 8 h periods prior to surgery. Gastric emptying is usually not impaired following burn injury unless sepsis develops later on. Enteral feeding can and should be continued up until the time of surgery. Some advocate feeding throughout the perioperative period. Aspiration of gastric contents from the nasogastric tube should be performed before induction of general anesthesia to reduce the risk of pulmonary aspiration during to intubation. In the ICU gastric emptying is monitored during enteral feeding by periodic measurement of gastric residual volume. An effect of sepsis is impairment of gastrointestinal motility as manifest by increasing volumes of fluid in the stomach. This should be noted during the preoperative evaluation and steps taken to avoid aspiration, such as reducing or stopping enteral feeding for a period preoperatively.

When the head and neck are not involved in the burn injury and there is no risk of inhalation injury, airway management is by conventional guidelines (with the exception that succinylcholine may be contraindicated). Cutaneous burns to the head and neck or evidence of inhalation injury may require special considerations. Cutaneous burns to the face can make mask ventilation difficult. Moderate to severe edema, or scar formation as wounds heal, may also make direct laryngoscopy difficult. When there is significant risk of inhalation injury, fiberoptic bronchoscopy (FOB) is indicated for evaluation of injury. During subsequent operations after initial excision FOB may be indicated as follow-up of the status of inhalation injury. For these reasons at our hospital nearly all acute burn patients are intubated fiberoptically. Intubation during spontaneous ventilation is the safest way to secure the airway when management is difficult. There are no contraindications to fiberoptic intubation. An additional advantage is that when this technique is used routinely under controlled conditions, it greatly increases the level of experience for all the involved personnel. As a result airway management in more urgent situations is facilitated and becomes more controlled. Fiberoptic intubation for adults can be accomplished in the awake state with topical local anesthetic and sedation. Children, however, will not cooperate and require deep sedation. As described above, ketamine provides nearly ideal conditions for FOB or fiberoptic intubation. An intravenous dosage of 1–2 mg/kg is usually adequate. Pretreatment with glycopyrrolate (0.1–0.2 mg intravenously) helps to decrease secretions.

As mentioned in the section on pharmacology, succinylcholine is contraindicated after large burns. It is generally agreed that succinylcholine can be used safely for approximately 48 h after the initial injury. After that it becomes controversial because there is so little evidence during the time period up to 2 weeks postburn. It is best to avoid succinylcholine after the first 48 h following burns up to about 1 year after wounds have healed.

Once the trachea has been intubated, the endotracheal tube must be secured. This can be difficult for patients with facial burns. Tape will not adhere to burned skin and cloth ties may cross the surgical field. When patients are intubated nasally, many burn centers utilize some modification of a tie that includes the nasal septum (Fig. 5). In our hospital, 8 or 10 Fr red rubber catheters are passed through each naris and retrieved from the pharynx by direct laryngoscopy and McGill forceps. A single length of one-eighth inch cotton umbilical tape is tied to each of the catheters and when the catheters are pulled back out of the nose, each end of the umbilical tape is pulled out its respective naris, producing a loop around the nasal septum. Before securing with a knot, care should be taken to

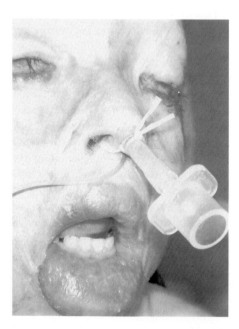

FIGURE 5   Using small catheters (8 Fr) a loop of ⅛ inch umbilical tape can be tied around the bony nasal septum. An endotracheal tube tied to this loop is quite secure, without tape or circumferential ties crossing facial burn wounds.

avoid capturing the uvula in the loop. A knot in the nasal septal tie should be snug enough to prevent excessive movement of the endotracheal tube but loose enough to avoid ischemic necrosis of the underlying tissues.

Airway management using a laryngeal mask airway has also been used successfully in children. Clinicians at the Cincinnati Shriners Burns Hospital reported that in 141 acute burn cases managed with laryngeal mask, there were no persistent sequelae from airway complications.

Ventilation of critically ill patients is at times challenging during the perioperative period. Patients with inhalation injury or acute respiratory distress syndrome (ARDS) may require support beyond the capabilities of anesthesia machine ventilators. This may necessitate moving an ICU ventilator into the operating room. This instrument, along the electrical and pneumatic connections, takes up considerable space and can interfere with access to the patient. In a hospital with a large population of burn patients this may be a frequent occurrence. We have solved this problem by attaching an ICU ventilator to our anesthesia machine (Fig. 6). This allows use of the same ventilation parameters that have been found effective for the patient in the burn ICU but with no inconvenience from added

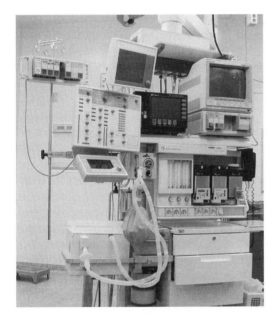

FIGURE 6   A full-service ventilator (such as the Servo 300A shown here) attached to the anesthesia machine can provide the same ventilator settings as used in the ICU, including pressure support and continuous positive airway pressure without the need to bring additional cumbersome equipment into the operating room.

equipment in the operating room. An added advantage is the ability to use pressure support ventilation during surgery. Spontaneous ventilation provides a margin of safety if the endotracheal tube is dislodged and reduced intrathoracic pressures minimize the hemodynamic effects of mechanical ventilation.

Selection of Anesthetic Technique

Many anesthetic agents have been used effectively in burn patients. Intravenous agents can be used for both induction and maintenance. The specific agent used will depend primarily on the patient's hemodynamic and pulmonary status as well as the potential difficulty in securing the patient's airway. Ketamine has many advantages for use in the burn patient for induction and maintenance of anesthesia. As an induction agent, ketamine can be administered at a dosage of 0.5–2.0 mg/kg. Except for patients who are depleted of catecholamines or are compensating with maximal sympathetic activity, ketamine generally preserves hemodynamic stability. In addition, ketamine preserves hypoxic and hypercapnic ventilatory responses and reduces airway resistance. Compared to other intravenous anesthetics, airway reflexes and patency remain intact after ketamine administration. Patients who do not require ventilatory support can be allowed to breathe spontaneously. This provides an additional margin of safety should inadvertent extubation occur. In fact, some clinicians have used ketamine anesthesia for burn surgery without intubating the trachea. Patients were allowed to breathe spontaneously and the airway complication rate was comparable to that of intubated patients. This technique may be especially beneficial for patients with laryngeal burns because it avoids potential mechanical injury to a larynx that has already been injured by heat. The use of intramuscular ketamine can be beneficial in securing the airway in pediatric burn patients or uncooperative adults who do not have vascular access. Because ketamine preserves spontaneous ventilation and induces dissociative anesthesia, it provides good conditions for securing the airway with a fiberoptic bronchoscope. Addition of other anesthetic agents, especially potent volatile agents or opioids, should be avoided until the airway is secured because these anesthetics depress respiratory drive and relax pharyngeal muscles, thus increasing the risk of apnea, upper airway obstruction, or laryngospasm. Ketamine can also be utilized, either alone or in combination with other anesthetics, for maintenance of anesthesia either by infusion or intermittent bolus. Ketamine has potent analgesic properties and is used extensively in the operating room as well as for painful dressing changes and patient manipulations. As mentioned earlier glycopyrrolate (0.1–0.2 mg) is commonly given in combination with ketamine to reduce ketamine-induced secretions. In addition, benzodiazepines are often recommended in older children and adults to reduce the incidence of dysphoria sometimes associated with ketamine administration. When used in this manner, benzodiazepines may be more effective during emergence.

Induction agents such as thiopental or proprofol are more commonly used in patients returning for reconstructive procedures than in the acute phase of injury, but are also sometimes chosen in patients with small burns or when there is no evidence of airway or facial involvement and direct laryngoscopy is planned.

Volatile anesthetics may be used for both induction and maintenance of anesthesia in burn patients. In pediatric patients, mask induction with either halothane or sevoflurane is commonly used if the patient does not have injuries that may make airway manipulation difficult. In the acute setting, an anesthetic technique involving nasotracheal intubation after mask induction with halothane, nitrous oxide, and oxygen has been described. The proponents of this method particularly emphasize that it avoids the potential dysphoria associated with the ketamine-based technique. However, volatile agents produce dose-dependent cardiac depression and vasodilation. In addition, hypoxic ventilatory drive is ablated by volatile anesthetics at low concentrations and a dose-dependent depression of hypercapnic drive also occurs. However, as maintenance agents volatile anesthetics have predictable wash-in and wash-out kinetics and are a useful adjunct to other agents when titrated to hemodynamic and ventilatory parameters. Of the volatile agents, nitrous oxide has the least impact on cardiovascular and respiratory function and can serve as a useful component of a balanced anesthetic if the patient's oxygen requirements permit.

Opioids are important analgesic agents for burn patients throughout the acute phase of injury and for postoperative analgesia during reconstructive procedures. The spectrum of opioids currently available provides a wide range of potencies, durations of action, and effects on the cardiopulmonary system. Burn patients experience intense pain in the absence of movement or procedures. Opioids provide the mainstay of analgesia in the acute phase of burn management. However, acute burn patients usually become tolerant to opioids because they receive continuous and prolonged administration of these drugs. Therefore, opioids should be titrated to effect in the acute burn patient. Most opioids have little effect on cardiovascular function, but they are potent respiratory depressants. Therefore, the ventilatory status of patients receiving opioids, particularly those with compromised airways, should be monitored closely.

Regional anesthesia can be used effectively in patients with small burns or who are undergoing reconstructive procedures. In pediatric or adult patients undergoing procedures confined to the lower extremities, lumbar epidural or caudal anesthesia can provide a useful adjunct for control of postoperative pain. In cooperative adult patients with injuries confined to the lower extremities, epidural or subarachnoid anesthesia may be used if contraindications do not exist. For upper extremity procedures, brachial plexus has been used both as primary anesthetic and to control postoperative pain.

Topical anesthesia has also been used successfully for acute burn surgery. Elderly and debilitated patients requiring full-thickness grafts have been cared for successfully under topical anesthesia with EMLA cream (eutectic mixture of local anesthetics, lidocaine, and prilocaine).

Fluid Management

End points used to titrate fluid administration intraoperatively are similar to those used during resuscitation of acute burns. In fact, because of the nature of surgical trauma associated with burn wound excision, management of anesthesia for these procedures is largely a resuscitation effort. This involves continuous assessment of volume status, titration of fluids to various physiological end points, and assessment of tissue perfusion. Evaluation of the effectiveness of intraoperative volume replacement is much the same as assessment of effectiveness of resuscitation of the acute burn.

For extensive wound excisions expected to involve substantial blood loss, it is prudent to minimize the volume of crystalloid fluids administered intraoperatively. In the early phase of the hospital course, a large amount of edema fluid from the initial resuscitation will be present. In addition, the surgeons will frequently inject dilute crystalloid solution subcutaneously (clysis solution) to facilitate debridement or harvest of split-thickness skin for autografts. The volume of this clysis solution used can be quite large (e.g., more than 50 ml/kg). Limiting crystalloid used for volume replacement can minimize the volume of extra fluid needed to be eliminated after these procedures.

Normal saline (0.9%) is a popular intravenous solution for volume replacement of surgical blood loss. Large amounts of normal saline administered intravenously, however, have been associated with hyperchloremic metabolic acidosis. By itself this metabolic derangement is relatively benign, but during resuscitation from major blood loss it can confuse assessment and/or exacerbate effects of acidosis due to poor tissue perfusion. Lactated Ringer's solution is not associated with such problems, but there is theoretical concern regarding diluting packed red blood cells with lactated Ringer's solution because of the latter's calcium content and the potential for formation of thrombi. Balanced salt solutions that do not contain calcium (e.g., Plasmalyte) can be used for volume replacement without this concern.

In our practice, blood loss during burn wound excision is replaced with packed red blood cells reconstituted with plasma. Plasmalyte is added as needed to reduce the viscosity of administered blood or when additional volume is needed but not more oxygen-carrying capacity. This minimizes crystalloid load and helps to prevent coagulopathy due to dilution of coagulation factors. When large volumes of blood loss are expected (e.g., greater than one total blood volume) it seems intuitive that prevention of coagulopathy is associated with less morbidity than treatment of coagulopathy after it is established. As a rule of thumb, once the blood loss exceeds the estimated total blood volume of the patient, it may be best to avoid further wound excision. In our experience at this point another total blood volume will be lost before the wounds are grafted and dressed. Blood loss in excess of two blood volumes in these patient is associated with increased risk of coagulopathy.

Titrating fluid replacement for blood shed during acute burn excision is a difficult task at present. No single monitor or physiological end point will accurately reflect volume needs or tissue perfusion. Although mean arterial blood pressure and urine output are most commonly cited as physiological end points for resuscitation of acutely burned patients, abundant data indicate that these variables do not adequately reflect cellular oxygen delivery.

It is also difficult to estimate blood loss intraoperatively. In most surgical procedures shed blood is removed from the field by suction and collected in reservoirs where it can be measured. During burn wound excision blood is lost over a potentially broad surface where it can flow under drapes or out through a drain on the table. Since the blood is not collected in a single reservoir or in sponges that can be examined, it is impossible to estimate accurately blood loss intraoperatively.

The anesthetist must base evaluations of the patient's volume status on several physiological variables. Since each of these variables lacks sensitivity, specificity, or both, several monitors of preload and perfusion must be followed and decisions regarding administration of volume are somewhat subjective in these cases.

Blood pressure and heart rate change with blood loss but many other causes of decreased blood pressure and increased heart rate during burn wound excision decrease the monitoring value of these variables. Among the confounding factors are anesthetic drugs, pain, and the effects of bacterial products or inflammatory mediators released by wound manipulation. In addition, even though cardiac output and tissue perfusion are reduced by hypovolemia, blood pressure can be maintained by vasoconstriction up to a point.

Much information is available from observation of the arterial wave form. The area under the each wave is related to the ejection volume and the slope of the upstroke is influenced by the heart's contractility. When blood loss exceeds replacement, preload falls and stroke volume is diminished. This is reflected by a reduction in the area under the arterial wave of the arterial blood pressure and a reduction in the pulse pressure. The wave appears dampened. Reduction of contractile force reduces the slope of the arterial wave upstroke. When hypovolemia is compensated by intense vasoconstriction, the ejection volume and the area under the arterial wave are still diminished but the waves are tall and narrow. This is because the pressure is maintained by increased afterload and the intense vasoconstriction reduces arterial compliance, leading to an increased pulse pressure. The result is tall, narrow, peaked arterial waves.

Directly monitoring blood pressure through an arterial catheter allows observation of beat-to-beat variation in pressure. In the presence of hypovolemia, hemodynamically significant beat-to-beat alterations in myocardial preload can result from phasic changes in venous return caused by changes of intrathoracic pressure during the respiratory cycle. These changes in preload result in beat-to-beat variation in ejection volume and, thus, systolic blood pressure. The relationship between respiratory-related changes in intrathoracic pressure and systolic blood pressure variation have been studied and quantitated to some extent for positive pressure ventilation. The relationship is more complex for spontaneous ventilation and has not been quantitated. Systolic pressure variation during spontaneous ventilation can increase with changes other than decreased preload such as increased respiratory effort or increased airway resistance. Still, hypovolemia can reduce preload to the point that changes in venous return during the respiratory cycle are enough to alter stroke volume noticeably, resulting in increased systolic pressure variation. When other causes are ruled out, respiratory variation in systolic blood pressure can, thus, be used as one of several imperfect indicators of hypovolemia that needs to be corrected.

Transfusions

There is no general agreement regarding the point at which transfusion may be indicated for burn patients. As a rule, currently accepted guidelines support transfusion almost always when the hemoglobin concentration falls below 6 g/100 ml but rarely when the hemoglobin concentration is 10 g/100 ml or greater. In the past, hemoglobin concentration has been maintained at 10 g/100 ml or higher in patients with significant burns. Several centers now recommend lowering the acceptable hemoglobin concentration in order to reduce exposure to blood products and to conserve the resource. Some have proposed a hemoglobin count of 6–6.5 g/100 ml for healthy patients with small burns, 8–8.5 g/100 ml for patients with more extensive burns, and 10 g/100 ml for those with pre-existing cardiac or pulmonary disease. There are few objective data on the optimal management strategy for blood transfusion during burn wound excision.

At present the most logical approach is to assess the needs of each patient individually and continually through the perioperative period. If preload is optimized as described earlier, then oxygen-carrying capacity can be increased as needed depending on the presence of acidosis or problems with oxygen delivery. Demonstration of acidosis, decreased mixed venous oxygen content, or evidence of myocardial ischemia despite adequate preload and blood pressure suggests a need for more oxygen-carrying capacity.

During excision of extensive burn wounds, patients will require transfusion of large amounts of blood, often an exchange volume or more. Massive blood transfusions are associated with a variety of complications, which can be minimized but not entirely avoided by careful practice.

A variety of techniques have been utilized to decrease surgical blood loss during burn excision. Limb tourniquets or compressive dressings at sites of wound excision or skin harvest help to minimize bleeding. Some centers use epinephrine-soaked dressings or topical epinephrine spray to induce local vasoconstriction. Epinephrine solution can also be injected subcutaneously or beneath the burn eschar. The epinephrine solutions appear to be well tolerated but the effectiveness of these maneuvers is uncertain. Another method is to spray topical thrombin solution (1000 U/ml) on bleeding surfaces before application of compressive dressings. Despite all these interventions, blood loss during extensive excisions is still prodigious.

Coagulopathy is one of the more prominent complications associated with massive blood transfusion. This is due to thrombocytopenia or depletion of coagulation factors. Packed red blood cell preparations (PRBCs) are essentially devoid of platelets and whole blood stored for more than 24 h does not possess significant numbers of functional platelets. Whole blood contains essentially normal levels of coagulation factors, with the exception of the volatile factors V and VIII. Because most plasma is removed from PRBCs, they provide a poor source of coagulation factors. Massive blood loss and transfusion with PRBCs or whole blood results in dilutional losses of both platelets and factors V and VIII.

Thrombocytopenia is the most common cause of nonsurgical bleeding after massive blood transfusion. In general, 2–4 blood volumes of blood or PRBCs must be transfused before bleeding due to thrombocytopenia will develop. Observed platelet counts usually remain higher than calculated values due to release of platelets from sites of sequestration. Bleeding due to thrombocytopenia usually develops when the platelet count drops below 50,000 platelets/μl. Replacement of platelets in adults usually requires transfusion of 6 units of whole blood platelets or 1 unit of single donor platelets in adults.

Development of coagulopathy due to depletion of coagulation factors is also possible during massive blood transfusion. Significant prolongation of the prothrombin (PT) and partial thromboplastin time (PTT) can result after transfusion of 10–12 units of packed red blood cells. In general, fresh frozen plasma should be given to correct dilutional coagulopathy if the PT and PTT exceed 1.5 times normal levels. It is also important to know the fibrinogen level in massively transfused patients, since hypofibrinogenemia can also result in prolongation of the PT and PTT. Fibrinogen may be replaced using cryoprecipitate.

Citrate toxicity is possible with rapid infusion of large volumes of blood products. Citrate is universally used as an anticoagulant in the storage of blood because of its ability to bind calcium that is required for activation of the coagulation cascade. Citrate is metabolized by the liver and excreted by the kidneys. Patients with normal liver and kidney function are able to respond to a large citrate load much better than patients with hepatic or renal insufficiency. During massive blood transfusion, citrate can accumulate in the circulation, resulting in a fall in ionized calcium. Hypocalcemia can result in hypotension, reduced cardiac function, and cardiac arrhythmias. Severe hypocalcemia can also result in clotting abnormalities. However, the level of calcium required for adequate coagulation is much lower than that necessary to maintain cardiovascular stability. Therefore, hypotension and decreased cardiac contractility occur long before coagulation abnormalities are seen. During massive blood transfusion it is generally prudent to monitor ionized calcium, especially if hemodynamic instability is present in the hypocalcemic patient.

During the storage of whole blood or packed red cells, potassium leaks from erythrocytes into the extracellular fluid and can accumulate at concentrations of 40–80 mEq/L. Once the RBCs are returned to the in vivo environment, the potassium quickly re-enters RBCs. However, during rapid blood transfusion transient hyperkalemia may result, particularly in patients with renal insufficiency. The transient hyperkalemia, particularly in the presence of hypocalcemia, can lead to cardiac dysfunction and arrhythmias. In patients with renal insufficiency, potassium load can be minimized by the use of either freshly obtained blood or washed packed RBCs.

Hypokalemia can also result from massive blood transfusion due to re-entry of potassium into RBCs and other cells during stress, alkalosis, or massive catecholamine release associated with large volume blood loss. Therefore, potassium levels should be monitored routinely during large-volume blood transfusions.

During the storage of whole blood, an acidic environment occurs due to the accumulation of lactate and citrate with a pH in the range of 6.5–6.7. Rapid transfusion of this acidic fluid can contribute to the metabolic acidosis observed during massive blood transfusion. However, metabolic acidosis in this setting is more commonly due to relative tissue hypoxia and anaerobic metabolism due to an imbalance of oxygen consumption and delivery. The anaerobic metabolism that occurs during states of hypovolemia and poor tissue perfusion results in lactic acidosis. Administration of sodium bicarbonate is generally not indicated. The re-establishment of tissue perfusion and homeostasis is a much more important factor in re-establishing acid–base balance.

In contrast, many patients receiving massive blood transfusion will experience a metabolic alkalosis during the posttransfusion phase. This is due to the conversion of citrate to sodium bicarbonate by the liver and is an additional reason to avoid sodium bicarbonate administration during massive blood transfusion, except in cases of severe metabolic acidosis (base deficit >12).

Rapid infusion of large volumes of cold (4°C) blood can result in significant hypothermia. When added to the already impaired thermoregulatory mechanisms in burn patients, this can result in significant hypothermia. Potential complications of hypothermia include altered citrate metabolism, coagulopathy, and cardiac dysfunction. During large-volume blood transfusion in burn patients, fluids should be actively warmed with systems designed to warm large volumes of rapidly transfused blood effectively. In addition, the room temperature should be elevated and the patient's extremities and head covered to minimize heat loss. Body temperature should be maintained at or above 37°C in burn patients.

Thermoregulation

The skin plays an important role in maintenance of body temperature. The skin contains sensory receptors to monitor surface temperature, subcutaneous fat that serves as insulation, blood vessels that dilate or contract to dissipate or retain heat, and it acts as a barrier to evaporation of body fluids, which is another potential source of heat loss. Cutaneous burns compromise all these functions. Large burn injuries also alter the central regulation of temperature control. The hypermetabolic state that occurs within days of burn injury is associated with an increase in the skin temperature that is perceived as cold and that elicits homeostatic reflexes to maintain body temperature. Burn patients respond to perceived cold with a brisk increase in heat generation by shivering and increased oxidative metabolism. Since the metabolic rate is already accelerated, this response causes additional catabolic stress. Hypothermia is poorly tolerated by these patients.

In the perioperative period burn patients are at increased risk for hypothermia, which is associated with more morbidity than in nonburned patients. Anesthetic agents may also impair thermoregulation. Large areas of the body surface area exposed and open wounds allow evaporative heat loss. Aggressive efforts to minimize heat loss are necessary to prevent hypothermia during burn surgery. The room should be heated and, if necessary, radiant heaters should be used. The head and extremities should be covered when not in the surgical field. Anesthetic gases and intravenous fluids should be warmed. Body temperature should be monitored closely and appropriate actions taken to avoid heat loss. Bladder temperature monitored with a Foley catheter equipped with a thermister probe is an accurate and convenient way to monitor body temperature during burn surgery.

POSTOPERATIVE CARE

One of the most important issues in the immediate postoperative period for burn patients is adequate analgesia and sedation, particularly for those who are intubated and mechanically ventilated. Debridement of burned tissue and the harvesting of skin grafts are painful procedures that merit ample analgesic dosages to ensure patient comfort. It is not uncommon for burn patients to be quite tolerant to narcotic analgesics, especially after they have had several operative procedures, and in this case higher dosages than normal are required.

Continuing blood loss is unfortunately a common problem after the excision and grafting of a large burn wound, even when strict attention is given to intraoperative hemostasis by surgical personnel. The burn wounds are necessarily excised down to bleeding tissue before skin grafts are applied. Massive intraoperative transfusion adds to the problem, with the potential for dilutional thrombocytopenia and coagulopathy. During postoperative transport from the operating room (OR) to the burn ICU, adequate monitoring to identify developing hypovolemia along with resources to resuscitate must be available. Diligent postoperative care is needed to assess continually any continuing blood loss and transfuse additional blood products as they are indicated by clinical course and results of laboratory studies. Monitoring of central venous pressure and urine output also helps in guiding postoperative blood and fluid therapy.

Ventilation may be impaired in the postoperative period whether breathing is spontaneous or mechanically controlled. Blood gases and oxygen saturation can be used as guides to ventilator management. Patients with inhalation injury benefit not only from rational ventilator management but also from a program of inhaled bronchodilators and mucolytics combined with judicious airway suctioning. Extubated patients require supplemental oxygen for at least the first few hours until the effects of general anesthetics resolve. Airway support may also be necessary initially in these patients until they are more alert and responsive.

Burn patients must recover in a warm environment. Postoperative hypothermia can result in vasoconstriction, hypoperfusion, and metabolic acidosis. Radiant heaters, blood and fluid warmers, warm blankets, heated humidifiers for gas delivery, and high room temperatures are all useful in the postoperative period to provide warmth to the recovering patient.

SUMMARY

The most important practical principles of anesthetic management of burn patients were described in the introduction but should be repeated for emphasis. Perioperative management of burned patients presents numerous challenges, both technical and cognitive. Safe and effective anesthetic management of these patients requires detailed knowledge of the continuum of pathophysiological changes associated with burn and inhalation injuries from resuscitation through healing of wounds. In addition, optimal patient care is possible only when it includes close communication with the surgeon. Modern advances in burn care rely on coordination of the efforts of a large team of specialists. The anesthetic plan should be compatible with the overall treatment goals for the patient. The anesthetist joins the burn care team when the anesthetic plan is coordinated with the overall treatment goals for the patient.

BIBLIOGRAPHY

1. Ahrenholz DH, Cope N, Dimick AR, Gamelli RL, Gillespie RW, Ragan RJ, Kealey GP, Peck MD, Pitts LH, Purdue GF, Saffle JR, Sheridan RL, Sundance P, Sweetser S, Tompkins RG, Wainwright DJ, Warden GD. Practice guidelines for burn care. J Burn Care Rehab 2001.
2. Woodson LC, Sherwood ER, Morvant EM, Peterson LA. Anesthesia for burned patients. In: Total Burn Care. 2nd Ed. Herndon DN(), Ed. London: W.B. Saunders, 2001:183–206.
3. MacLennan N, Heimbach DM, Cullen BF. Anesthesia for major thermal injury. Anesthesiology 1998; 89:749–770.
4. Szyfelbein BK, Martyn JAJ, Sheridan RL, Coté CJ. Anesthesia for children with burn injuries. In: A Practice of Anesthesia for Infants and ChildrenCoté CJ, Todres ID, Ryan JF, Goudsouzian NG, Eds. London: W. B. Saunders, 2001:522–543.
5. Porter JM, Ivatury RR. In search of the optimal end points of resuscitation in trauma patients: a review. J Trauma 1998; 44(5):908–914.
6. Deitch EA, Rutan RL. The challenges of children: the first 48 hours. J Burn Care Rehab 2000; 21(5):424–431.
7. Saffle JR, Davis B, Williams P. The American Burn Association Registry Participant Group. Recent outcomes in the treatment of burn injury in the United States: a report from the American Burn Association Patient Registry. J Burn Care Rehab 1995; 16 (3 part 1):219–232.
8. Wallace BH, Caldwell FT, Cone JB. The interrelationships between wound management, thermal stress, energy metabolism, and temperature profiles of patients with burns. J Burn Care Rehab 1994; 15(6):499–506.
9. McLellan SA, McLelland DB, Walsh TS. Anaemia and red blood cell transfusion in the critically ill patient. Blood Rev 2003; 17:195–208.
10. Maldini B. Ketamine anesthesia in children with acute burns and scalds. Acta Anaesthesiol Scand 1996; 40:1108–1111.
11. McCall JE, Fischer CG, Schomaker E, and Young JM. Laryngeal Mask airway use in children with acute burns: intra-operative airway management. Paediatric Anaesthesia 1999; 9:515–520.

6

Principles of Burn Surgery

David M. Heimbach and Lee D. Faucher
University of Washington Burn Center, Seattle, Washington, U.S.A.

HISTORY OF BURN EXCISION

Although early excision and grafting has been considered a procedure of the late 20th century; it was actually first described by Lustgarten in 1891. The fire at the Cocoanut Grove Nightclub in Boston in November, 1942, brought new insight into many aspects of the care of burned patients. Cope suggested then that patients with early wound closure had improved survival [1]. Several reports are scattered throughout the literature over the next 30 years [2–4], but results were discouraging since they showed little clinical improvement from the usual practice of waiting for spontaneous eschar separation followed by grafting on granulation tissue. Janezekovic reported good results in 1970 with sequential shaving of burns of varying depths in [5]. The surgical community began to take notice; however, the need to estimate the depth of burn and ancillary support required for a major burn excision made acceptance of this technique difficult.

The University of Washington Burn Center was formed in 1974. In 1978, a major change in approach to burn care was instituted: burns judged to require more than 3 weeks to heal were to be managed by excision and grafting. Before that, all burns were treated in the nonoperative manner. A study was done to compare the two methods using matched subjects. The patients who underwent excision and grafting had significantly shorter hospital stay, lower hospital charges, and fewer infectious complications [6]. Based on that information, a randomized prospective study was done in patients with burns of indeterminate depth. The results again found that those with excision had shorter hospital stay, lower hospital charges, fewer reconstruction surgeries, and returned to work sooner [7].

PATIENT SELECTION FOR SURGERY

Burns involving the superficial dermis heal within 3 weeks, generally without hypertrophic scarring. Since these burns generally cause no functional and little cosmetic impairment, primary skin grafting does not reduce morbidity or improve appearance and function. Full-thickness burns do not present a decision problem either. They will eventually need skin grafting and the sooner they are grafted the sooner the wounds will be healed.

Many burns, however, cannot be defined into either of these categories. Burns that are very large, of indeterminate depth, or very deep, pose difficult questions. The decision of what to excise and when is crucial. Extensive burns can be too large for complete excision and grafting in one operation. This leaves a large open surface that must be covered temporarily. Tools to evaluate indeterminate wounds are being sought. The use of immunohistochemisty [8], infrared fluorescence [9], and laser Doppler studies [10] all show promise in vitro, but a trained surgeon has been shown to be at least as good [11]. This leaves a surgeon with the decision based on clinical grounds. The cause of the burn, inspection and palpation of the wound, and sensory nerve function are all important clues. Finally, excision of very deep burns over joints, tendons, and bones may leave a wound that may not accept a skin graft.

Some truisms regarding burns and burn care include the following:

Burns in patients at the extremes of age are not shallow.

Immersion burns are not shallow.

Except for contact burns, most burns of the palms and soles heal within 3 weeks.

Patients whose clothing or bedding has been on fire rarely escape without some full-thickness burns.

All electrical burns are full-thickness and should be assumed to be fourth-degree.

Flash burns are rarely full-thickness, except in areas of very thin skin.

Burns are dynamic and deepen over the first 48 h. Wounds that appear shallow on day 1 may be indeterminate on day 3. Burns never get shallower.

Burns from hot soups and sauces are deeper than those from hot water alone.

Burns resulting from direct contact with a tar pot are usually very deep dermal or full-thickness burns, while those from tar that has been transferred into a bucket or spread on a surface are usually shallow.

Small burns that will eventually heal present little threat to life if allowed to heal over several weeks. If small burns are excised, operative mortality should be zero.

Early excision requires an experienced surgeon. Inadequate excision with skin grafting on a poor bed leads to skin graft loss, adds the size of the donor site to the total area of open wounds, and may necessitate another operation.

Non-life-threatening burns in patients with associated medical problems or injuries should not be excised until the associated problems are under control and the operation can be done with low morbidity and essentially no mortality.

Patients with burns of the hands and feet will be able to return to work sooner if their burns are excised and skin grafted shortly after hospital admission.

Large, superficial burns with scattered small deeper components are best treated nonoperatively until the shallow areas have healed.

Early excision decreases the need for wound cleansing and daily debridement. If pain management becomes a significant problem, this in itself is an indication for excision.

A patient with a small burn who can continue to work despite the burn and who can manage the wound at home will have the least expensive care and, in the long run, will miss much less work than if the burn is excised.

Small deep burns can be treated initially on an outpatient basis and then excised and skin grafted electively on a day surgery schedule.

PATIENT PREPARATION FOR SURGERY

Complete resuscitation

Before a patient is taken to the operating room for excision of a burn wound, we recommend that he or she be completely resuscitated. That is, he or she should have adequate urine output receiving only maintenance intravenous fluid administration or in combination with enteral nutrition. This allows us to begin excision about postburn day 3. There are always exceptions to the rules. In patients with extensive full-thickness burns, who still require large volume fluid resuscitation beyond the first 48 h excision of some of their burn before resuscitation is complete may be necessary. These patients have a very high mortality rate.

Nutrition

It is well known that early and aggressive enteral nutrition in the thermally injured patient improves mortality, decreases complications, optimizes wound healing, and diminishes the catastrophic effects of protein catabolism. Nutritional support should be instituted immediately upon admission and continued throughout the acute phase of burn care. It has been shown in a randomized study that nearly continuous nutrition throughout the perioperative period maintained nitrogen balance and improved outcome [13,14]. Jenkins also showed that continuous feeding throughout the perioperative period does not risk aspiration in intubated patients [14]. Intubated patients taken to the operating room do not need to have their feedings discontinued before or during surgery [14]. It is the practice at our institution to continue tube feedings for intubated patients throughout the perioperative period. We stop tube feedings and allow nothing orally in nonintubated patients for 4 hours prior to induction.

Preoperative laboratory evaluation

Our daily laboratory evaluation of patients consists of a full electrolyte panel and complete blood count. Prothrombin and partial thromboplastin times are checked only if there is concern based on the patient history that they could be abnormal. We ensure that all electrolytes are in within the normal range prior to operative intervention. Over the past 20 years, we have become better at limiting blood loss during surgery. This will be discussed later. In 1980, a patient with a 50% burn would receive roughly 15 units of blood during their hospital course, now this same patient averages 1.5 units during their stay. The reasons are twofold: we tolerate lower hematocrit levels and intraoperative blood loss is less. For an excision of 20% total body surface area, we will have 2 units of blood ready to use.

OPERATING ROOM PREPARATION

Excision of major burns

Life-threatening burns should be excised only in a specialized burn treatment facility, where the entire burn team is experienced in excision techniques and has a thorough understanding of burn pathophysiology, critical care, nutrition, and monitoring. Excision of a burn should be an elective procedure and done in a timely fashion. We generally schedule the first excision in an otherwise stable patient for postburn day 3. We continue excisions every 2 or more days and excise at most 20% total body surface area at a time. This allows almost all burns to be excised before bacterial burn wound sepsis begins.

In patients with very large total body surface area (TBSA) burns, the highest priority is to diminish overall burn size. The trunk and extremities are excised first, followed by face and hands. In our patients with extensive burns that include bilateral hands, who also have donor sites available to provide sheet grafts to cover both hands, we will excise and graft the hands very early. We have found that this practice allows our patients to have their hands available to assist in activities and therapy earlier.

The overall strategy for excision should be designed upon admission. Excision of the obviously full-thickness areas should be done first and indeterminate areas allowed to declare themselves. Excision of the posterior trunk requires the patient to be in the prone position, the most dangerous of all anesthetic positions; therefore it should be done when the patient is most stable medically. This is generally postburn day 3, after resuscitation is complete. Pulmonary complications that occur later in a patient's course may inhibit placing him or her in the prone position. If anterior burns are excised and grafted before those on the posterior trunk, there is a risk of graft shearing when the patient is placed in the prone position to have the back burns excised. Proper dressings (to be discussed later) minimize shear, permit excellent graft take, and allow the patient to resume normal activities.

We performed a retrospective review and did not find a difference in postoperative complications when compared to length of operation [15]. However, our experience dictates that it is best to limit operating time to 2 h for stable patients with major burns. This keeps a critically ill patient out of the intensive care unit for about 3 h. We will limit operating time to 1 h for patients in more tenuous medical condition. The ambient temperature of the operating room is at least 80°F, forced air warming devices are placed over the patient if possible, and all fluids are warmed.

Tangential excision

The principle of tangential excision is to shave very thin layers of eschar sequentially until viable tissue is reached. Even though this concept is extraordinarily simple, the technique requires considerable experience and excellent operating room support.

Excision can be done with a variety of power or handheld instruments. Power dermatomes may be more precise in depth setting but can dull rapidly and become clogged with debris. Changing blades is time-consuming and tedious, and this time is crucial while the patient continues to bleed. For these reasons, we prefer the use of Watson (Fig. 1) and Goulian (Fig. 2) knives for tangential excision.

Proper skin tension above and below the area to be excised is necessary in order to use a manual dermatome properly. Broad slices are taken with the knife and the back of the instrument is then used to wipe the area to inspect the bed. If the bed does not bleed briskly, another slice of the same depth is taken. Healthy dermis appears white and shiny, therefore if the area is dull and gray or if clotted blood vessels are seen, the excision needs to be carried deeper.

As excision continues to the deeper layers of the dermis and into fat, vessels with pulsatile flow may be transected. Any fat that has brownish discoloration

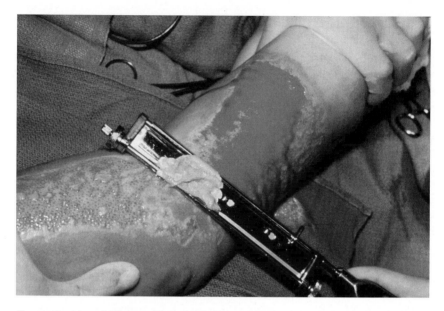

FIGURE 1   Use of Watson blade for burn excision

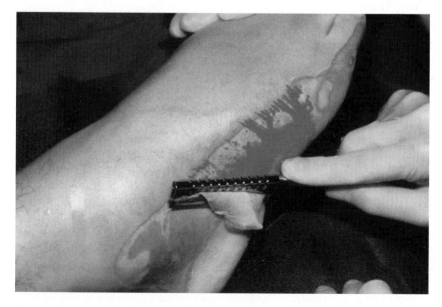

FIGURE 2   Use of Goulian blade for burn excision.

or bloodstaining will not support a skin graft and needs to be excised. Fat should appear uniformly yellow with briskly bleeding vessels.

Pulsatile blood vessels are controlled with electrocautery and the wound is then covered with a Telfa dressing soaked in 1:10,000 epinephrine solution before the surgeon moves on to the next area. The Telfa dressing is applied cellophane-side down to minimize adherence to the wound, with removal this may stimulate bleeding that was under control. When the burn to be excised is completed (Fig. 3), epinephrine-soaked Telfa is applied, then an epinephrine-soaked laparotomy pad is added on top of the Telfa. Extremities are wrapped in elastic bandages and suspended. Direct pressure is applied to areas that cannot be suspended. These dressings are left undisturbed for 10 min. The outer wraps are carefully removed and the Telfa dressing is removed after being soaked in saline. Any persistent bleeding points can be controlled with electrocautery. This process is repeated until the wound bed is hemostatic (Fig. 4). Summarized Below are several points about the use of epinephrine to stop bleeding:

> Substantial amounts of epinephrine are absorbed systemically from the wound. We have measured blood levels as high as 4,000 µg/dl 100 ml after a major excision. Systemic manifestations of any consequence are very rare in patients with acute burns. Systolic blood pressure and pulse

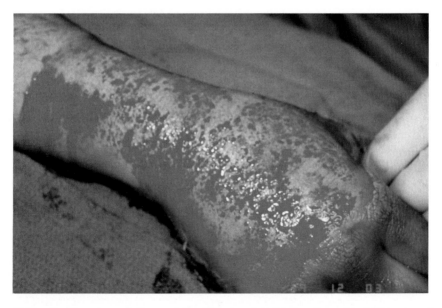

FIGURE 3 Burn wound after excision with pinpoint bleeding throughout. This wound is adequately excised.

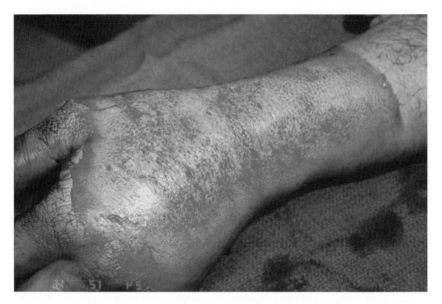

FIGURE 4   Hemostatic burn wound ready for grafting after application of epinephrine.

rate may be elevated slightly. We have used this technique in thousands
of patients without significant complications. We still suggest caution
when using epinephrine to stop bleeding after burn excision in patients
with pre-existing hypertension or cardiac arrhythmias.

The surgeon must be sure the bed is adequately excised prior to the application of epinephrine. Once the dressings are removed, the bed appears
avascular and further excision risks removal of viable tissue.

The fear that reactive vasodilatation would cause postoperative bleeding
has not been realized. Major bleeding has been extremely rare and its
occurrence was a result of inadequate cauterization of a pulsatile vessel.
Minor bleeding is vented into the dressings through the interstices of
mesh grafts. Sheet grafts need to be inspected frequently during the postoperative period and any hematomas evacuated.

Extremities should be excised under tourniquet, but the cadaver-like appearance of the dermis and lack of brisk bleeding make this technique more
difficult. One should acquire considerable expertise prior to using this
technique.

Fascial Excision

Fascial excision is reserved for patients with very deep burns or very large, life-
threatening, full-thickness burns.

Our fascial excision technique uses electrocautery for excision. Inflatable tourniquets are placed as high as possible on the affected extremity and inflated. The initial incision is made around the periphery of the tourniquet and carried down to the investing fascia. The flap is grasped with penetrating clamps and pulled by an assistant (Fig. 5). The eschar flap is the separated at the level just above the fascia, with great care being taken to identify perforating vessels and coagulate them appropriately. All fat tissue should be removed, with the exception of areas of tendons and bony prominences. We leave a thin layer of fat over these areas to ensure that the tenuous vascular supply is left intact to support a skin graft.

Epinephrine-soaked Telfa sponges are applied as the excision progresses. When the excision is completed, the extremity is wrapped with epinephrine-soaked Telfa sponges and laparotomy pads held in place by an elastic bandage. The tourniquet is deflated and the dressings are left intact for 10 min. Hemostasis is achieved using the same technique of removal of the sponges as described above. There have been many techniques described for fascial excision, but in our experience, the electrocautery is quick, less expensive, and can successfully provide a viable bed for grafting.

The advantages of fascial excision over tangential excision include the following:

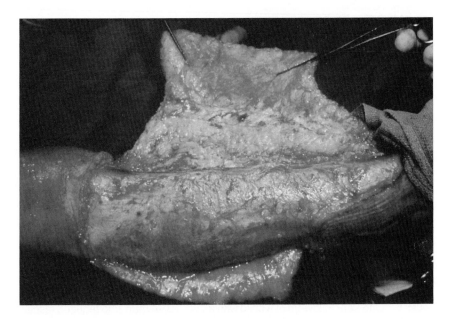

FIGURE 5 Large flaps raised during fascial excision.

1. A reliable bed of known viability is provided.
2. Tourniquets may be used routinely for extremities.
3. Operative blood loss is less.
4. Less experience is required to obtain an optimal bed.

The disadvantages of fascial excision include the following:

1. Operative time is longer.
2. Severe cosmetic deformity is possible (Fig. 6), especially in obese patients.
3. The incidence of distal edema is higher when excision is circumferential.
4. Risk of damage to superficial tendons and nerves is greater.
5. Cutaneous denervation occurs and sensation may not return.
6. Skin graft loss may occur from the relatively avascular fascia over joints, may lead to an ungraftable bed, and may require eventual flap coverage.

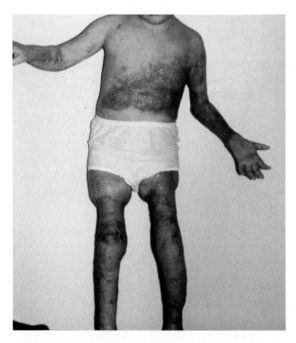

FIGURE 6   One-year follow-up of a child with a 75% TBSA burn who required fascial excision.

The risks and benefits must be weighed carefully, and each burned area on each patient reviewed to identify the optimal excision technique to provide the best result.

Donor sites

When treating a patient with extensive burns, the decision of where to create donor sites is easy: You take what you can get. In those with lesser burns, the decision is slightly more complicated. Since all donor sites scar to some degree, it is best to take skin from an area that will be otherwise hidden under most circumstances. Donors should also be taken from an area that allows ease in harvesting and donor site care.

Our first choice of donor site for children still in diapers is the buttocks. This allows for a hidden donor site and use of the diaper to hold the silver sulfadiazine in place for wound care. The use of the buttocks in others is not forbidden, but we have found that it is more painful in older patients than other sites and wound care is more difficult. The thighs are excellent sites for donors. It is less difficult to harvest because the femur provides excellent support during harvesting and there is minimal motion even with ambulation so that the dressings remain intact during the healing period.

The lower back is another area that is less difficult to harvest and provides ample skin. It also tends to be hidden with most clothing. The difficulty with using the lower back is that most often it requires a patient to change position during the operation.

The key points in harvesting donors are traction and countertraction. The use of clysis can help provide support to the area to be excised so that the best donor may be harvested. We use lactated Ringer's solution to inject and use clysis on any site that needs additional support, especially the abdomen and chest. Using assistants to provide traction to the skin and surgical soap for lubrication can also help.

Donor site dressings

Before we started our process of early excision of indeterminate burns, many patients endured weeks of daily debridement and donor sites were not a problem. With the pain of daily debridements gone, since the burns were excised, this left larger donor sites to cover the excised wound and now the patients focused on their donor site pain.

Over the past 20 years, our institution has used many donor site coverings. Fine-mesh gauze and scarlet red dressings were popular early on. We also went through periods using petroleum-jelly-impregnated gauze, adhesive polyurethane sheets, calcium alginate, Biobrane (Bertek Pharmaceuticals, Inc), and others. We now most commonly use Acticoat (Smith and Nephew) for most donor sites. We use silver sulfadiazine cream on buttock donors of children in diapers and on donor sites near unexcised burns treated with silver sulfadiazine. We have found Acticoat to be more cost-effective, provide better patient tolerance, and better pain control than other dressings we have tried.

To use Acticoat effectively, we follow the application technique for small donor sites as follows:

1. Ensure that the donor site is hemostatic.
2. Cut Acticoat to cover the entire donor site to include at least a 2 inch border covering normal skin and place the dry Acticoat on the donor site.
3. Spray the edges of Acticoat and skin with tincture of benzoin or Mastisol and allow to dry.
4. Tape edges of Acticoat to skin using Hypafix (Smith and Nephew) tape. There should be no wrinkles in the Acticoat.
5. The site is wrapped in a Kerlex gauze followed by an elastic bandage. This is left in place for 24 h, then removed, and the dressing is allowed to dry.
6. After 7 days, the tape is removed and the edges of Acticoat trimmed.
7. The patient may now shower and continue to trim the edges of Acticoat as the donor site heals and the scab falls away.
8. If the Acticoat does not dry properly or become adherent, we will then remove the Acticoat completely and treat with silver sulfadiazine and daily dressing changes.

Some specific findings regarding donor site techniques include the following:

1. An air-driven dermatome is our instrument of choice. Grafts to cover Integra (Integra Life Sciences Corporation, Plainsboro, NJ, USA) are taken at 0.006 inch and all others at 0.010 inch. Sheet grafts are always used on hands and faces. They are used whenever possible on children and burns over joints, tendons, and small burns. Grafts are meshed when donor sites are limited, and the use of Integra avoids the need for a mesh wider than 2:1 mesh. We try never to mesh greater than a 3:1 ratio.
2. The posterior trunk is the only donor site with skin thick enough to heal reliable in elderly patients. It should be used preferentially for skin grafts in all patients over age 60.
3. We recommend the use of scalp donor for all face, neck, and upper anterior chest grafts. Donor sites need to be kept within the hairline and clysis should be used to assist harvesting. We will not use the scalp in bald individuals.

4.   Clysis should be used for harvesting skin over the ribs, back, and abdomen. It may be used anywhere to assist in making a broad, flat surface for harvesting. The anesthesia team needs to be aware of the volume injected so that they may decrease the amount of intravenous fluid given.
5.   When taking skin from the abdomen, we first inject the clysis solution and then set the dermatome to twice the depth we want. The skin is harvested by applying almost no pressure to the dermatome. Great care must be taken to avoid a full-thickness excision.
6.   If the sole of the foot is used for a donor site, the first 0.010–0.015 inch must be excised and discarded as it contains only dead epithelium that is not suitable for grafting.
7.   Pigmented people tend to experience hypertrophic donor sites as well as hypertrophic burn scars. In dark-skinned patients, both burns and donor sites frequently become darker than the surrounding normal skin, even if they do not hypertrophy.

Our general findings regarding excision and donor sites include the following [12]:

Most nonshallow burns should be excised to diminish the likelihood of burn wound sepsis.

The maximum area that should be excised at one sitting is about 20% TBSA, and the maximum operating time should be about 2 h.

Donor skin left as sheet graft will shrink by about one-third. Meshing 1.5:1 will leave it only slightly larger than the original size. Meshing 3:1 will leave it about twice the original size.

Donor sites taken at a depth of 0.010 inch take 10–14 days to heal to a point that they can be taken again.

Scalp is the premier donor site for face and neck. The face should never be grafted with expanded skin.

Sheet grafts should always be used on the fingers and hands.

The posterior trunk is a premier donor site. Skin is easy to take, and the skin is very thick, which allows numerous harvests.

Wound Coverage

Autograft

Sheet autograft is the ideal covering for all excised burn wounds. Its use is necessarily limited as the burn size becomes larger. Many of our ideas about the use of sheet grafts have already been discussed, but their use can not be overemphasized for those special areas. It is our opinion that sheet grafts for hands, fingers, and faces are the only way to cover those excised areas. The use of sheet grafts on the face will give the best functional and most cosmetically pleasing result. The hands and fingers require skin with excellent pliability to achieve full range of motion of all joints, which is necessary to perform most activities of daily living.

When using sheet graft for primary coverage after excision, the wound bed must be hemostatic. Fluid collections that form under the graft do not allow graft adherence and thus lead to graft failure in those areas. Frequent inspection of the grafted area is necessary in the early postoperative period is necessary to achieve the best result. Any collections of fluid found can be drained by incising the skin graft with a surgical blade and expressing the fluid with cotton-tipped applicators. If a large hematoma develops, return to the operating room is most likely necessary.

There are many ways to secure sheet grafts, including various suture materials and staples. In our center, we then dress the wound with a petroleum-jelly-impregnated gauze, wrap with cotton gauze, and support with elastic wraps. The dressing is taken down the following day and the wound inspected for fluid collections that are drained if present. This is continued on a daily basis until no fluid collections are found, at which point the dressing is left intact until postoperative day 5. If the graft appears intact, the mechanical holding devices are removed, and range-of-motion exercises are begun.

Over the past year, we have begun to use a different method of securing sheet and meshed autograft that covers smaller areas. The use of Hypafix, tape was first discussed by Cassey in 1989, and he demonstrated its success in a small series of patients [16]. We have also found the Hypafix, along with spray adhesive, holds grafts securely and allows drainage of fluid collections. In most cases, it entirely eliminates the need for staples or sutures.

Allograft

The decision to excise burns early led to the need to find a suitable, temporary covering until autograft was available. The first reported use of cadaveric skin was in 1881 to cover a burn wound. This might also be the first reported case of possible rejection: what was termed erysipelatous inflammation occurred and the graft was lost in the second week [17]. Many burn centers, including ours, use allograft as a temporary wound covering; to test the bed of an infected area; to provide temporary coverage for large nonburned, open wounds; and to provide protection for widely meshed autograft. Allograft rejection begins about 14 days after application: replacement or final closure is needed before that time. There are published reports of the successful use of allograft with systemic immunosuppression to achieve wound closure [18,19]. This idea has not been widely accepted up to now.

Many centers have tissue banks closely associated with them so that unfrozen allograft is readily available. We routinely use frozen allograft and find that it suits our needs. Our most common use of allograft is to test a questionable wound bed. In excisions that need to be carried down near tendons, bone, or fascia of questionable viability, we will cover the area with allograft; if the allograft takes, we can assume the bed is viable and will accept autograft. Our overall use of allograft has diminished because we have had tremendous success with the use of Integra as our primary, temporary wound coverage.

Integra

Integra is a bilayer material: the inner layer is a combination of bovine collagen and glycosaminoglycan chondroitin-6-sulfate; the outer layer is a polysiloxane polymer that functions as a temporary epidermis. Integra was developed in the early 1980s by researchers from the Massachusetts General Hospital and Massachusetts Institute of Technology [20], and is now approved by the US Food and Drug Administration for use in life-threatening burns. Early studies of its use found no significant immunoreactivity [21,22], which led to its adoption as a viable temporary wound coverage. Many studies support tout its is for massive burns [23,24], purpura fulminans [25], neck contracture [26], burn scars [27,28], and other complex wounds [29–31].

At the University of Washington Burn Center we have used Integra on over 100 patients and have placed it on every part of the body except the face, palms, and soles of the feet. We believe it provides our patients with better long-term skin integrity, pliability, durability, and cosmetic results.

Our process for the application of Integra on an excised burn wound is outlined below:

1. Integra is prepared for use in the operating room following the manufacturers recommendations.
2. It is then meshed 1:1 and applied to an excised bed that is clean and hemostatic. It is imperative that all areas of the bed be able to provide an adequate blood supply to the Integra. Excision to fascia is often necessary in obese and elderly patients.
3. The meshed Integra is then applied without opening the interstices of the mesh, and great care is taken to ensure that no wrinkles are present. This is especially important in areas around joints. Edges are overlapped about 5 mm.
4. The sheets of Integra are held in place with staples, then Spandage (Medi-Tech International Corp., Brooklyn, NY) is stretched tightly over the Integra and also stapled in place (Fig. 7).
5. The areas are then covered with gauze dressings and 5% mafenide acetate is applied immediately, and added every 4 h to keep the dressing soaked.
6. Areas where Integra is over joints are splinted with temporary devices that allow the 5% mafenide acetate to be applied.
7. On postoperative day 4, the dressings are removed down to the Spandage and any fluid under the Integra is expelled.

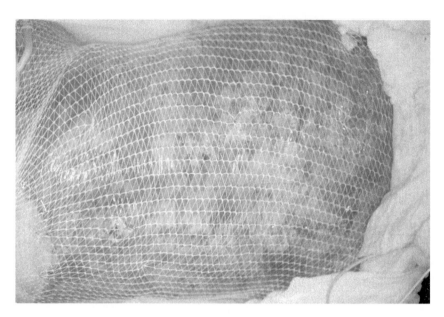

Figure 7 Integra applied to wound after tangential excision. Spandage is in place to help hold the Integra securely.

      8.   Dressings are changed every 3 days and administration of 5% mafenide acetate continues until autograft is applied.

On or about postoperative day 14 Integra is usually ready to be grafted. It will be adherent, have a somewhat contracted appearance, and will have a pink tone of varying degrees throughout.

      Integra is grafted with autograft taken at a depth of 0.006 inch and meshed 3:1 after careful removal of the silastic covering (Fig. 8). Grafts are secured with staples. A synthetic, meshed dressing (Conformant, Smith & Nephew, Largo, FL) is used to cover the grafted area and is held in place with staples.

      Dressings, as described above, with 5% mafenide acetate then cover the Conformant. By postoperative day 7, good graft take is appreciated and range-of-motion exercises are begun.

      Thinly meshed autograft gives us excellent results with minimal residual mesh pattern, good skin durability, excellent skin pliability, and happy patients (Fig. 9).

TREATMENT OF SPECIFIC AREAS OF THE BODY

Not all areas of the body are as easy to excise and graft as others. It is fortunate that the perineum and perianal areas are burned infrequently as these are the most

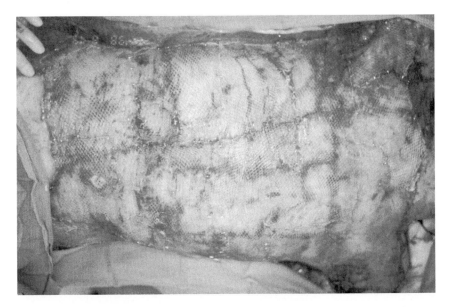

FIGURE 8   Autograft meshed 2:1 placed on the Integra™ after removal of the Silastic membrane. The grafts are held in place with staples.

difficult areas to care for. Integra is an option for wound coverage in all of the areas described below. The following sections outline how we care for specific body areas.

Posterior Trunk

Treatment of the posterior trunks includes the following:

Shallow burns are allowed to heal spontaneously.

If the overall burn size is less than 30%, indeterminate and full-thickness burns should be excised and grafted.

In larger burns, the back needing excision and grafting can have 3:1 meshed skin applied since this is a relatively low-priority area cosmetically.

Charred burns to the back should be excised to the fascia. The removal of all fat of questionable viability improves the chances of graft take.

Dressing the back can be difficult. Prone positioning is not recommended because this can lead to problematic airway and facial edema. Physical therapy is nearly impossible, which is also detrimental to the patient. Shear can be limited with the use of Biobrane to cover the grafts and hold them in place. The grafted area is then allowed to dry and the

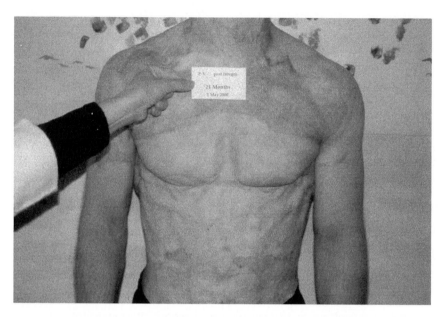

FIGURE 9 Patient 21 months after excision and grafting using Integra. Note the better appearance of the lower chest and abdomen compared to the upper chest, where Integra was not used.

Biobrane removed after the area heals. If wet dressings are desired, the use of a quilt dressing as described by Sheridan [32] and others is also an option.

Buttocks

Burned buttock can be very difficult to manage because continued fecal soilage facilitates early bacterial invasion of deep burns. This can lead to infectious graft loss as well. We follow the principles listed below:

Remove necrotic tissue early to diminish burn wound sepsis.
In patients with large burns, allow partial-thickness burns to remain unexcised. Meticulous wound debridement is needed.
Skin graft take over the inferior gluteal creases is poor as a result of shearing. This area is fortunately narrow enough to heal from the periphery.
If fascial excision is required for deep burns to the buttocks, do not excise the fat from the perirectal spaces because the resulting defect is nearly ungraftable.

Biobrane makes an excellent skin graft dressing because it conforms well. Frequent evaluation is needed: the dressing should be removed if fecal soilage occurs.

Preoperative mechanical bowel preparation, followed by a somewhat constipating diet, may give up to 5 days of avoidance of fecal soilage. This may be enough time for graft take that is more resistant to infection.

Chest and Abdomen

We follow these principles in treating patients with burns to the chest and abdomen:

Fascial excision of the chest and abdomen is reserved for char burns and patients with massive burns. Excision in the early postburn course allows easier excision: the fluid under the eschar facilitates sequential excision without the use of clysis.

Care must be taken with excision near the umbilicus: many patients have asymptomatic defects in the abdominal wall. Inattentive excision in this area could lead to invasion of the peritoneal cavity that would carry an increased risk of peritoneal infection.

Breast

The management of the burned breast depends on the total burn size, depth of burn, age of the patient, and occasionally the social circumstances of the patient. Below list some of our management principles.

The most common burn to the breast we see is a scald burn in a preadolescent girl. Partial-thickness burns should be allowed to heal. Deeper burns, if allowed to heal, can lead to significant scarring and later displacement of the breast. When excision is indicated, great care should be taken to avoid excision of the subareolar tissue, as it contains the breast bud.

Sheet grafts should be applied when possible.

Deep flame burns of the chest should be managed in the same way.

Burns needing excision of the developed female breast are difficult to treat. Sheet and meshed grafts give equally poor cosmetic results. Grafts need to be held in place with Biobrane.

Extensive burns with limited donor sites and involved breasts are often an indication for simple mastectomy: this will lessen the need for skin to cover the anterior chest.

Severe breast burns in the elderly woman most often are caused when a nightgown or bathrobe catches fire and this leads to deep burns. We have a much lower threshold for recommending mastectomy in these patients.

Axilla

Fascial excision of the axilla can lead to neurovascular disruption and a very poor bed to allow good skin graft take. We try to use tangential excision whenever possible. This area also tends to contract easily, which leads to functional deficits. Grafts are held in place with tie-over dressings or Biobrane. Arms are abducted to 90 degrees and splinted in position until graft take, and then range-of-motion exercises are begun. Physical therapy is crucial to achieve adequate arm function and avoid contraction.

Perineum

The perineum is spared in almost all but the most extensive burns. Scald burns to the genitalia frequently heal without operative intervention. Meticulous hygiene is paramount to good wound healing. Most of our experience with skin grafts to the perineum is in patients with necrotizing soft tissue infections. Many full-thickness burns to the penis and scrotum will heal with minimal deformity. Skin grafts to the penis heal without resultant chordae or voiding difficulty.

Lower Extremities

Thighs

For circumferential burns to the thighs, excision is carried out under tourniquet that is placed as high as possible on the thigh. The lower extremity is suspended from ceiling hooks to allow access to the entire thigh.

If fascial excision is deemed necessary, the fascia lata should probably also be removed. In our experience, this nearly avascular fascia usually fails to support a skin graft.

Legs

The legs have several areas that can be troublesome should they have deep burns. Great care needs to be taken when excising near the anterior tibia, the medial and lateral maleolus, and the Achilles tendon. It is best to leave as much viable fat as possible to protect the tenuous blood supply.

In patients with deep burns to the Achilles tendon and heel, we often will excise only to the area just above the ankle and allow the area surrounding the ankle and tendon to granulate. The patient with more extensive burns is usually suspended at all times using balanced skeletal traction pins to keep the area free from any pressure while he or she is lying in bed.

Another area of concern, especially during fascial excision of the leg, is the proximal fibular region. Damage to the peroneal nerve can easily occur, even without evidence of direct nerve damage with excision. This overall incidence of neurological deficits in the lower extremity is quite high in patients with lower extremity burns [33]. Foot drop can occur postoperatively with improper use of splints and foot positioning, as well as generalized weakness from intensive care unit neuropathy.

Feet

Burns to the feet are the most difficult of all burns to treat on an outpatient basis. Patients are usually unwilling or unable to keep their feet elevated, and the incidence of edema and cellulitis leading to hospital admission is quite high. Burns that do not require grafting often blister significantly from friction caused by normal footwear. We try to sheet graft the feet whenever possible to provide a more durable covering.

In patients with extensive burns and severe burns to the toes, we generally will graft the great toe and leave the others to granulate or autoamputate. If burns to the feet are part of less extensive burns, the toes can be excised and grafted in a manner similar to fingers.

Full-thickness burns to the sole of the foot are rare in patients with survivable burns. Electrical burns, immersion scalds, and contact burns are the exceptions. Unless the burn is obviously full-thickness, we give burns of the sole every opportunity to heal on their own.

Upper Extremities

Hand

There is more written about the treatment of burns to the hands than any other area of the body. Proper care of hand burns is essential to get a patient back to his or her preburn level of activity. The care of the badly burned hand should be reserved for those who understand the technical and treatment aspects of properly caring for such patients.

Arms

As described for lower extremities, excision of burns to the arms requires great care in areas near tendons and bony prominences. We use tourniquets to assist in tangential and fascial excision of the arms. Fascial excision is reserved for char burns and does carry a significant risk of chronic hand edema.

Our general findings regarding burns of the upper extremities include the following [12]:

Patients with indeterminate burns to the hands have a shorter hospital stay and return to work more quickly after early excision and grafting than will patients with managed non surgically.

Sheet grafts to the hands offer superior functional and cosmetic results to meshed grafts.

Excision and grafting of two badly burned hands may take 3–4 h. It is therefore best to devise an operative plan so that no other procedures are included.

Most palm burns should be allowed to heal without operative intervention. Very deep burns to the dorsum of the hand may require flaps to provide coverage.

The use of tourniquets allows for less intraoperative blood loss, but may lead to excision of unnecessary tissue by less experienced surgeons.

Head and Neck

Face

We have been aggressive in the treatment of facial burns since 1979. All burns to the face are treated with daily dressing changes until day 10, when a judgment is made whether the burn will heal by day 14. If it is judged that the burn will not be healed, plans for surgery are made. Our results have been encouraging even in patients with extensive burns (Figs. 10, 11).

Excision is the first stage. Tangential excision is performed following aesthetic units [34] that can include small areas of unburned skin. Blood loss can be excessive and is minimized with the liberal use of epinephrine-soaked nonadherent sponges. Electrocautery can be used with caution to stop bleeding that is uncontrollable with epinephrine sponges.

The area is then grafted with sheet allograft sewn tautly into position. The grafts are covered with petroleum-jelly-impregnated gauze, followed by a conforming, elastic head dressing. A padded neck splint is also used to prevent head movement. The grafts are checked at least daily to drain any fluid collections.

The patient can return to the operating room between postoperative days 7 and 10 for autografting if the allograft is stuck and intact.

Scalp provides the best color match for face grafts and should be used when possible. The head should be shaved and the hairline clearly marked. The needed donor should then be outlined and harvested after the scalp is injected with clysis solution. The sheet autograft is then sutured to the hemostatic wound bed with slight tension on the graft. The same dressing plan is then done as outlined above.

Scalp

Most scalp burns are treated nonoperatively. For burns to the skull, flaps are often needed. The more traditional method of drilling holes in the skull table to allow granulation tissue to develop with subsequent grafting usually leaves less than ideal skin. These grafts are susceptible to loss from shear forces. We have been able to cover large defects with Integra after ensuring a viable bed by testing with allograft.

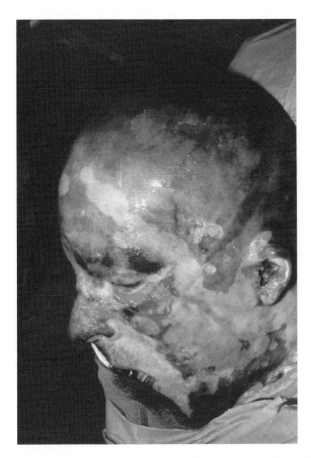

FIGURE 10 A 33-year-old man with severe facial flame burn.

We will very often apply a neurosurgical halo device to avoid any pressure to the skull with the patient in a supine position.

OPERATING ROOM SET-UP

The operating room should be as large as possible and staffed with personnel familiar with all equipment and procedures for burn excision. A room with its own thermostat is also preferable since patients are usually greatly exposed; keeping the ambient temperature about 80°F can help maintain the patient's temperature.

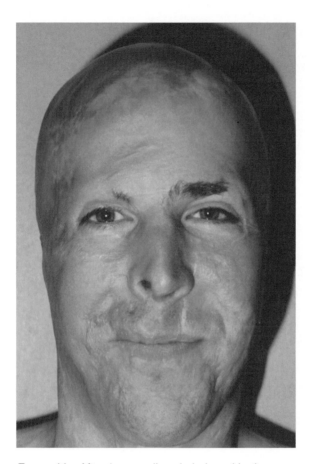

FIGURE 11 After 1 year, all scalp hair and both ears were destroyed. The overall appearance of the face is good.

Adjustable ceiling hooks are necessary (Fig. 12). These can be easily added to any existing room and many other services have also found uses for these hooks. The extremity can then be suspended with a sterile soft restraint and rope.

Instruments

The instruments we have available for a tangential excision include the following:

2 #3 knife handles
Ruler
Thumb forceps

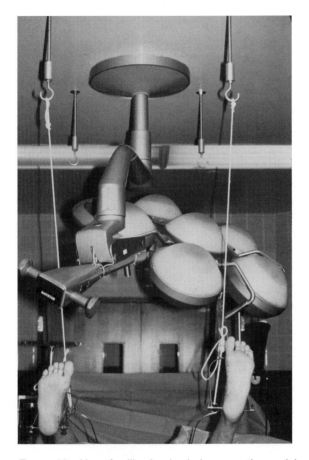

FIGURE 12 Use of ceiling hooks during operative excision of lower-extremity burns.

    2 Adson with teeth
    2 Adson without teeth
    4 with teeth
    4 without teeth
Scissors
    2 straight Mayo
    2 curved Mayo
    2 Metzenbaum
    2 serrated Metzenbaum
Clamps
    2 mosquitoes
    4 hemostats

2 Allis
2 Kocher
2 nonperforating towel clips
6 needle holders
6 perforating towel clips
Other
3 Watson knives
3 Goulian handles with guards
2 metal staplers
1 small bowl
3 medication cups
3 dressing shears
For fascial excision the following instruments are added:
8 Kocher clamps
8 Lahey clamps
8 mosquitoes

Equipment

In addition to the general instruments listed above, two electrocautery units, two arm tables, and furniture for two prep sets can speed up the procedure. We have also found it easier to have a rolling cart with multiple sterile and nonsterile supplies since we tend to operate in various operating rooms.

Our general findings regarding the operating room include the following [12]:

The operating room personnel must be familiar with the procedure before the excision starts.

The room must be large and warm.

Duplicate chuck keys and wrenches should be kept sterile to save time if one becomes contaminated.

Checklists should be available if inexperienced operating room personnel are present.

Ensure that blood is available prior to beginning a major excision.

REFERENCES

1. Cope O, Laugohr J, Moore F, Webster R Expeditious care of full thickness burn wounds by surgical excision and grafting. Ann Surg 1947; 25:1.
2. Switzer W, Jones J, Moncrief J. Evaluation of early excision of burns in children. J Trauma 1965; 5:540.

3. Jackson D, Topley E, Cason J, Lowbury E. Primary excision and grafting of large burns. Ann Surg 1960; 152:167.
4. Taylor P, Moncrief J, Pugsley L. The management of extensively burned patients by staged excision. Surg Gynecol Obstet 1962.
5. Janzekovic Z. A new concept in the early excision and immediate grafting of burns. J Trauma 1970; 10:1103.
6. Gray D, Pine R, Harner T. Early excision versus conventional therapy in patients with 20 to 40 percent burns. Am J Surg 1982; 144:76.
7. Engrav L, Heimbach D, Reus J, Harner T, Marvin JA. Early excision and grafting vs. nonoperative treatment of burns of indeterminant depth: a randomized prospective study. J. Trauma 1983; 23:1001.
8. Ho-Asjoe M, Chronnell CM, Frame JD, Leigh IM, Carver N. Immunohistochemical analysis of burn depth. J Burn Care Rehab 1999; 20:207–11.
9. Svaasand LO, Spott T, Fishkin JB, Pham T, Tromberg BJ, Berns MW. Reflectance measurements of layered media with diffuse photon-density waves: a potential tool for evaluating deep burns and subcutaneous lesions. Phys Med Biol 1999; 44:801–13.
10. Park DH, Hwang JW, Jang KS, Han DG, Ahn KY, Baik BS. Use of laser Doppler flowmetry for estimation of the depth of burns. Plast Reconstr Surg 1998; 101: 1516–23.
11. Heimbach D, Afromowitz M, Engrav L, Marvin J, Perry B. Burn depth estimation—man or machine? J Trauma 1984; 24:373–8.
12. Heimbach D, Engrav L. Surgical Management of the Burn Wound. New York. NY: Raven Press, 1984:161.
13. Wilmore DW. Postoperative protein sparing. World J Surg 1999; 23:545–52.
14. Jenkins ME, Gottschlich MM, Warden GD. Enteral feeding during operative procedures in thermal injuries. J Burn Care Rehab 1994; 15:199–205.
15. Foy HM, Pavlin ED, Heimbach DM. Excision and grafting of large burns: operation length not related to increased morbidity. J Trauma 1986; 26:51–3.
16. Cassey JG, Davey RB, Wallis KA. 'Hypafix': new technique of skin graft fixation. Aust NZ J Surg 1989; 59:479–83.
17. Girdner JH. Skin grafting with grafts from a dead subject. Med Rec NY 1888; 20: 119–120.
18. Mindikoglu AN, Cetinkale O. Prolonged allograft survival in a patient with extensive burns using cyclosporin. Burns 1993; 19:70–2.
19. Wendt JR, Ulich TR, Ruzics EP, Hostetler JR. Indefinite survival of human skin allografts in patients with long-term immunosuppression. Ann Plast Surg 1994; 32: 411–7.
20. Tompkins R, Burke J. Progress in burn treatment and the use of artificial skin. World J Surg 1990; 14:819–24.
21. Michaeli D, McPherson M. Immunologic study of artificial skin used in the treatment of thermal injuries. J Burn Care Rehab 1990; 11:21–6.
22. Stern R, McPherson M, Longaker M. Histologic study of artificial skin used in the treatment of full-thickness thermal injury. J Burn Care Rehab 1990; 11:7–13.
23. Dantzer E, Queruel P, Salinier L, Palmier B, Quinot JF. Integra, a new surgical alternative for the treatment of massive burns. Clinical evaluation of acute and reconstructive surgery: 39 cases. Ann Chir Plast Esthet 2001; 46:173–89.

24. Loss M, Wedler V, Kunzi W, Meuli-Simmen C, Meyer VE. Artificial skin, split-thickness autograft and cultured autologous keratinocytes combined to treat a severe burn injury of 93% of TBSA. Burns 2000; 26:644–52.

25. Besner GE, Klamar JE. Integra Artificial Skin as a useful adjunct in the treatment of purpura fulminans. J Burn Care Rehab 1998; 19:324–9.

26. Hunt JA, Moisidis E, Haertsch P. Initial experience of Integra in the treatment of post-burn anterior cervical neck contracture. Br J Plast Surg 2000; 53:652–8.

27. Chou TD, Chen SL, Lee TW, et al. Reconstruction of burn scar of the upper extremities with artificial skin. Plast Reconstr Surg 2001; 108:378–85.

28. Berger A, Tanzella U, Machens HG, Liebau J. Administration of Integra on primary burn wounds and unstable secondary scars. Chirurgie 2000; 71:558–63.

29. Wang JC, To EW. Application of dermal substitute (Integra) to donor site defect of forehead flap. Br J Plast Surg 2000; 53:70–2.

30. Moiemen NS, Staiano JJ, Ojeh NO, Thway Y, Frame JD. Reconstructive surgery with a dermal regeneration template: clinical and histologic study. Plast Reconstr Surg 2001; 108:93–103.

31. Dantzer E, Braye FM. Reconstructive surgery using an artificial dermis (Integra): results with 39 grafts. Br J Plast Surg 2001; 54:659–64.

32. Sheridan RLB. Effective postoperative protection for grafted posterior surfaces: the quilted dressing. J Burn Care Rehab 1995; 16:607–9.

33. Helm P, Pandian G, Heck E. Neuromuscular problems in the burn patient: cause and prevention. Arch Phys Med Rehab 1985; 66:451–3.

34. Maillard G, Clavel P. Aesthetic units in skin grafting of the face. Ann Plast Surg 1991; 26:347–52.

7

Management of Superficial Burns

Juan P. Barret and Peter Dziewulski
Broomfield Hospital, Chelmsford, Essex, United Kingdom

Current therapy for burn care is organized into three stages:

1. Assessment
2. Management
3. Rehabilitation

Although the time course of each of these phases may vary, they are essential to obtain perfect outcomes.

The assessment stage involves determining the extent and depth of the injury. This is the most important part of the management process because decisions made during this stage will affect the therapeutic outcome. It is particularly true in the superficial burn. An accurate diagnosis and treatment plan needs to be implemented to provided the expected outcome. Superficial burns (termed either as superficial second-degree burns or superficial partial-thickness burns) usually heal within 2 weeks with conservative treatment. Burns that heal within 3 weeks do not exhibit hypertrophic scarring or cause functional impairment. Therefore, any therapeutic protocol to treat superficial burns should provide complete healing without any cosmetic or functional impairment.

The hallmark of a partial-thickness burn is a weeping, blistering, painful wound that will potentially heal within 2–3 weeks and involves variable amounts of dermis. The appearance is that of a mottled red/pink, moist wound that blanches with pressure. Such wounds blister, and edema and serous exudate (Fig. 1) accom-

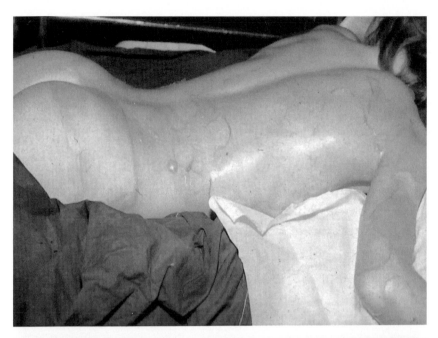

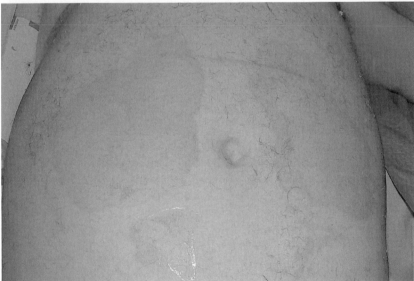

FIGURE 1 Typical appearance of superficial second-degree burns. Note the red/pink moist appearance. They blanch with pressure. Pain is very intense, and good procedural pain control must be achieved during superficial debridement.

pany them. Pain is intense; therefore good pain control regimen and wound dressings that reduce pain are mandatory.

Once the extent of burn injury has been established, an individual management plan should be instituted. After the burn wound has been cleansed and debrided, an appropriate dressing is placed. A burn dressing should serve three principal functions:

1. It must protect the damaged skin and should isolate the wound from the surrounding normal tissue. It should also provide appropriate splinting or allow early mobilization, depending on the extent and anatomical site.
2. The dressing should be occlusive to reduce evaporation heat loss and minimize cold stress.
3. The dressing should provide comfort

Superficial burns have been treated conservatively in the past with daily or twice-daily application of topical antimicrobials. A good alternative, and the author's preference, is the utilization of biological or synthetic materials to dress the burn wound.

TOPICAL ANTIMICROBIAL AGENTS

A number of topical agents are available to assist in antimicrobial control of the burn wound. The most commonly used antimicrobials are listed in Table 1. No single agent is totally effective, and each has advantages and disadvantages.

Silver sulfadiazine is the most commonly used topical antimicrobial agent in the treatment of burns. Its antimicrobial properties are derived from the dual

TABLE 1 Commonly used topical antimicrobials

– Silver sulfadiazine
– Mafenide acetate
– 0.5% Silver nitrate solution
– Cerium nitrate–silver sulfadiazine
– Acticoat
– Nitrofurantoin
– Chorhexidine
– Povidone–iodine
– Nystatin
– 0.025% Sodium hypochlorite
– Gentamycin sulfate
– Mupirocin
– Bacitracin/polymyxin
– Combination therapy

mechanisms of its silver and sulfonamide components, and it has a broad spectrum of antimicrobial coverage, including gram-positive bacteria, most gram-negative bacteria, and some yeast forms. Silver sulfadiazine does not hinder epithelialization, but it does hamper contraction of fibroblasts and retards wound healing. It is a white, highly insoluble compound synthesized from silver nitrate and sodium sulfadiazine. It is available in 1% concentration in a water-soluble cream base. The cream is relatively painless to apply and does not stain bed linens or other objects. The most common toxicity is a transient leukopenia, which typically recovers spontaneously, whether or not the agent has been discontinued. The agent is usually applied on a daily or twice-daily basis (antibacterial activity lasts up to 24 h, unless a slough exudate appears on the wound, when a more frequent application is needed). When it is used on superficial burns, a yellow–grey pseudoeschar typically forms after several days, which can be confusing and misleading to inexperienced surgeons. A good diagnosis and treatment plan must be established before its application, because pseudoeschar may pose difficulties in future management decisions. This film of pseudoeschar, which is several millimeters thick, results from interaction between the cream and the wound exudate (Fig. 2). It is harmless and can be easily lifted; however that action may prolong healing time and is accompanied by different degrees of procedural pain.

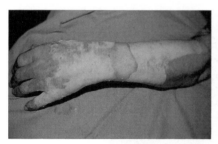
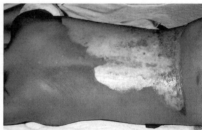

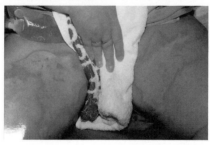

Figure 2 Pseudoeschar formed on a superficial burn treated with silver sulfadiazine. Although harmless, it can be misleading in inexperienced hands and diagnosed as full-thickness eschar. If lifted away, a healthy superficial wound bed is revealed beneath it.

Cerium nitrate–silver sulfadiazine was introduced in the mid-1970s, but its popularity increased 10 years later. It is frequently used in Europe, especially in centers where deep burns are managed with a more conservative approach. Cerium is one of the lanthanide rare earth series of elements that has antimicrobial activity in vitro and is relatively nontoxic. Wound bacteriostasis may be more efficient with its use in major burns than with silver sulfadiazine. The efficacy of cerium nitrate–silver sulfadiazine may be due in part to an effect on immune function. Methemoglobinemia due to nitrate reduction and absorption has been rarely observed with this agent. Initial application of cerium nitrate–silver sulfadiazine can be painful, but this problem resolves after few applications. Perilesional rash may also appear on initial application and it may be difficult to differentiate from true cellulitis. A leathery hard eschar with deposition of calcium occurs in deep dermal and full-thickness burns, which prevents bacterial invasion and permits easy delayed tangential excision (Fig. 3). Conversion of partial-thickness wound to full-thickness skin loss has occurred as well as deepening of donor sites with the use of this agent. It should be reserved for use in cases of deep partial and full-thickness burns awaiting excision. It is a good alternative in elderly patients who are not candidates for surgical intervention. Facial burns can also be treated with cerium nitrate–silver sulfadiazine. After regular application

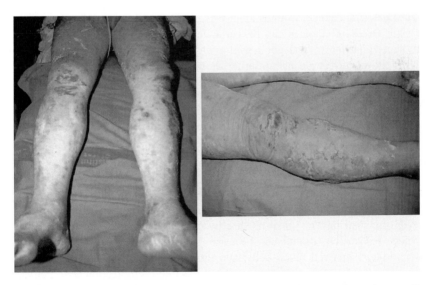

Figure 3 Typical appearance of burn wounds treated with cerium nitrate–silver sulfadiazine. Note the leathery hard scar with deposition of calcium, which often prevents invasive burn wound infections. It creates a wound that is easily treated with delayed tangential excision.

for 48–72 h, the pseudoeschar is left in place without new applications of the agents. Superficial and deep partial burns heal uneventfully and separate the pseudoeschar.

The use of many other topical antimicrobials depends on the surgeon's choice, characteristics of the wound, and anatomical site of the burn. Nevertheless, the most commonly used topical antimicrobial in partial-thickness wounds continues to be 1% silver sulfadiazine. Antimicrobial activity differs depending on the agent. Mafenide acetate is the only agent with good eschar penetration, and it is particularly suited for infected wounds. However, it presents with systemic toxicity since it is a potent carbonic anhydrase inhibitor. It produces considerable pain on application, and it should be reserved for short-term control of invasive burn wound infections.

Topical antimicrobial creams are generally used with closed dressings. This provides for greater patient comfort and less desiccation than with use of the open technique. The creams are spread on fine-mesh gauze, applied on the wounds, and then covered with bulky protective gauze dressings and an elastic compressive wrap. As an alternative, silver sulfadiazine cream can be directly applied on the wound and then wrapped accordingly. When a program of early mobilization can be instituted, light dressings should be used to permit good range of motion. Dressings are changed based on the antimicrobial activity of the agent. When silver sulfadiazine is used, dressings should be changed ideally every 12–24 h. At each dressing change, wounds are gently cleaned prior to reapplication of the dressing. Dressing changes can be particularly painful, especially for patients with superficial burns, and good pain control regimen should be instituted in order to allow correct cleansing during showering or tub bathing.

SYNTHETIC AND BIOLOGICAL DRESSINGS

Topical antimicrobial agents are used to limit proliferation and fungal colonization of wounds, with the ultimate goal of preventing invasive infection until the burn wound re-epithelializes or can be excised and grafted. All topical antimicrobial agents, however, adversely affect wound healing, alter the metabolic rate, and require reapplication and daily maintenance. Synthetic and biological dressing are an excellent alternative to topical antimicrobial agents. Temporary skin substitutes provide transient physiological closure by creating a wound environment that prevents desiccation; diminishes bacterial proliferation; reduces loss of heat, water, protein, and red blood cells; and promotes more rapid wound healing. Such temporary physiological closure of wounds implies protection from trauma, vapor transmission characteristics similar to skin, and a physical barrier to bacteria. These membranes create a moist wound environment with a low bacterial density and they also reduce burn wound pain. These materials may be organic or synthetic in origin, but good wound adherence is the key to their function

(Table 2). The most commonly used organic or biological materials are skin allograft from donors and xenograft (pigskin). Among synthetic materials Biobrane, Transcyte, and Mepitel are used regularly.

Human allograft (also called homograft) (Figs. 4, 5) is generally used as a split-thickness graft after being procured from organ donors. It remains the gold standard of temporary wound closures. It can be refrigerated for up to 7 days, but can be stored for extended periods when cryopreserved. It is also used in a nonviable state after preservation in glycerol or after lyophilization. Numerous laboratory tests to exclude the possibility of viral disease transmission are followed, and with modern screening techniques the risk of viral disease transmission is exceedingly small. When used in deep excised burns, viable and cryopreserved allografts vascularize (this usually does not occur when used in superficial burns), providing durable biological cover until the patient's own skin has regenerated under the skin allograft.

Porcine xenograft (Fig. 6) is commonly distributed as a reconstituted product consisting of homogenized porcine dermis fashioned into sheets and also meshed. It is nonviable, adheres more poorly than allograft, and does not undergo revascularization by the recipient bed. Xenografts undergo progressive degenerative necrosis rather than classic rejection. They do not provide the same level of protection from infection as allograft, and so they often contain embedded salts of antimicrobial agents. Porcine xenograft or pigskin is well suited for temporary coverage of partial-thickness wounds to allow spontaneous healing. It is less expensive than allograft and more readily available. Other uses include temporary cover of clean granulating wound beds awaiting autografting, and use as a test graft to determine suitability for autografting. When used in partial-thickness burns, it is applied after cleansing and superficial debridement of the wound. It

TABLE 2 Synthetic and biological materials commonly used in superficial burns

---

Biological materials
  Human allograft
  Human amnion
  Allogenic epithelial sheets
  Xenografts (pig skin)
Synthetic materials
  Biobrane
  Transcyte
  Mepitel
  Opsite
  Duoderm

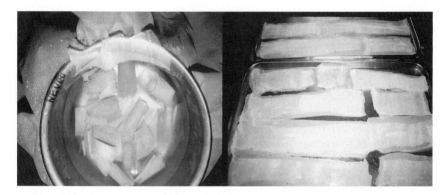

FIGURE 4 Human allografts are easily thawed in the operating room and ready for use within minutes.

is secured with tape and a light dressing for 24 h, leaving it exposed when it appears well fixed to wound. The patient is allowed to shower and pigskin is left in place until complete wound healing is achieved, when the porcine xenograft would be completely detached from the wound.

Synthetic biological dressings also provide wound protection from desiccation and contamination, increase the rate of wound healing, and reduce patient discomfort. Good wound adherence is needed, and any necrotic tissue needs to be debrided to prevent infection. Diligence in application is essential. It should

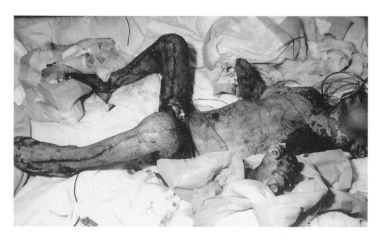

FIGURE 5 A patient with 80% TBSA full-thickness burns covered with human allografts.

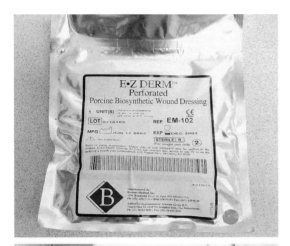

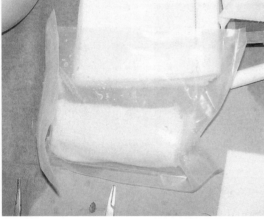

FIGURE 6 Porcine xenografts are available meshed and unmeshed. They are easily stored and ready to use.

be applied as soon as possible before bacterial colonization has taken place. When used to cover partial-thickness burns, the dressing detaches as re-epithelialization and keratinization occur underneath. A number of semipermeable membrane dressings can provide a vapor and bacterial barrier and reduce pain while the underlying wound heals. These synthetic materials typically consist of a single semipermeable layer that provides a mechanical barrier to bacteria and has physiological vapor transmission characteristics. All synthetic membranes are occlusive and can foster infection. Appropriate monitoring is essential to their proper use.

Biobrane is a synthetic, bilaminate membrane with an outer semipermeable silicone layer bonded to an inner collagen-nylon matrix (Fig. 7). Its elasticity and

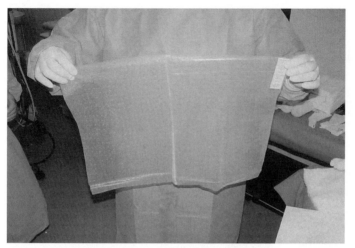

A

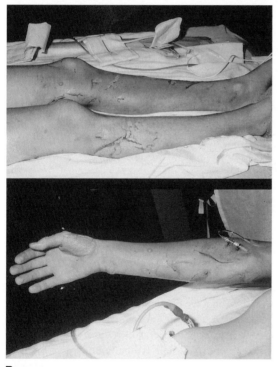

B

FIGURE 7 A. Biobrane is a synthetic, bilaminate membrane with an outer semipermeable silicone layer bonded to an inner collagen-nylon matrix. Its elasticity and transparency allow early mobilization and easy wound inspection

172

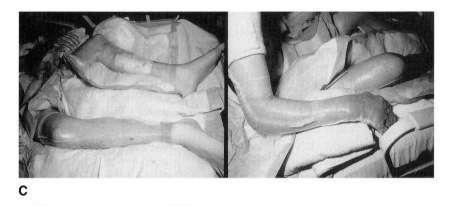

C

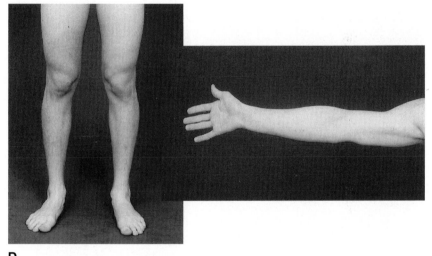

D

Figure 7 (**Cont.**) (B–D). A patient with 25% superficial partial-thickness burns TBSA was treated with superficial debridement and Biobrane application. Biobrane must be stapled to itself to prevent granuloma formation.

transparency allow easy drapability, full range of movement, and easy wound inspection. It is widely used to provide temporary closure of superficial burns and donor sites. It significantly reduces pain and allows early discharge of patients. Biobrane gloves on superficial hand burns reduce discomfort and increase motion, allowing earlier aggressive physiotherapy. The major problems with Biobrane are its expense and its lack of inherent antimicrobial properties. Wound infections with its use are not uncommon.

TransCyte (Smith & Nephew, Inc. Largo, FL) is a bioengineered human fibroblast-derived temporary skin substitute that has similar properties to Biobrane and can be used in a similar way (Fig. 8). The outer layer of TransCyte, the synthetic epidermal layer of nonporous silicone net, is biocompatible and protects the wound surface from detrimental environmental effects. It is semi-permeable to allow fluid and gas exchange, which keeps a healthy moist, wound healing environment. The inner layer, the bioengineered human dermal matrix, adheres quickly to the wound surface and contains the dermal components known to promote healing of the burn. The product contains essential human structural and provisional matrix proteins, glycosaminoglycans, and growth factors known

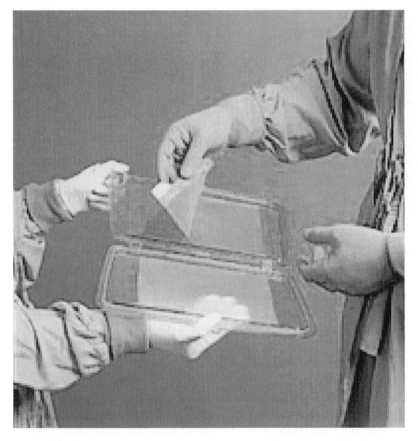

FIGURE 8 TransCyte is a bioengineered human fibroblast-derived temporary skin substitute with similar properties to Biobrane that can be used in a similar way (Adapted from Smith + Nephew)

to facilitate healing. The patient's epithelial cells proliferate and migrate across the wound, resulting in rapid wound healing. TransCyte presents with physical properties, risks, and complications similar to those of Biobrane.

Mepitel (Fig. 9) is made of an elastic, transparent polyamide net enclosed by a soft silicone layer. This layer is inert and adheres only to dry healthy skin and not to the moist wound bed. The release film is transparent, allowing the wound to be visible during application. The structure of Mepitel allows exudate to pass into an outer absorbent dressing. Mepitel prevents the outer dressing from sticking to the wound and therefore minimizes trauma and pain during dressing changes. Dressings can be left in place for several days, avoiding repetitive dressing changes and minimizing pain. It provides a moist wound environment that promotes re-epithelialization. It is very useful for the treatment of small partial-thickness burns in the outpatient setting.

A variety of hydrocolloid dressings are currently available in the market for the treatment of burns. These dressings are generally designed with a three-layer structure:

A porous adherent inner layer
A middle layer composed of a methyl cellulose absorbent material
A semipermeable outer layer

They provide a moist environment, which has been shown to favor wound healing, while absorbing exudate. They require repeated application every 2–4 days depending on the agent, although patient comfort with their use is high.

MANAGEMENT OF SUPERFICIAL PARTIAL-THICKNESS WOUNDS

The aim of management of superficial partial-thickness burns (or superficial second-degree burns) is to promote rapid spontaneous re-epithelialization with the minimum number of painful dressing changes and to allow early mobilization and early discharge from the hospital. At the same time treatment of superficial burns should prevent infection, which can convert the injury to a deeper one that requires grafting. It is the authors' belief that all the former can only be accomplished with the extensive use of biological and synthetic materials. These dressings are easy to apply and allow inspection of the burn wound without the need for repetitive dressing changes. They improve wound healing, and decrease pain significantly. Even though these agents are more expensive than topical creams, patients treated with these dressings need one application and they are usually discharged home sooner than patients treated with the traditional topical antimicrobial creams. When hospital costs are included in the whole treatment budget, the extensive use of biological and synthetic temporary skin substitutes is more cost-effective than the traditional method.

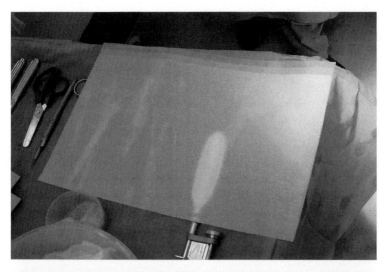

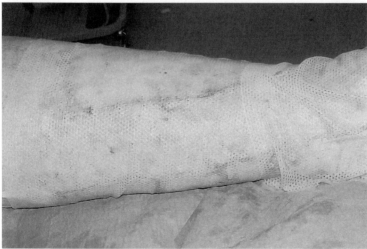

FIGURE 9   Mepitel is made of elastic, transparent polyamide net enclosed by a soft silicone layer. Its structure allows exudate to pass into an outer absorbent dressing. Mepitel prevents the outer dressing from sticking to the wound and therefore minimizes trauma and pain during dressing changing.

Treatment of Small and Medium Superficial Partial-Thickness Wounds (Up to 30% Total Body Surface Area)

Biobrane Temporary Skin Substitute

For patients admitted within 24 h of their injury, the preferred method that renders, in the authors' opinion, the best outcome with short hospital stay and rapid wound healing is the application of Biobrane as temporary skin substitute (Fig. 10).

After the patient is admitted and stabilized, all burn blisters are cleaned and debrided and all burned epithelium is removed. Debridement of all burned epithelium in superficial partial thickness burns is an extremely painful procedure. Therefore, sedation or general anesthesia is required in order to perform a complete cleaning of burn wounds. Burns under 15% total body surface area (TBSA) can be managed under sedation. Full monitoring is essential, including pulse oximetry, continuous cardiac monitoring, and blood pressure monitoring. Patients should receive oxygen supplementation during the procedure. Children can be easily sedated with ketamine (1–2 mg/kg intravenously, 3–7 mg/kg intramuscularly, 6–10 mg/kg orally). For older children, a benzodiazepine can be added to avoid postprocedural nightmares. For adults either midazolam or propofol can be used. Medium-sized partial-thickness burns are best managed in the operating room with the patient under general anesthesia. This allows good access to all anatomical locations, proper analgesia, and good cleansing.

After monitoring and administration of proper sedation or anesthesia, burn blisters are cleaned, and all burned epithelium is removed with a superficial and gentle debridement. All burned areas are exposed and the patient is cleaned with antiseptic solution. Alcohol-based solutions should be avoided to prevent desiccation and conversion to deep partial- or full-thickness burns. All fluids employed should be warmed to maintain appropriate core temperatures. Biobrane is then applied to the wound. It should be applied under slight tension so wrinkles are avoided. Excessive tension may result in a constrictive band, and, in the worst scenario, in true compartment syndrome. Therefore, the distensibility of Biobrane should permit enough elasticity to allow the natural swelling of burn wounds. Biobrane is applied in a circumferential fashion around the limb or trunk so that is tight and closely adherent to the wound. The Biobrane is secured by stapling it to itself. In burn wounds with large areas of normal skin, Biobrane can be stapled to fabric dressings or secured with wide tape on normal skin. Care is taken not to staple the Biobrane to the patient because this can cause granulomas and the staples are painful to remove. The Biobrane is then wrapped with a standard dressing of fine-mesh petroleum jelly gauze or fine-mesh gauze impregnated with Polysporin/Mycostatin and covered with elastic bandages. Burn areas are elevated and the patient is allowed to exercise. Patients receive preoperative antibiotic prophylaxis with staphylococcal/streptococcal coverage that is continued for 24 h. The dressings are removed at 24–48 h to inspect the wound. If

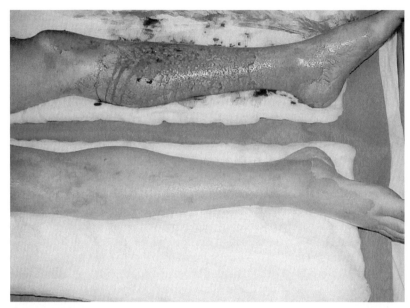

A

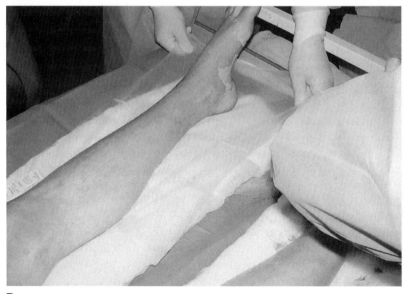

B

FIGURE 10   Biobrane is the treatment of choice for small and medium-sized burn injuries. A. Burns are cleaned with antiseptic solutions and debrided B.

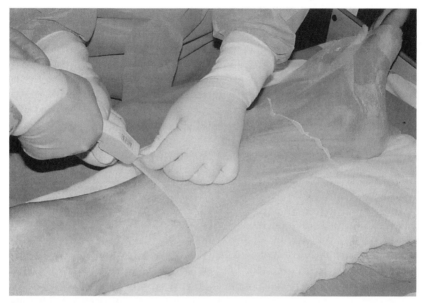

C

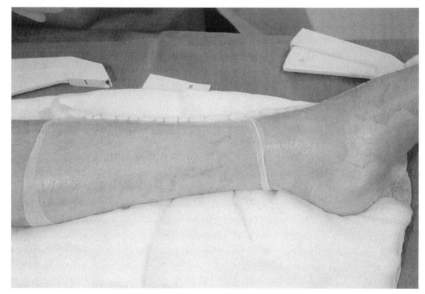

D

FIGURE 10 (**Cont.**)   C. Biobrane is then applied (it must be stapled to itself) and (D) dressed with petrolatum-soaked fine-mesh gauze or standard burn dressing.

Biobrane is adherent, no further dressings are required. As re-epithelialization occurs in 10–14 days, Biobrane spontaneously separates from the healed wound. Patients are allowed to bathe, although the dressing must be kept dry, which is usually accomplished by exposing it to room air. If wound infection supervenes, the Biobrane rapidly becomes nonadherent and can trap any exudate by the wound. For this reason it is not used in patients presenting more than 24–36 h following their injury. In larger wounds (> 30% TBSA) it must be used with caution, since collections under the Biobrane may extend and the patient become septic. If the Biobrane appears nonadherent in some areas, it should be trimmed and a topical antimicrobial or Mepitel applied. If left in place it can become infected. When infection is present, patients can become rapidly sick and septic. This is particularly true in children, who must be managed quickly to prevent any septic episode. After the first Biobrane check, patients are discharged home and monitored in the burn outpatients department. Patients with small superficial burns can be discharged soon after the injury (usually between 24 and 48 h). A more cautious approach is advised for patients with larger superficial burns, which are usually discharged between the third and fourth day, after a second Biobrane check to rule out any deeper area or infection. A good outpatient setting, however, is necessary. Experienced nurses well-versed in the care of open wounds must staff it and burn specialists and surgeons should be available 24 h a day. The burn outpatient department should function as an extension of the burn unit, with availability to manage patients 7 days a week.

Alternative temporary skin substitutes

Xenograft skin (porcine skin or pigskin) can be used in similar fashion to Biobrane. It closes the wound physiologically while re-epithelialization occurs. Its application follows the same criteria as Biobrane. After proper cleansing, it is applied to the raw surface and affixed in place with a light dressing. After 24 h the porcine xenograft is stable and it can be exposed. Patients are allowed to wash the areas and it separates when complete re-epithelialization has occurred. It forms a dry surface that can be uncomfortable for some patients (Fig. 11). Another good alternative for small- and medium-size superficial burns is Mepitel. It is a silicone sheet that sticks to normal skin but not to the wounds. Its application and removal are painless with excellent patient satisfaction. After gentle debridement, wounds are covered with the silicone sheet and protected with a light dressing. Topical antimicrobials are not necessary. The dressing is left in place for 5 days, and it is replaced until complete re-epithelization has occurred. Other synthetic dressings such as Duoderm and hydrocolloids have all been used with some success to dress such wounds. They provide a moist environment that promotes wound healing.

Another semisynthetic biological dressing that is very effective in this type of wound is TransCyte. Its properties are similar to that of Biobrane. Their inner

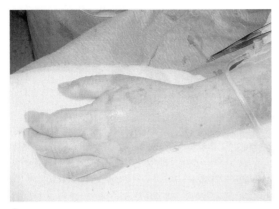

A

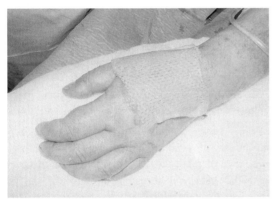

B

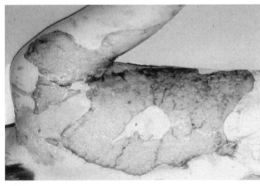

C

FIGURE 11   Superficial burns (A) can be treated with pig skin application (B). It is less expensive than Biobrane, but patients may experience more discomfort when it desiccates (C). The same treatment protocols apply as for Biobrane.

surface is coated with neonatal fibroblast, which adheres to the wound and promotes wound healing by producing growth factors. It is much more expensive than Biobrane, so we reserve its use for neonatal and infant burns.

Topical Antimicrobial Creams

The usual alternative for superficial burns that has been the standard and traditional method for the last 30 years is the application of topical antimicrobial creams. The treatment of choice in many burn centers around the world is 1% silver sulfadiazine (Silvadene, Flammazine). After the wound is cleaned and the blisters, debrided, silver sulfadiazine is applied topically to the wound. It is then covered with a roll of fine mesh gauze and elastic bandage. Dressings are changed once or twice daily until re-epithelialization occurs and the wound has healed. This method requires frequent dressing changes, which can be painful and produce severe discomfort and anxiety. We reserve this method for the following situations:

> Plantar burns
> Perineal burns
> Patients presenting late after injury with a colonized or infected wound

Plantar burns are frequently colonized soon after the injury. Our experience is that management of this type of burns with synthetic dressings results in a high rate of infection. Therefore, we believe that daily wash with application of silver sulfadiazine is the treatment of choice. Perineal burns are likewise difficult to dress and keep clean. Patients are best managed with daily wash of the area and application of silver sulfadiazine until complete re-epithelialization has occurred. Pain is very low, and patients feel very comfortable with this dressing. Another type of burns that can benefit of silver sulfadiazine application are some hand burns not suitable for Biobrane or Mepitel application (geographical burns with large nonburned areas, hand–palm burns, finger burns). The application of hand bags with silver sulfadiazine is painless and allows easy and early mobilization of the involved anatomical areas.

Treatment of Large Superficial Partial-Thickness Burns (> 30% TBSA)

Homograft

These are uncommon injuries that can lead to a high morbidity and mortality rate. They are more prone to contamination and infection than medium-sized superficial burns, large amounts of fluid resuscitation are necessary, and intense swelling often occurs. Cardiogenic and noncardiogenic pulmonary edema are complications that carry a high risk of mortality in patients with these injuries.

Best results are achieved if homograft is applied within 24 h of the injury. Under general anesthesia the wound is cleaned and all blisters and nonadherent epidermis removed. It is not uncommon to observe mixed areas of superficial and indeterminate depth in these large injuries. Areas of indeterminate depth are shaved superficially with the Zimmer or Padget powered dermatome with depth settings of 8–10/1000 inch. Cryopreserved or fresh homograft split-skin grafts are placed over the open dermal wound and secured with staples. If homografts are meshed, it is important not to open the mesh on the homograft: this can lead to desiccation, infection, and deepening of the underlying wound. A standard dressing is applied. Wounds are inspected at 48–72 h unless the condition of the patient dictates otherwise. When homografts are stable, the wound can be left open with petroleum jelly gauze covering to prevent desiccation or a light dressing applied (Fig. 12). Wounds heal spontaneously without incorporation or homograft rejection. As the healing process progresses, homografts separate after leaving a completely re-epithelialized wound. When homografts are stable, patients can be gently showered or bathed; all areas that start to separate can be trimmed. Big dressing changes are not necessary, and pain control is easily achieved.

Alternative temporary skin substitutes

Biobrane can be used in the same way as for smaller injuries. There is a higher rate of wound infection, which can lead to loss of the Biobrane and deepening of the burn wound. Given the large surface area covered with Biobrane, if purulent collections develop under the synthetic membrane, patients can experience severe sepsis and septic shock. Therefore, we do not advise treatment of large areas with Biobrane unless human cadaver skin is not available. If Biobrane is chosen, daily inspection is absolutely necessary, with aggressive intervention and trimming of all nonadherent areas should the patients become unwell and septic. TransCyte can be used in a similar manner to Biobrane, and, as with medium size superficial burns, it is particularly helpful in neonates and small infants.

Xenograft skin can be used in a similar fashion as homograft. Such skin does not adhere as well, and desiccation can lead to infection and deepening of the burn wound, requiring formal excision and autografting. It is our belief that homografts provide the best treatment for these injuries, because the grafts are viable and protect the healing wound by creating a permanent moist environment with the benefit of growth factors produced by dermal fibroblasts.

Topical Antimicrobial Creams

The traditional method of treatment for massive superficial partial-thickness burns has been for many decades the application of topical antimicrobials daily. Among them, 1% silver sulfadiazine has been the gold standard for many years. Patients require daily dressing changes, which are such a painful ordeal for patients that

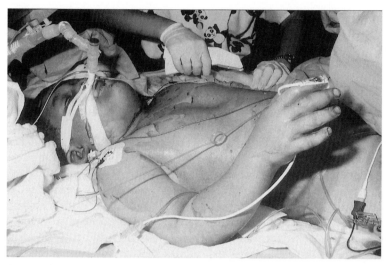

A

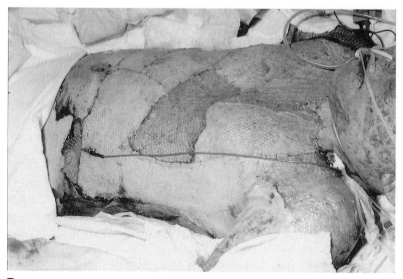

B

FIGURE 12   Treatment of massive superficial partial-thickness burns with superficial debridement and homograft application leads to a perfect outcome. Homograft skin does not vascularize, allowing re-epithelialization underneath. The layers separate after complete wound healing has occurred.

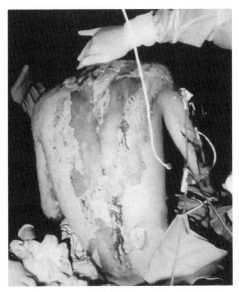

A

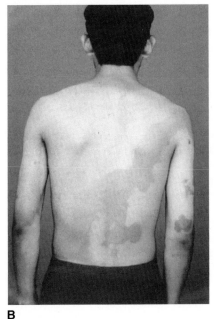

B

FIGURE 13 A. Silver sulfadiazine has been the traditional treatment for partial-thickness burns. It requires daily dressing changes, which create significant stress and procedural pain. B. It produces good outcomes is an ordeal to the patient and required hospital stay is significantly longer than with skin substitutes.

they may require sedation and even general anesthesia (Fig. 13). Management of patients using topical antimicrobials can be much more difficult than with homograft application, but it is an ordeal for the patient and the hospital stay is much longer. They are often more catabolic than patients treated with human cadaver skin, probably due to the pain involved in dressing changes and the bacterial contamination of wounds. There is also a higher incidence of wound sepsis, which can lead to deepening of the burn wound, and may then necessitate skin grafting. Even though daily application of topical antimicrobials is a good alternative to homograft application, in our hands the latter present with lesser incidence of wound infections and patients' management and recovery are much improved. We therefore strongly recommend the treatment of massive superficial partial-thickness burns with superficial debridement and application of viable homografts.

BIBLIOGRAPHY

1. Fox CL. Silver sulfadiazine: a new topical therapy for *Pseudomonas* in burns. Arch Surg 1968; 96:184–188.
2. Wasserman D, Schlotterer M, Lebreton F, et al. Use of topically applied silver sulfadiazine plus cerium nitrate in major burns. Burns 1989; 15:257–260.
3. Barret JP, Dziewulski P, Ramzy PI, Wolf SE, Desai MH, Herndon DN. Biobrane vs. 1% silver sulfadiazine in second degree pediatric burns. Plast Reconstr Surg 2000; 105:62–65.
4. Lal S, Barrow RE, Wolf SE, Chinkes DL, Hart DW, Heggers JP, Herndon DN. Biobrane improves wound healing in burned children without increased risk of infection. Shock 2000; 14(3):314–319.
5. Rose JK, Desai MH, Mlakar JM, Herndon DN. Allograft is superior to topical antimicrobial therapy in the treatment of partial-thickness scald burns in children. J Burn Care Rehabil 1997; 18(4):338–341.
6. Dziewulski P, Barret J. Assessment, operative planning and surgery for burn wound closure. In: Burn Care Wolf Steven E , Herndon David N, Eds. Austin. TX: Landes Bioscience, 1999.
7. Barret JP, Heggers JP. Wound care. In: Color Atlas of Burn Care Barret Juan P, Herndon David N, Eds. London. UK: WB Saunders, 2001.
8. Lawrence JC. Dressing for burns. In: Principles and Practice of Burn Management Settle John AD, Ed. Edinburgh. UK: Churchill Livingstone, 1996.

8

The Small Burn

Juan P. Barret
Broomfield Hospital, Chelmsford, Essex, United Kingdom

Small burns and superficial burns are the most common injuries in patients admitted to burn centers around the world. In most centers, they account for more than 80–90% of all admissions. Thanks to prevention programs and the increasing awareness of society regarding burn injuries, the incidence of massive, life-threatening burns is declining. Advances in critical care and wound closure have led to improved mortality. Many research efforts and passion have been devoted to the care of major burns, which, no doubt, remains a model for the study of deranged physiology, cytokine production, metabolism, immune response, and infection. Few efforts have been carried out in the minor burn arena despite these injuries representing more than 80% of admissions. Many of them, however, represent major burns according to the American Burn Association criteria because they usually are deep burns of hands, face, feet, perineum, or major joints. Quality of life and improved outcomes are now more than ever an issue in modern societies, and these can only be achieved with excellence in burn care. Although surgery is the central treatment of minor deep burns, all members of the burn team are necessary to provide the best outcome and reintegration of patients into society. Discharge planning has to be started from admission, and a full functioning outpatient department is extremely important to manage these patients in the best possible way.

GENERAL CONSIDERATIONS

Deep minor burns, either partial-thickness or full-thickness burns, have significant morbidity in terms of time to healing, infective complications, and subsequent scarring. Conservative management leading to spontaneous healing usually involves prolonged and painful dressing changes and the resultant scar is invariably hypertrophic, leading to cosmetic and functional debility. Thus an early surgical approach that tries to preserve dermis and achieve wound healing is preferred. This is particularly true in full-thickness burns, which, if managed conservatively, tend to heal by granulation tissue formation, loss of parts, and chronic wounds (Fig. 1). In general, unless the physiological and medical condition of the patient dictates otherwise, deep partial-thickness and full-thickness burns are treated with early excision and autografting. These wounds include the following:

1. Wounds that will take more than 3 weeks to heal
2. Full-thickness burns
3. Infected wounds unless very superficial on admission

Timing of surgery in minor burns differs somewhat from that in cases of life-threatening burns. Although an aggressive approach is favored in the latter, with programs of immediate (in the first 24 h) or early (within 48–72 h) burn wound excision, a more conservative and individualized approach is preferred in the management of minor burns. However, unjustified delays in definitive treatment do not add any benefit, prolong hospital stay, and delay early discharges, which challenges the final outcome and the patient's early reintegration in society. It is the author's belief and that of many others that as soon as a final diagnosis is reached and the burn wound is deemed to be treatable surgically, definitive treatment should not be delayed.

The following is our general therapeutic plan for minor burns:

Deep burns with clear indication for surgery on admission: surgery in the first week (preferably within 48–72 h)
Indeterminate-depth burns: allow 10–14 days for second look and final decision
Scalds: allow re-epithelialization to occur, and graft within a 3 week window

It is important to note, however, that burns in patients at the extremes of age (infants and the elderly) are not shallow. Their dermis is significantly thinner that that of adults, resulting in deeper burns with the same type of injury. Burns in this group of patients should be treated more aggressively, because infants tend to react with a more florid and profound systemic inflammatory response, making them more prone to sepsis; older patients have small metabolic reserves. It is not uncommon for them to experience delayed multiple organ dysfunction and failure after days or weeks of conservative treatment.

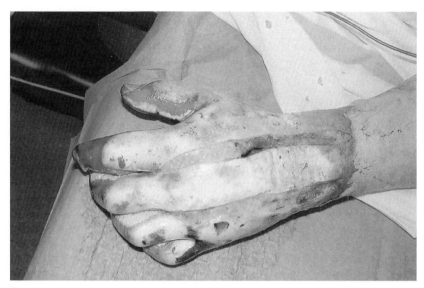

A

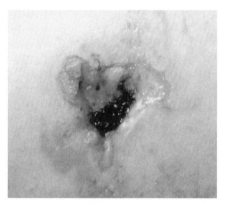

B

FIGURE 1   A. Full-thickness burns present with total destruction of skin and different degrees of soft tissues. B.

Surgical treatment of minor burns should be considered an elective operation, and, as such, intraoperative mortality should be 0%. Experienced anesthetists and surgeons should perform early excision and grafting, with operating teams well versed in these sort of operations and a burn unit and burn team readily available to cope with any patient need. To achieve low morbidity and negligible

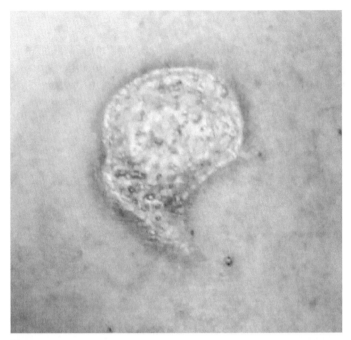

C

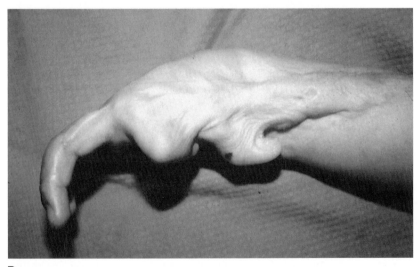

D

Figure 1 (**Cont.**)   C. They usually heal by secondary intention, although chronic wounds and loss of parts are not uncommon (D).

operative mortality, the patient's medical condition and premorbid status must be assessed and corrected. Although some injuries may be considered major burns due to anatomical location, minor burns are not life-threatening conditions. Therefore complete assessment and physiological correction come first.

PREPARATION FOR SURGERY

Full medical history, physical assessment, and full blood count and biochemistry must be obtained. Past medical history, medications, drug allergies, nutrition, and physical and psychological premorbid status has to be noted. All information regarding past operations and administration of anesthesia must be obtained. Social services should be contacted to assess the psychosocial status of the patient and any needs for intervention to allow early discharge. The physiotherapy and occupational therapy departments should be informed to start early aggressive intervention and assess individual needs. Full anesthetic review is mandatory.

After complete workup and definitive diagnosis of the patient, the surgical plan is established. The patient is inspected and the choice of donor site is made together with patient's wishes and expectations. Surgery is explained to the patient and guardians, including review of preoperative and postoperative needs and interventions. Based on the patient's diagnosis, premorbid status, and social circumstances, the treatment plan and discharge plan are established. The operating room team and members of the surgical team are informed of the proposed operation and all necessary arrangements are made. The blood bank is informed and the need for skin substitutes determined. Scrub nurses need to be informed of all special equipment needed, including instruments for flap elevation, operative microscopes, sterile tourniquets, dermatomes, and others. If the surgeon is planning to splint the patient at the end of the procedure, physiotherapy and occupation therapy specialists should be available during surgery.

Minor burns, depending on their anatomical location and individual characteristics, can be managed successfully as outpatient procedures. To make a final decision as to whether the patient can be managed as an outpatient, we need to differentiate between two patient populations:

Those with minor burns managed initially as inpatients
Those with minor burns managed as outpatients

Patients admitted to the burn unit and managed initially as inpatients are assessed by the whole burn team and a final diagnosis and treatment plan are established. A careful and accurate determination of the patient's social situation and comorbidity is necessary to ascertain whether the patient is suitable for outpatient management after surgery. Patients without any significant pre-existing medical condition who have family or social support at home can be managed as outpatients, provided the anatomical location of the burn injury does not necessitate special

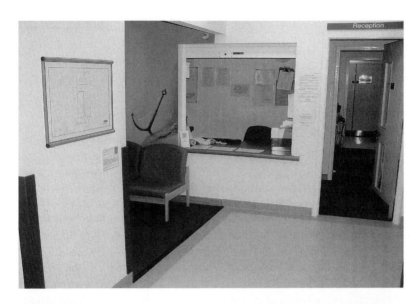

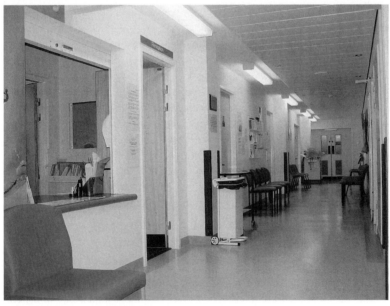

FIGURE 2   A full operating outpatient department staffed by experienced nurses is necessary for successful day-case burn surgery.

nursing care or strict immobilization. Patients who present with indeterminate-depth burns are usually discharged and evaluated as outpatients until a decision on final treatment: either surgery or continuation of conservative treatment. Those who present on admission with deep partial-thickness or full-thickness burns are kept as inpatients and surgery is carried out. A careful analysis is also necessary prior to surgery to ascertain whether the patient will be suitable for outpatient management after surgery. For those patients treated initially as outpatients who need surgical intervention to achieve complete wound closure, full assessment is performed in the outpatient department. Patients are prepared for surgery and the burn team and operating room informed of the proposed date and special requirements. If the patient can be managed as an outpatient, he or she is invited to come to the burn unit on the day of surgery. After full recovery he or she is sent home and followed up in the outpatient department. Staff nurses should contact the patient the next morning to assess his or her postoperative course, pain control, and any other needs. Patients who need a short hospital stay after surgery (based on the anatomical location and the wound care required) are also invited to come the day of surgery and are admitted to the ward after the operation. They usually stay 3–5 days.

A full operating, state-of-the-art burn outpatient department is necessary to perform burn surgery as day surgery (Figs. 2,3). It must be staffed by experienced nurses 7 days a week. Physicians must be readily available to assess and treat patients, should a problem arise. It is important to maintain a good flow of information between patients and carers, and patients should be able to reach the outpatient department at any time. After discharge, patients should be contacted via phone to evaluate their postoperative course, including pain control. All questions can be then addressed, and patients are asked to return to the department if staff deem that necessary. If there is any doubt regarding patient safety, he or she should not be discharged or should be asked to return to the burn center to be managed as inpatient. Patients and relatives are informed about the operation and what to expect before, during, and after surgery. They need to be informed about any special treatments that may be necessary, such as the intervention of rehabilitation services. It is very helpful to provide patients with written information, in the form of pamphlets and booklets, in which all relevant information as well as contact information should be included.

SURGICAL TECHNIQUE

Surgical treatment of minor burns requires perfect coordination among all specialities to achieve a good outcome. Minor burn surgery is an elective procedure, and as such, a comprehensive preoperative plan must be outlined to provide the

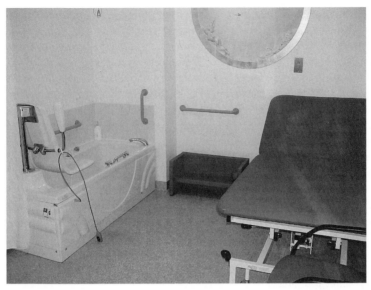

A

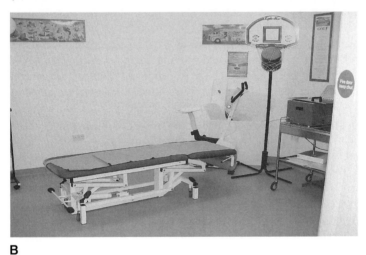

B

FIGURE 3   Proper burn care in the outpatient setting requires spacious rooms with availability of hydrotherapy (A) physiotherapy, and occupational therapy (B).

best result with minimal morbidity. Planning the surgical procedure includes all of the following:

1. Choice of skin graft
2. Choice of donor sites
3. Type of excision
4. Hemostasis
5. Fixation of skin grafts and splinting
6. Dressings

Although excision and grafting of minor burns may seem easy and straightforward operations to novices, the final outcome in terms of cosmesis and function depends on the experience and proficiency of the burn surgeon. Extreme finesse and excellence in technique are required to obtain a good result, and burn patients deserve a well-dedicated burn team. Minor burn surgery should not be considered a minor procedure. It is delicate, precise work that will show in the patient's scars for the rest of his or her life. It is no longer a small skin graft but a complex procedure that commences with good preoperative planning and ends after months of intensive rehabilitation intervention.

Choice of Skin Grafts

Patients with minor burns present with many donor sites. There is plenty of skin to use as skin grafts. Therefore, minor burns should be grafted with sheet skin autografts. There are no reasons or excuses to mesh skin grafts in these patients. Expansion of skin grafts should be condemned. The only excuse for their use is surgeons' comfort, to avoid postoperative hematoma and serum collections under the skin graft. Surgeons who mesh grafts tend to forget that our goal is the patient's well being. A meshed graft will show the scar pattern for the rest of the patient's life and is completely unacceptable (Fig. 4). Every little cut that is made on the surface of a skin graft will become scar; thus it should be avoided. It is also the author's belief that there it is not necessary to make drain cuts on the surface of the skin graft. Good hemostasis can be achieved with topical and subcutaneous epinephrine solutions and tourniquets. There is no rebound effect and skin grafts heal uneventfully without the need for any other intervention (Fig. 5). Split-skin grafts are normally used, but small full-thickness skin grafts may be necessary in specific areas (lips, eyelids, nose, hand/fingers, toes, and genitalia). In general, medium-thickness split-skin autografts are used (14–16/1000 inch), which provide a good color and texture to the grafted site. Donor sites heal in 10–14 days with no scarring.

As soon as the burn wound has been excised, the defect is measured and a drawing that resembles the excised burn wound is created on the donor site. It must be taken into account that skin grafts will shrink after harvesting due to skin relaxation. Therefore, it is advised to make the drawing 10–15% bigger than

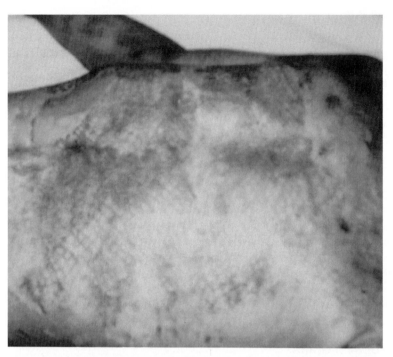

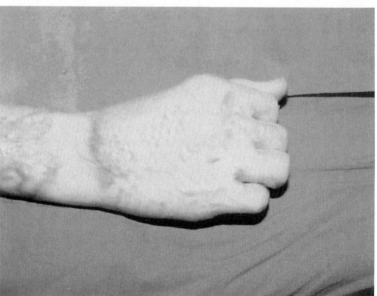

Figure 4 Meshed skin grafts should be avoided in minor and medium-sized (up to 40% TBSA) burns. The scars and mesh pattern are permanent marks and re-minders of the injury.

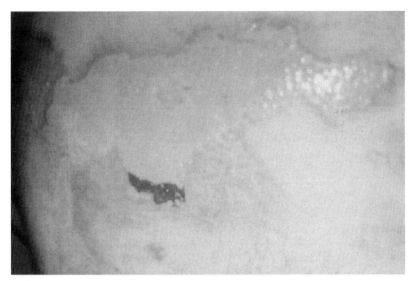

A

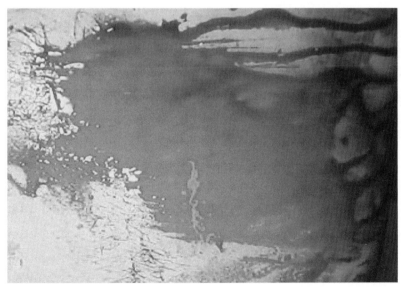

B

FIGURE 5 A–D. After complete hemostasis has been achieved, sheet skin grafts can be applied to the wound. Drain cuts are not necessary.

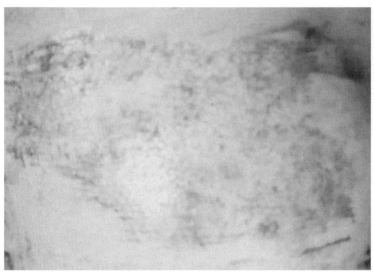

C

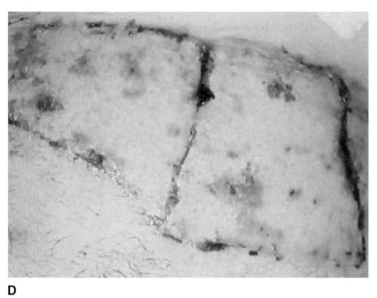

D

Figure 5 (Cont.)

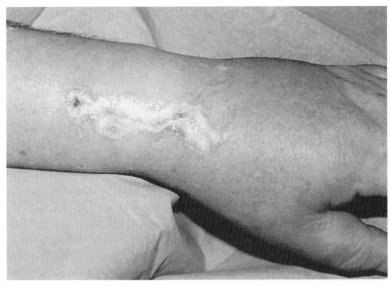

E

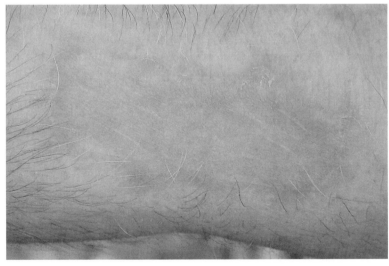

F

FIGURE 5 (Cont.) E, F. When performed, they will leave a permanent scar.

the defect to avoid excessive stretching of skin grafts when they are fixated on the wound. Donor sites are infiltrated with normal saline with epinephrine 1/200,000. An infiltrating pump is very useful. Other useful techniques include the Pipkin's syringe and infiltration through a pressurized system (a manometer commonly used for arterial lines will suffice) (Fig. 6). Enough tension must be obtained to immobilize the skin and produce an even surface that avoids bony structures. It is very helpful in donor sites on the scalp, torso, and back. Powered dermatomes should be used. Although skin grafts can be taken with a hand dermatome, thickness is not as predictable as with powered dermatomes. Hand dermatomes leave also an uneven contour around the donor site that will show in the postoperative result. Zimmer and Padgett air- or electrically powered dermatomes can be used. Donor site is moistened and the skin graft is taken. Liquid paraffin is normally used to moisten the skin surface but it is the author's preference to use normal saline, which provides better friction. The dermatome is then applied at 45 degrees with pressure and started. It should not be turned on before its application on the skin to avoid uncontrolled pressure and skipping. It is very helpful to hold the body of the dermatome with one hand and apply gentle pressure with the other hand on the head of the dermatome to get perfect control of the device. The surgeon should concentrate on the harvesting while the assistant holds and fixates the donor site. An operating assistant should hold the skin graft that is being taken with a pair of forceps to prevent any rolling on the drum and to let the surgeon check the thickness of the skin graft. Tension should not be applied to prevent deepening the plane of harvest.

When harvesting is complete, the angle of the dermatome is diminished to let the blade cut through the skin graft. This will leave the final portion of the skin graft thinner than the rest. If a uniform skin graft is desired, the surgeon can either discard the final part or stop the dermatome while maintaining its angle. The thickness of the drum is then opened to maximum aperture and the dermatome is gently withdrawn, exposing the final part of the skin graft. The graft is then trimmed with Metzenbaum scissors. Epinephrine-soaked (1:10,000) Telfa dressings are then applied to the surface of the donor site to allow good hemostasis. After 10 min, the donor site is dressed (Fig. 7).

Specific Donor Sites

Patients with minor burns present with many donor sites. Choice of donor site depends on graft requirements, anatomical location, extent of burn, patient's characteristics, and patient's preference.

The most commonly used donor sites for small- and medium-sized burns are:

Scalp
Thigh
Back

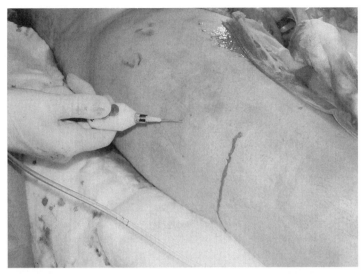

A

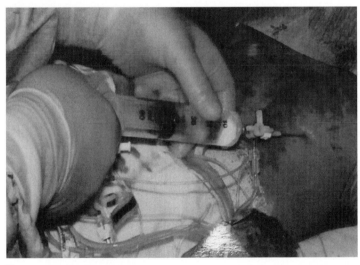

B

FIGURE 6 Donor sites are infiltrated with normal saline with epinephrine 1/200,000 to promote hemostasis, provide enough tension to immobilize the skin, and produce an even surface. Infiltrating pumps (A) or the Pipkin's syringe (B) can be used.

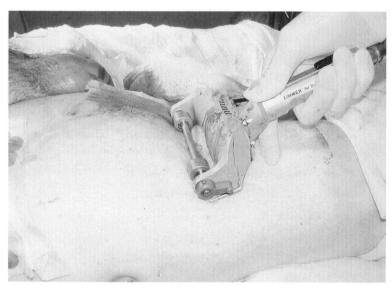

A

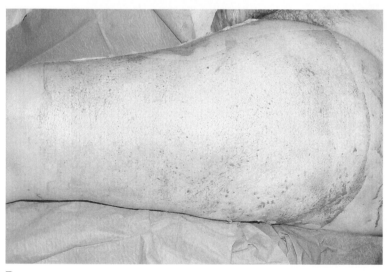

B

FIGURE 7 A. Powered dermatomes should be used to harvest the skin, which provide the best quality of skin by a reproducible means. B. Donor sites are infiltrated before harvest, which provide good blood loss control. Donor sites are then dressed with epinephrine-soaked Telfa dressings for 10 min. and dressed in the standard fashion.

The scalp provides the surgeon with the best quality of skin for burn surgery. The harvesting is practically painless and the donor site remains concealed provided the hairline is not crossed. The scalp should be considered the first choice in infants and small children and when excision and grafting of face burns are considered. The following are some of the principles for successful harvesting of scalp donor sites:

1. Draw the hair line prior to shaving (Fig. 8).
2. Infiltrate the area to be harvested with 1:200,000 epinephrine solution. Provide enough tension to facilitate the harvest by achieving a flat surface.
3. Powered dermatomes should be used. Avoid handheld dermatomes.
4. Blades become blunt after few harvests. Change the blade after every two or three strips of skin are harvested.
5. The head should be fixated by an assistant to allow control and good exposure
6. A scrubbed anesthetist should hold the endotracheal tube and protect the airway (Fig. 9).
7. Apply epinephrine-soaked (1:10,000) Telfa dressings when harvesting is completed.
8. Apply definitive dressing after 10 min.

When the scalp is not an option as a donor site (either due to concomitant scalp burns or lack of parent or patient's consent), the buttocks are the second choice in small children who are still in diapers. For older children, the thigh or back provides the surgeon with plenty of skin grafts.

The thigh is probably the most common donor site in burn surgery. It is more painful to harvest than the scalp, but it is easy to dress and care for, and it heals properly in few days. Infiltration of subcutaneous epinephrine solutions should be considered to obtain good hemostasis, although it is not necessary to use tumescent technique to provide good tension. An assistant should hold the limb in good position and the muscles should be positioned in tension. The thigh is then serially harvested until enough quantity of skin grafts has been obtained. Epinephrine-soaked Telfa dressings are then applied to the donor site and the thigh is dressed after 10 min.

Medium-sized burn injuries present with extensive graft requirements beyond those available from scalp or thigh donor sites. Even though some medium-sized burns can be grafted by using both thighs, the back is usually the best donor site for these injuries. Large amounts of skin grafts with excellent quality are readily available from this area. However, many surgeons dislike using skin from the back because the patient has to be positioned prone. The use of a second operating table to roll the patient and on which to harvest the back can solve this problem.

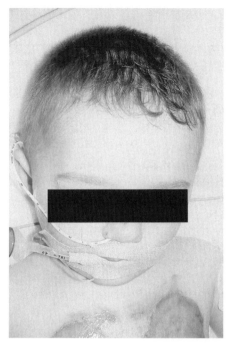

A

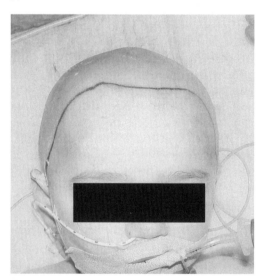

B

Figure 8 The scalp is an excellent donor site for split-thickness skin autograft. The hairline should be drawn before shaving to avoid inadvertent harvest of skin in the upper neck posterior neck and on the forehead.

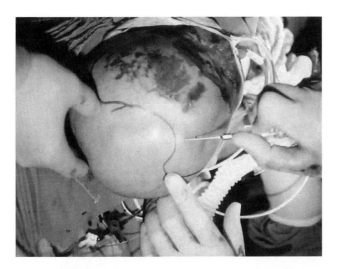

FIGURE 8 (Cont.)

Before graft harvest, the areas that will be excised and grafted are measured. A second operating table is placed parallel to the main operating table and sterile drapes are prepared. The patient is then rolled onto the second operating table and the main operating table is moved aside. The back is prepped in the standard fashion and the area infiltrated with 1:200,000 epinephrine solution. It is imperative to infiltrate the back, because good tissue tension is needed to provide good-quality skin grafts. Moreover, an even surface is needed, since all bony structures (especially ribs) preclude any good grafting technique unless Pipkin's technique is used. Graft requirements are then drawn onto the back surface according to burn wound measurements and long strips of medium-thickness skin grafts are harvested. It is necessary to change the blade of the dermatome very often: it becomes dull very quickly due to the thickness of the dermis. Epinephrine-soaked Telfa dressings are then applied to the wound and the donor site is covered with the definitive donor site dressing after 10 min.

When the harvest is completed, the main operating table is placed parallel to the second operating table again. It is draped sterile, and padded burn wound dressings are placed on the surface. Exu-Dry dressings or absorbing cotton-based materials should suffice. The patient is rolled back onto the main operating table and the second operating table is removed. The patient's wounds are prepped in sterile fashion again and the excision starts.

Type of Excision

In general, minor burns are treated with tangential or sequential excision. Fascial excision may be needed in few instances, especially in contact, chemical, and

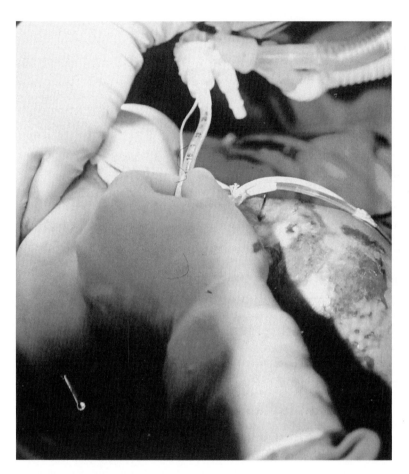

FIGURE 9 During scalp donor harvest and face burns excision, a scrubbed anaesthetist should hold the endotracheal tube and protect the airway.

electrical injuries. Tangential excision should be considered first unless gross, mass destruction of soft tissues is obvious. Tourniquets are strongly advised. Their use minimizes blood loss and increases the control of burn wound excision. Sequential slices of burn wound are excised until living tissue is seen. Punctate bleeding is absent under tourniquet control and the completeness of the excision is dependent on the surgeon's experience. Living dermis appears as a shiny ivory net without hemorrhages or discolorations. Living fat appears as pale yellow fatty tissue without hemorrhages or brownish discoloration. In inexperienced hands, it is advised to deflate the tourniquet briefly to assess punctate bleeding. The tourniquet is inflated afterwards and further excision of nonviable tissue, if present, is performed. After completion of excision, epinephrine-soaked Telfa dressings are applied. Burn wounds on the torso, back, and face are tangentially excised until punctate bleeding is observed. Epinephrine-soaked Telfa dressings are applied afterwards. Burn wounds may be infiltrated with epinephrine solutions (1:200,000). However, it must be used in experienced hands, because the burn wound may acquire a cadaveric appearance that makes the assessment of excision very difficult.

Hand dermatomes are commonly used for excision of burned tissue (Fig. 10). The Watson dermatome is used to excise large areas, whereas the Goulian dermatome, which comes with different guards to accommodate the depth of excision, is used in small areas and specific anatomical sites such as face, hands, and feet. A back-and-forth action is essential to achieve good control of the excision. The dermatome should be handled like the arch of a violin. A gentle forward push must be maintained during the excision, but the real action of the dermatome is determined by the delicate back-and-forth action of the body of the dermatome. The complete width of the dermatome must be used in the action, while maintaining the excision in its precise location. Pressure must be avoided, and all muscles in the hand and forearm must be relaxed to allow precise control of the instrument (Fig. 11). An assistant should hold the burned tissue being excised, allowing the surgeon total control over the progression of the excision. Pressure must not be applied while holding the burned tissue because this deepens the plane of excision. It must only be considered when dealing with full-thickness burns in which it is imperative to excise the complete thickness of the skin to graft on subcutaneous tissue. The use of powered dermatomes provides an even excised surface. They are helpful in the management of large minor burns, but the excised surface must be inspected to identify nonviable tissue. Small areas of nonvital tissue must be then excised with the handheld dermatome to avoid excision of surrounding vital tissue.

Fascial excision is rarely necessary in minor burns. When gross destruction of soft tissues is present, en bloc resection of the damaged area is recommended. The resection does not differ from any other fascial resection; and the reader is referred to Chapter 6. When this type of resection is performed, flap coverage may be necessary in selected anatomical locations.

Hemostasis

Extensive bleeding may occur during burn surgery that challenges the patient's hemodynamic stability during and after surgery and graft take. The recommended hemostatic measures during burn surgery include the following:

Tourniquets
Topical epinephrine solution
Subcutaneous infiltration of epinephrine solution

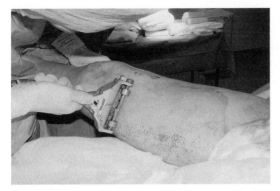

A

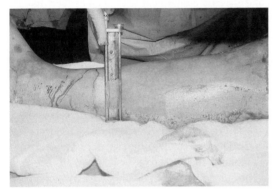

B

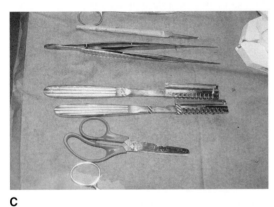

C

FIGURE 10   A. Hand dermatomes are commonly used for excision of burned tissue, although large flat surfaces may benefit from excision with powered dermatomes. Hand dermatomes include the Watson (B) and Goulian (C) dermatomes. The Watson knife is used to excise large areas; the Goulian dermatome is used in small areas and face, hands, and feet.

208

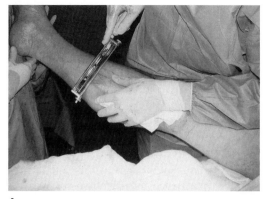

A

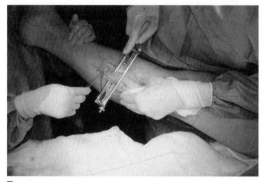

B

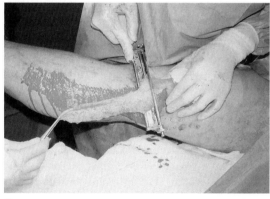

C

FIGURE 11 The dermatome is handled like the arch of a violin, a back-and-forth action is executed. A gentle forward push must be maintained, but the back-and-forth movement, which should accommodate the complete length of the instrument, determines the real action.

The use of sterile tourniquets with or without limb exsanguination creates excellent blood loss control. Limbs are prepped sterile and tourniquets applied. If the burns extend to the area where the tourniquet is to be applied, the area is excised first and covered with epinephrine-soaked Telfa dressings. Tourniquets are inflated and excision is started. After completion of the burn excision, the area is dressed with epinephrine-soaked Telfa dressings and the tourniquet is deflated. If the burn surgeon lacks the necessary experience with excision under tourniquet control, tourniquets may be briefly deflated to assess accurate excision of all devitalized tissue and inflated again. Any nonvital tissue is excised and dressed with Telfa. When the surgeon has enough experience, the operations may proceed without tourniquet deflation (Fig. 12).

The application of epinephrine-soaked (1:10,000) Telfa dressings has proved very effective in achieving complete hemostasis of excised burn wounds. Telfa dressings are cotton-based dressings with a nonadherent side. The nonadherent side must be always put into contact with the wound. This allows removal of the dressing without starting new bleeding points. The surgeon must be confident that all nonvital tissue has been removed before the epinephrine is applied to the wound because the wound acquires a cadaveric appearance after the application and it is not longer possible to assess the extent of the excision. Epinephrine-soaked laparotomy pads are placed on top of the Telfa dressings and then wrapped with elastic bandages. The dressing is left in place for 10 min and then removed. All blood clots are wiped with the Telfa dressings and evident arterial bleeding points are controlled with diathermy. Any other dermal bleeders are not coagulated at this point. New fresh Telfa dressings are applied again and wrapped in same manner. The dressing is left in place for another 7 min and removed. If complete hemostasis is not achieved, a third dressing application is considered. After removal of the dressings, the wound surface is rinsed with saline. Any minor remaining bleeders are controlled with diathermy. The wound must not be wiped with compresses but cleaned with saline irrigation. When a complete dry surface has been obtained, the wound is then ready to be grafted (Fig. 13).

The third main principle of hemostasis during burn surgery is the infiltration of subcutaneous tissue with epinephrine (1:200,000) solutions. The infiltration of donor sites should be universally adopted. This controls bleeding very effectively, is not associated with any side effect, and does not affect wound healing. On the other hand, the infiltration of burn wound before formal excision should be reserved for unequivocally full thickness burns. The infiltration of deep partial-thickness burns may lead to excision of vital tissue in inexperienced hands. Dermis becomes congested and acquires a cadaveric appearance after infiltration. Vast experience is needed with this technique to avoid extending the excision to deeper planes of living tissue.

Other techniques that have been explored to control blood loss during burn surgery include use of fibrin sealant and bovine thrombin. These agents are very

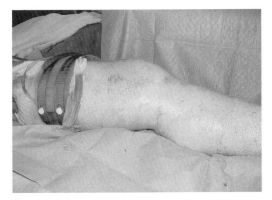

A

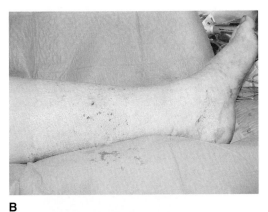

B

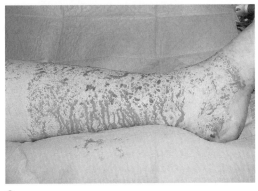

C

FIGURE 12 The use of sterile tourniquets provides excellent blood loss control. A. The tourniquet is inflated before excision and (B) excision is performed. Epinephrine-soaked Telfa dressings are applied after completion. As an alternative, the tourniquet can be deflated to assess the depth of excision and then reinflated (C).

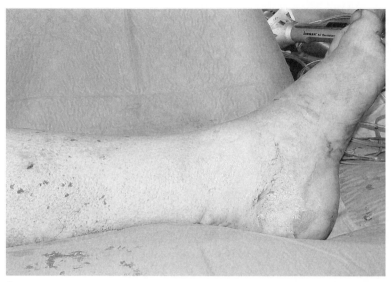

A

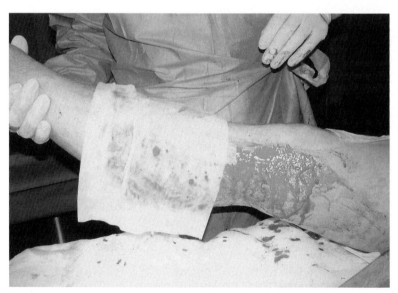

B

FIGURE 13 Epinephrine-soaked (1:10,000) Telfa dressings are very effective in achieving complete hemostasis. A, B, C.

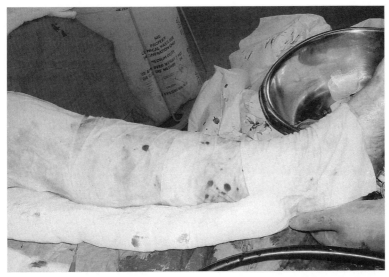

C

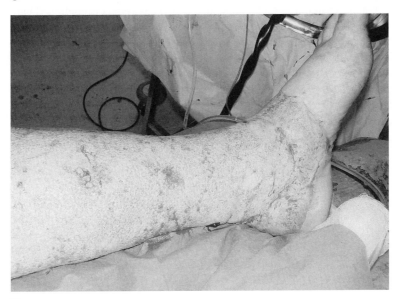

D

FIGURE 13 (**Cont.**)   Telfa dressings are applied with the nonadherent surface facing the wound. When epinephrine-soaked dressings have been applied to the wound, it is not longer possible to assess the extent of the excision because the wound acquires a cadaveric appearance (D).

expensive and their use must be rationalized to control the burn unit's budget. Some studies have shown a significant decrease in blood loss during burn surgery with their use, although combination with topical or subcutaneous epinephrine renders the best hemostatic effect.

Fixation of Skin Grafts and Splinting

Many techniques for skin graft fixation are documented in the medical literature. The methods extends from paper tape to fibrin glue, but the most frequently used are metallic staples, resolvable sutures, and bolsters or tie-overs.

In general, skin grafts are fixed with metallic staples. Skin grafts must not extend over normal skin because that will lead to desiccation and infection. Graft seams need to be overlapped a few millimeters to provide good coaptation and avoid open wounds during the rehabilitation phase. One edge is fixed first, and the graft is then stretched until full tension has been achieved. If the wound is small enough to be covered with one single skin autograft, the opposite edge is fixed before the rest of the graft is sutured. When more than one graft is needed, the next graft is placed beside the previous graft and they are fixed together to provide enough tension to the first skin autograft. The process is continued until the wound is covered completely (Fig. 14). Drain cuts are not necessary if good hemostasis has been achieved.

A good alternative to staples, although time-consuming, are resolvable stitches. Commonly used suture material is 4/0–5/0 Vycril rapide and Chromic Catgut. They are particularly useful in children (suture removal is not necessary) and in selected anatomical locations (face, hands, feet, genitalia). Key stitches are placed at the corners of the skin graft to maintain tension and location of the skin graft. The rest of the skin graft is then sutured with a running suture technique (with the so-called surgette technique), which provides a good seal of the wound.

Bolsters, or tie-over dressings, are often necessary in selected anatomical locations where shearing forces and tridimensional configuration challenge the skin graft's stabilization. Staples or resolvable suture may be used to fix the skin graft on the wound. 2/0–3/0 silk stitches are placed 2 cm apart around the skin graft. Tethering must be avoided. The bolster stitches must hold together the skin graft and the surrounding normal skin and the knot should be tighten in the ordinary fashion. Petrolatum-based fine-mesh gauze is applied on the skin graft overlapping 3–4 cm and a cotton bolster embedded in normal saline and liquid paraffin is secured with the bolster stitches. The bolster is then removed in 5 days (7 days for full-thickness grafts) unless purulent discharges are detected before the planned day of removal (Fig. 15). Other techniques that have been used for graft fixation include fibrin glue, resolvable staples, and tape.

Perfect positioning of graft site is essential for proper healing in a good functional position. The intervention of rehabilitation services is a key issue to

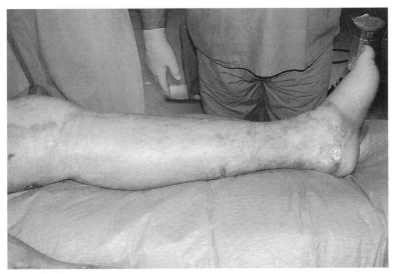

A

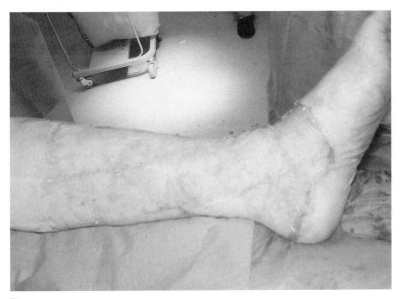

B

FIGURE 14   Donor sites are extensive in minor and medium-sized burns, therefore wounds should be always covered with sheet autografts.

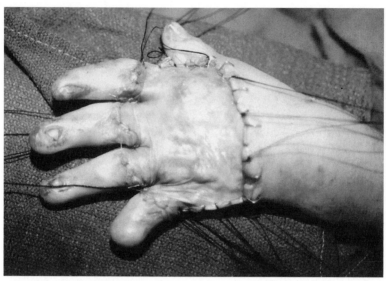

A

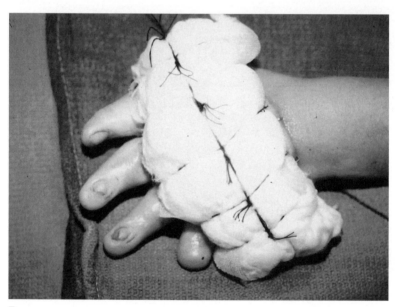

B

Figure 15   Bolsters, or tie-over dressings, are often necessary in selected anatomical locations where shearing forces and tridimensional configuration challenge the skin graft's stabilization.

achieve this goal. Good preoperative planning should include postoperative positioning and splinting. Grafts that extend over joints and other anatomical locations (hands, feet, and neck) need proper splinting. A comprehensive plan should be made before surgery, and preliminary splints should be tailored for postoperative positioning. Experts in physiotherapy and occupational therapy are invited to assist and intervene at the end of the operation. After a light protective dressing has been applied, the splints are then molded again to adapt to the anatomical configuration. After completion, they are hold in place with a second external dressing. Splints are revised during the first and consecutive dressing changes and tailored to the specific patient's needs. Interim pressure garments should be applied as soon as possible when grafts are deemed to be stable (usually within 7 days).

Dressings

After excision, donor site harvest, hemostasis, and graft fixation are completed, the most crucial part of the operation still must occur. Proper application of protective dressings requires a mastery that can only be acquired through experience and proper training. Burn dressings serve four main purposes:

Graft protection
Fluid and exudate absorption
Creation of a microenvironment that promotes wound healing
Patient comfort

An ill-dressed burn graft may not serve any of these purposes and, conversely, may promote shearing forces and graft dislodgement. As with any other surgical discipline, it can not be overemphasised that the art of dressing is the final touch that completes the excellence of surgical technique. In general, patients are ignorant regarding surgery and medicine, and they can not assess the excellence in technique as physicians measure it. They can only assess our mastery in terms of pain control, good outcome (i.e., freedom from disease), superficial scars, and outer dressing. A sloppy dressing means a sloppy surgeon and a sloppy surgical technique in the eyes of our patients. During the early postoperative period, the only way patients have to assess a successful operation is to watch the perfection of the dressing and the care that they receive. Dressings that do not match patients' expectation will ruin their trust. Also, and more important, dressings that are not properly applied may ruin the operation. Therefore, the application of dressings should be unhurried, follow a precise plan and technique, and be thoroughly inspected to avoid postoperative problems before the patient awakens.

For didactic purposes, burn dressings can be classified as to their two main anatomical locations:

1. Donor sites
2. Graft sites

Donor site dressings should provide a microenvironment that promotes wound healing and reduces pain. For small donor sites that have surrounding normal skin, the best choice is the application of Opsite or Tegaderm, a polyurethane occlusive film. It can be secured in place with the application of benzoine to normal skin, which increases fixation of the film. The dressing is completed with a compressive bandage to protect the inner film and provide patient comfort. The dressing is left in place until complete re-epithelialization has occurred. If fluid collections are detected under the film, they can be aspirated and the hole sealed with a small adherent film. This dressing can be complemented with the application of calcium alginate dressings, which absorb fluid collections and promote wound healing. The polyurethane film is applied on top of the calcium alginate and dressed in the standard fashion. Early separation of the polyurethane film may occur before complete healing has occurred. In this case, the dressing should then be removed and petrolatum-based fine mesh gauze or Mepitel applied until re-epithelialization has occurred, which is generally complete in few days.

Larger donor sites can be dressed either with Biobrane or Acticoat. Biobrane is particularly useful in donor sites on the trunk (front or back). It is placed in a circular fashion and covered with petrolatum-impregnated fine-mesh gauze. After 2 days it can be exposed and separates from the wound when complete re-epithelialization has occurred. Patient may bathe with Biobrane in place, but it should be dried afterwards. A good alternative to Biobrane is Acticoat, a specially tailored fine-mesh gauze impregnated with nanocrystalline silver nitrate. Acticoat is applied in direct contact with the wound and dressed with a standard dressing. Antimicrobial properties of Acticoat remain active for a minimum of 3 days.

Scalp donor sites deserve a special attention. Small donor sites in infants and small children can be managed successfully with Opsite or Tegaderm dressings with or without calcium alginate. Re-epithelialization occurs very rapidly. A protective head dressing is necessary to avoid trauma to the polyurethane film. Extensive scalp donor sites are best managed with the application of Biobrane. It is virtually painless and can be exposed on the second postoperative day, allowing good hygiene. A standard head dressing is also necessary during the initial postoperative period. Acticoat can be used in a similar fashion, although it does not allow for good hygiene and is more difficult to care for. Porcine xenograft can be used as donor sites dressing, although it is not the standard of care.

Skin grafts are generally dressed with protective bandages that provide good environmental properties to expedite vascular inosculation. Shearing forces must be avoided to prevent graft loss. It is necessary to place hands, feet, and joints in good functional position to allow graft take in maximum range of motion. Splinting may be necessary; therefore good communication with rehabilitation services is a must. Following graft fixation, a petrolatum-impregnated fine mesh gauze is placed in direct contact with the graft, and a soft dressing with soft gauze, Kerlix (if limbs are involved), and compressive bandages are applied. Excessive pressure should not be applied in order to avoid postoperative hematomas due to excessive venous pressure and the development of compartment syndrome. Mepitel can be used as an alternative to fine-mesh gauze. It does not stick to the wound, and removal of dressing is easy with minimal pain.

The main purpose of all dressings is to provide protection and immobilization of the graft site. When grafts are in close vicinity to superficial burns and donor sites, Biobrane should be considered. It allows for satisfactory wound healing for both grafts and superficial wounds. Biobrane is secured in place as described for superficial wounds, including the graft site in the dressing. Biobrane is then dressed in the standard fashion. Acticoat can be used in similar fashion. In cooperative patients and on special locations (face, hands) grafts can be left exposed. Antimicrobial creams (bacitracin or polysporin) should be applied on the surface of the grafts to prevent contamination of graft seams and graft desiccation. If the exposed method is used in hand grafts, the ukulele splint should be considered to allow full range of motion and good graft positioning. When all dressings have been applied, the anatomical location should be elevated and protected. Postoperative instructions are given to the nursing staff and on call team, and the patient and relatives are informed of the postoperative wound care plan. Grafts are inspected 5–7 days after surgery unless the clinical picture of the patient dictates otherwise.

BIBLIOGRAPHY

1. Heimbach DMBurn patients, then and now. Burns 1999; 25:1–2.
2. Heimbach DM. Editorial: who speaks for the little burn? Burns 1996; 26.
3. Dziewulski P, Barret J. Assessment, operative planning and surgery for burn wound Closure. In: Burn care. Wolf SE, Herndon DN, Eds. Austin, TX: Landes Bioscience, 1999.
4. Klasen HJ. Early excision and grafting. In: Principles and Practice of Burn Management. Settle JAD, Ed. Edinburgh, UK: Churchill-Livingstone, 1996.
5. Klasen HJ. Skin grafting. In: Principles and Practice of Burn Management. Settle JAD, Ed. Edinburgh, UK: Churchill-Livingstone, 1996.
6. Heimbach DM. Early burn excision and grafting. Surg Clin North Am 1987; 67: 93–107.
7. Muller MJ, Herndon DN. Operative wound management. In: Total Burn Care. Second Edition. Herndon DN, Saunders WB, Eds. London, UK: 2002.
8. Heimbach DM, Engrav LE. Surgical Management of the Burn Wound. New York: Raven Press, 1984.
9. Barret JP. Surgical closure of the burn wound. In: Color Atlas of Burn Care. Barret JP, Herndon DN, Eds. London, UK: WB Saunders, 2001.

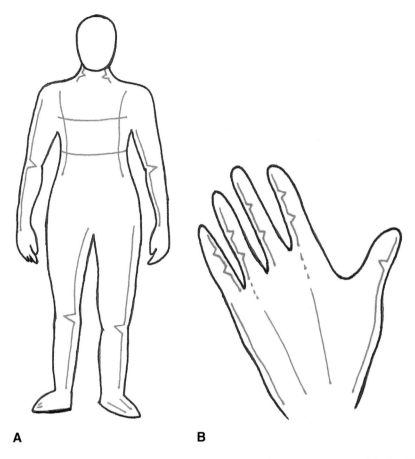

A   **B**

Figure 1-1: Suggested placement of escharotomies in the trunk and limbs (A) and on the hand (B). Note that darts should be included so that linear hypertrophic scar do not result.

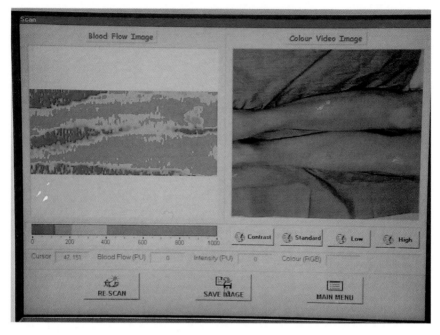

FIGURE 1-6: Areas that are colored in red are superficial burns with strong dermal vascularisation whereas areas colored in blue are full thickness burns. Air and normal skin show as blue colored areas.

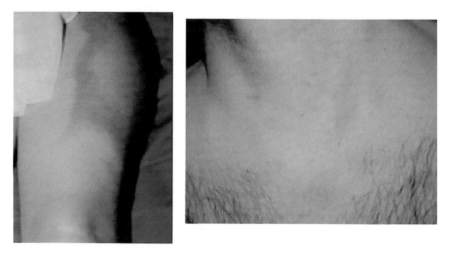

FIGURE 1-7: First degree burns. Only the epidermis has been damaged. Typical appearance is that of a hyperemic area with severe discomfort and hyperestesia. They do not blister, and they generally desquamate between 4 to 7 days after injury.

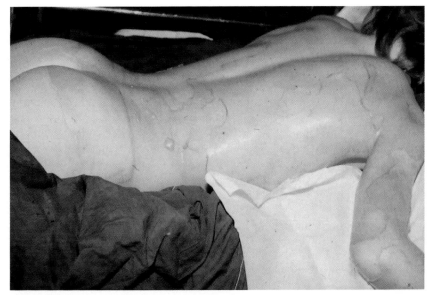

A

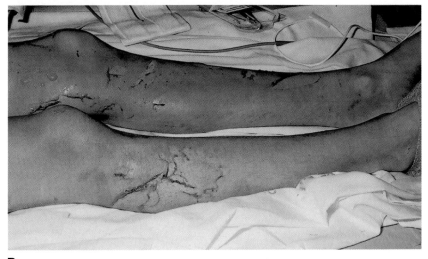

B

FIGURE 1-8: Second degree-burn injuries (or partial thickness burns) present with different degrees of damage to the dermis. Pain is very intense in superficial second-degree burns (A and B). They usually blanch with pressure and do not tend to leave any permanent scarring. On the other hand, deep second degree burns present with lesser degrees of pain and they tend to present with a prolonged healing time. Deep portions of the dermis have been damaged and they tend to leave permanent changes on the skin (C and D). *(Figure continues)*

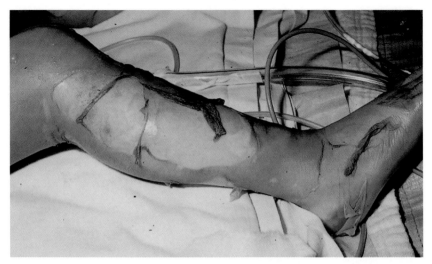

C

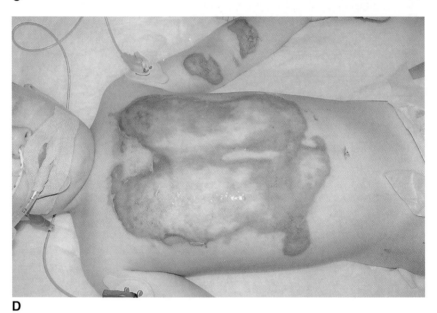

D

FIGURE 1-8: *Continued.*

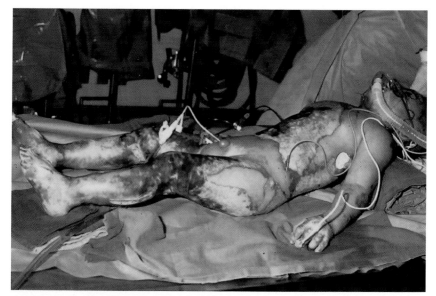

A

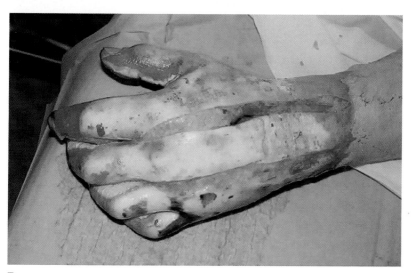

B

FIGURE 1-9: Third degree burns present with complete destruction of the skin and different degrees of soft tissues (A). Their appearance ranges from white non-blanching leathery look (B) to non-blanching red discoloration due to hemoglobin denaturation (C). A charred leathery dry eschar is typical of flame burns, more obvious in ignited liquid flammables.

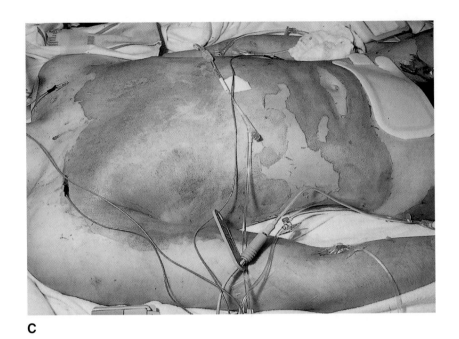

C

FIGURE 1-9: *Continued.*

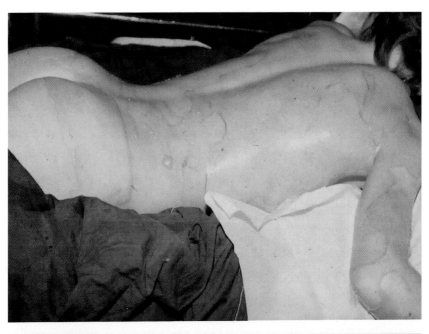

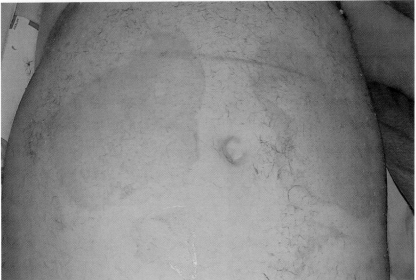

FIGURE 7-1: Typical appearance of superficial second-degree burns. Note the red/pink moist appearance. They blanch with pressure. Pain is very intense, and good procedural pain control must be achieved during superficial debridement.

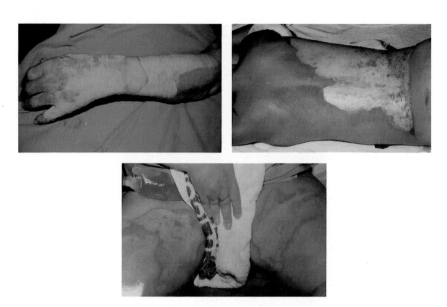

FIGURE 7-2: Pseudo-eschar formed on a superficial treated with silver sulfadiazine. Although harmless, it can be misleading in inexperience hands and diagnosed as full thickness eschar. If lifted away, reveals a healthy superficial wound bed beneath it.

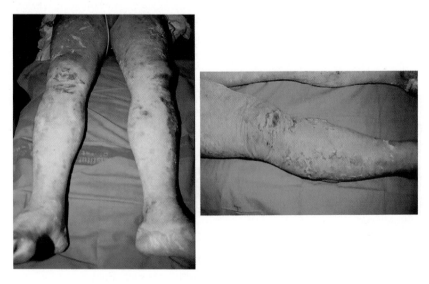

FIGURE 7-3: Typical appearance of burn wounds treated with cerium nitrate silver sulfadiazine. Note the leathery hard scar with deposition of calcium, which often prevents invasive burn wound infections. It provides a wound that is easily treated with delayed tangential excision.

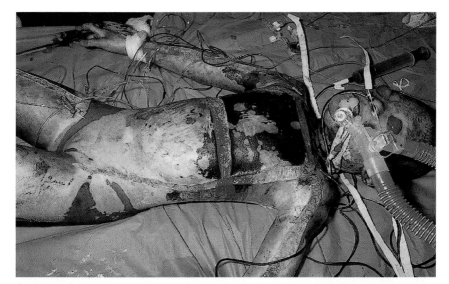

A

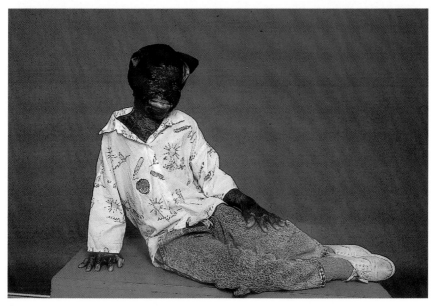

B

FIGURE 10-1: 95% TBSA burns (1-A) treated with immediate burn wound excision and grafting. Currently, all children and young adults are candidates for survival. No matter the surgical approach utilised, the aim should be to obtain LD50 over 90% TBSA burned. (B)

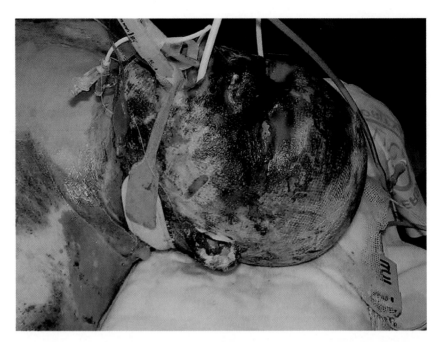

FIGURE 12-1: Full thickness burns to the face. Skin and soft tissues have been severely damaged by thermal injury. Early escharectomy is indicated. Patients with mixtures of deep dermal and indeterminate depth burns benefit of conservative treatment for 10 days followed by excision of true full thickness areas.

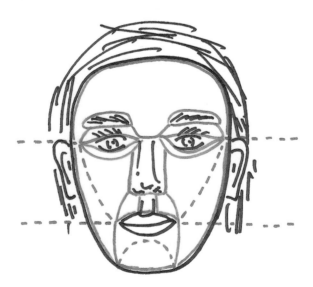

FIGURE 12-2: Excision of face burns must adapt to aesthetic units. The areas included in any given aesthetic unit are excised as a whole to provide optimal outcomes.

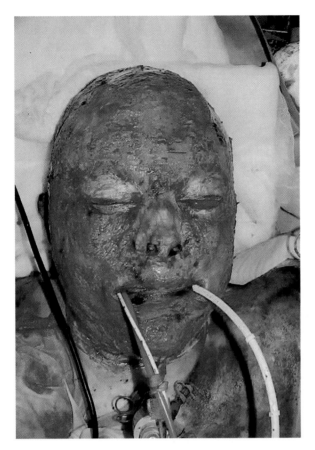

Figure 12-3: Total face excision in a patient affected of full thickness burn.

9

The Major Burn

Steven E. Wolf
The University of Texas Medical Branch, Galveston, Texas, U.S.A.

INTRODUCTION

Over 1 million people are burned in the United States every year, most of which injuries are minor and treated on an outpatient basis. Almost all of these treated as outpatients do not require operative treatment. However, approximately 60,000 burns per year are more severe and require hospitalization, and roughly 3000 of these patients die.[1] Most of these will require operations for timely burn wound closure to prevent infection as well as allow return to normal function.

Between 1971 and 1991, burn deaths in the United States decreased by 40%, with a concomitant 12% decrease in deaths associated with inhalation injury.[2] Since 1991, burn deaths per capita have decreased another 25% according to Centers for Disease Control statistics (*www.cdc.gov/ncipc/wisqars*). These improvements were probably due to prevention strategies resulting in fewer burns of lesser severity, as well as significant progress in treatment techniques.

Improved patient care in the severely burned, including operative strategy and techniques, has undoubtedly improved survival, particularly in children. Bull and Fisher first reported in 1952 the expected 50% mortality rate for burn sizes in several age groups based upon data from their unit. They reported that approximately one-half of children aged 0–14 with burns of 49% total body surface area (TBSA) would die, 46% TBSA for patients aged 15–44, 27% TBSA for those of age 45–64, and 10% TBSA for those 65 and older.[3] These dismal statistics have drastically improved, with the latest reports indicating 50% mortality for 98% TBSA burns in children under 15, and 75% TBSA burns in other young age groups.[4,5] Therefore, a healthy young patient with any size burn might be expected to survive.[6] The same cannot be said, however, for those aged 45 years or older, among whom the improvements have been much more modest, especially in the elderly.[7]

Reasons for these dramatic improvements in mortality after burn that are related to treatment include increased understanding of resuscitation, better support of the hypermetabolic response to injury, improved treatment of inhalation injuries, and, probably most important, control of wound complications through aggressive operative excision and closure of the burn wound. The dramatic effect of the practice of early wound excision on burn mortality cannot be overemphasized. This single advancement has led, in my opinion, to the routine survival of patients with massive burns in centers with experience in their care.

Burn wounds can be roughly categorized into two classes: partial-thickness and full-thickness. Partial-thickness wounds will generally heal by local treatment with skin substitutes or topical antimicrobials, and therefore do not require operative treatment. Full-thickness and very deep partial-thickness wounds, however, will require other treatments to affect timely wound healing. Since all the elements of the epidermis have been obliterated in full-thickness wounds, healing can occur only through wound contraction and/or spreading epithelialization from the wound edges. In a sizable wound, this process will take weeks to months to years to complete. To accelerate this process, skin grafting with the necessary keratinocytes from other parts of the body can be used. Alert patients do not generally tolerate this procedure, so anesthesia is necessary. Therefore, these procedures to accelerate burn wound closure are performed in the operating room. This chapter reviews the general principles of burn surgery, defines which patients should receive operations for burn wound closure, discusses necessary equipment and skills including patient preparation, reviews an excision and grafting procedure for a major burn, and discusses the techniques generally chosen based on the patient and injury characteristics. The discussion is general and therefore applicable to all specialists doing burn surgery. However, some of this information is by necessity an opinion and should be treated as such. Some local practices followed at different institutions may differ significantly from what is espoused here; however, they all should adhere to the general principles of burn surgery.

GENERAL PRINCIPLES

The intent of burn wound operations is twofold: to remove devitalized tissue and restore skin continuity. These are the only two things that must be accomplished.

The techniques used to achieve these goals are numerous; the choice of which is the challenge and art of burn surgery.

Excision

In concept, the first part of the operation involves removal of devitalized tissue injured in the burn. This tissue by definition does not receive blood supply and provides an excellent environment for the proliferation of micro-organisms. Therefore, no advantage exists in leaving this eschar in place on a burn wound, and it should be removed. The removal of eschar to viable tissue provides a wound base that can be used for wound closure with skin grafts or flaps. However, aggressive debridement that removes otherwise viable tissue under the eschar should be discouraged, because all tissue layers, including fat layers, provide function and cosmesis. The intent of excision, therefore, is to remove the burn eschar to the level of viability without disturbing underlying structures.

Wound Closure

Once a viable wound bed is achieved, the next goal is wound closure. This should be accomplished while minimizing scarring both in the excised wound and in donor sites from which skin grafts are taken (if this approach is used). The selection of method will therefore depend on the size of the wound and availability of donor site, and the functional and cosmetic importance of the wounded area. For example, a burn on the face is of great cosmetic and functional importance: Therefore, any skin grafts used there should be taken from a part of the body that will provide a good color match. Treatment and application of the autograft skin should be such that minimal disruption in all layers of the skin occurs, and lines in the grafts are minimized. In my practice, I use relatively thick skin grafts taken from the scalp applied in sheets and fashioned to the cosmetic units of the face for such injuries to address all of these concerns. This allows for minimized scarring of the wound, and donor site scarring is lessened in significance because the autograft is taken from the scalp, which will have natural camouflage if there is normal hair growth. This is an example of how the operative plan may change based on the area of the burn.

Once the techniques for excision and closure of the wound are chosen, care must be taken to provide a technically sound result. Although in small burns local flaps can be used for wound closure, most significant burn wounds will require closure with skin grafts. These are applied to wound beds where the cells of the graft are kept alive by nutrients in the serum produced by the wound bed until vascularization takes place (1–4 days after application). For this process to take place and for the skin graft to take, four things are required:

A viable wound bed
No accumulation of fluid between the graft and the wound bed

No shear stresses on the wound
Avoidance of massive micro-organism proliferation

Performance of the selected technique must be reliable to ensure adequate outcome. Emphasis must be placed on adequate excision to a viable wound bed. Then meticulous attention should be paid to placing the grafts and adhering them to the wound bed. Consideration should be given to the lines inherent in placing grafts either from the meshing or the grafts themselves in order to minimize cosmetic scarring. Selection and application of the dressing are equally important: the dressing should apply pressure to the wound to minimize dead space under the graft, minimize shear stress, and provide antimicrobial properties. This portion of the operation is often overlooked, and if performed inadequately will lead to poor results.

Wound Healing and Scarring

The skin is made up of two distinct layers: the epidermis and dermis; function of the skin depends on the presence of both. The epidermis, made primarily of keratinocytes, provides a continuous moisture and antimicrobial barrier. The underlying dermis is responsible for most of the other functions of the skin, including shear strength, pliability, contour, eccrine function, hair production, sensation, and so on. When the skin is lost from injury, the wound is closed by contraction, keratinocyte migration, and/or skin grafts. Most of the modern techniques of wound closure involve replacement of the epidermis to re-establish barrier continuity, which is generally successful. What is absent after closure is most of the dermal layer that is responsible for all the other functions. In its stead a neodermis of disorganized fibroblasts, macrophages, and collagen forms under the epidermal layer. This layer provides for continued wound contraction, hypertrophic collagen deposition, and is a nonpliable surface, which we typically associate with scarring.

It was found long ago that wound closure with full-thickness skin grafts containing a complete epidermis and dermis provides for the best outcomes in terms of wound contraction, appearance, and pliability. As a general principle, therefore, a graft with increasing levels of dermis should provide the best functional and cosmetic outcomes. Split-thickness donor sites can be taken at many depths, the deeper of which contain more dermis. When these are used as autografts, these sites will have decreased scarring. The limitation to this is that deep donor sites leave significantly increased scarring at the donor site. This should be kept in mind during operative planning and the use of donor sites.

OPERATIVE INDICATIONS AND PLANNING

Once the initial urgent measures for burn resuscitation have been undertaken, a plan of action for further management of the wound is necessary. This management plan can include conservative and operative measures depending on the patient's age and condition, burn depth, burn size, and burn wound location.

Wound Depth

Burn wounds are classified by depth of injury. This assessment is very important: it will dictate the proper treatment, including the need for operative treatment and the planning thereof. Burn depth is most accurately judged by the appearance of the wound to experienced practitioners. However, new technologies such as the heatable laser Doppler flowmeter with multiple sensors hold promise for quantitatively determining burn depth. These measurements may give objective evidence of tissue loss, and thus assist the treating physician in the proper choice of treatment (Fig. 1).[8]

First-degree burns are, by definition, partial-thickness injuries confined to the epidermis. These burns are painful, erythematous, and blanch to the touch with an intact epidermal barrier. Examples include sunburn or a minor scald from a kitchen accident. These burns will heal spontaneously, will not require operative treatment, and will not result in scarring. Treatment is aimed at comfort with the

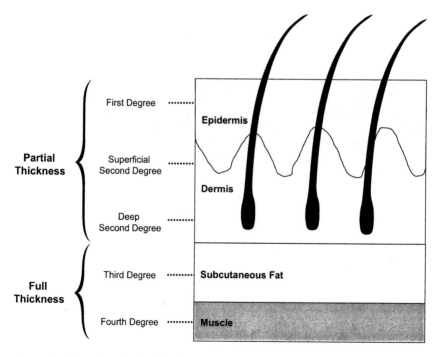

FIGURE 1 Burn depth classification.

use of soothing topical salves with or without aloe and oral nonsteroidal anti-inflammatory agents. Surgery should not be considered in these patients.

Second-degree injuries are partial-thickness injuries classified into two types: superficial and deep. All second-degree injuries involve some amount of dermal damage, and the division is based on the depth of injury into this structure. Superficial dermal burns are erythematous, painful, may blanch to touch, and often blister. Examples include scald injuries from overheated bathtub water and flash flame burns from open carburetors. These wounds will spontaneously re-epithelialize from retained epidermal structures in the rete ridges, hair follicles, and sweat glands in 7–14 days. The injury will cause some slight skin discoloration over the long term. Deep dermal burns into the reticular dermis will appear more pale and mottled, will not blanch to touch, but will remain painful to pinprick. These burns will heal in 14–28 days by re-epithelialization from hair follicles and sweat gland keratinocytes, often with severe scarring. Some of these may require surgical treatment.

Third-degree burns are full-thickness through the dermis, and are characterized by a hard leathery eschar that is painless and black, white, or cherry red. No epidermal or dermal appendages remain, and thus these wounds must heal by re-epithelialization from the wound edges. Deep dermal and full-thickness burns require excision and grafting with autograft skin to heal the wounds in a timely fashion. Fourth-degree burns involve other organs beneath the skin, such as muscle, bone, and the brain.

Initial examination of the wounds will reveal many of the signs consistent with burn depth descriptions above. However, at times the wounds characteristics will change, making it difficult even for experienced examiners to determine burn wound depth accurately. This is often associated with advancing microorganism growth and wound infection or inadequate resuscitation and systemic problems. For this reason, operative planning should be finalized only after examination of the wound just before excision.

Wound Size

The wound must also be assessed for burn size, which has a substantial impact on operative planning. The rule of 9s is generally used in adults, and Lund-Browder charts for children. These diagrams can be found in other parts of this book. The importance of this determination is discussed in the last section of this chapter.

Operative Indications

The principal indication for burn operations is the presence of a deep partial-thickness wound or a full-thickness wound that will not heal spontaneously in a timely fashion, and if it heals will leave an unsightly scar. Other indications are the presence of a massive partial-thickness burn that requires wound coverage to improve wound care and survival. The caveats to these notions are two. Patients who are elderly or otherwise infirm may not tolerate operative procedures well due to comorbidities. In this instance, the risks and benefits of the procedure must be weighed, and it may be found that performing dressing changes to await spontaneous wound closure may be preferable to the operative risks. However, the open wound will provide a source of infection and inflammation that may itself be more risky than the operation. No hard and fast recommendations can be given in this regard, and the decision to operate should be made on an individual basis by an experienced practitioner. The other caveat is in a wound that is delayed in presentation by 3–10 days from the time of injury. In this instance, often a pseudoeschar has formed on the wound from protein exudate that makes the determination of wound depth difficult even for the most experienced observers. For this reason, it may be more beneficial to wait until 14 days after the injury to allow for spontaneous separation of the eschar to determine whether the wound will heal spontaneously or an operation will be required.

NECESSARY EQUIPMENT

Before the patient is brought to the operating room, the equipment necessary for the operation must be ready. Some or all of the equipment mentioned below will be used in these operations. Thought should be given as to which are necessary and arrangements made for their presence. This will minimize time spent in the operating theater and improve the dynamics between the operating team and the other personnel in the room (anesthesia and nursing staff).

The equipment and instruments required for burn-related operations are described in detail in the following sections.

Operating Table

Burn operations can be performed on standard operating tables, but other types of tables that allow for full patient mobility while anesthetized are preferable. We use autopsy tables, which have several advantages (Picture 1). They are wider than standard operating tables so that patients may be moved from the supine position to the prone position safely. Each table has an edge and a drainage hole with tubing at the end of the table which can be used to drain irrigant during skin preparation as well as bodily fluids. The head and foot can be raised and lowered to allow for optimal patient position. We generally lay the patient on a waterproof foam pad to avoid pressure neuropathies. We also position an electro-cautery pad under the patient so that these need not be applied to the patient directly, again improving patient mobility. If these type of grounding pads are not available, grounding plates can be placed directly under the patient, or adhesive

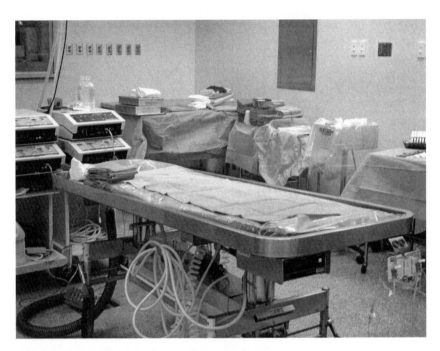

PICTURE 1   Burn operating table and operating room set-up.

grounding pads can be applied directly to nonburned areas of the skin. The soles of the feet work best in this regard, as these are rarely used as donor sites.

Drapes and Positioning Devices

The entire patient is usually prepped for these operations. The skin can be prepared using iodine solutions (e.g., Betadine) or chlorhexidine 1%. The patient is then placed on standard drape sheets. A thick roll (4–6 inches in diameter) should be available to place under the shoulders to extend the neck while the patient is in the supine position. Additional rolls should be available to place under the hips and ankles if the patient must be rolled to the prone position. Hooks or other devices that can be attached to the ceiling should be available to tie raised extremities. I prefer to fix the digits in a loop of cotton gauze, which can then be tied to hooks or loops attached to the ceiling. This allows for circumferential placement of grafts on the extremities while the patient is in the supine position.

Electrocautery Units

Standard pencil-held units can be used. In burn surgery at least two and preferably more separate units should be used at each operation so that hemostasis can be accomplished as quickly as possible.

Pitkin's Device

This is used for clysis of fluid underneath an eschar or donor site to decrease bleeding by increasing tissue pressure, and provides a flat contour to optimize donor site excision. Two different types of devices are available. One is a hand-driven syringe with an automatic fill mechanism connected to a bag of infusate. The other is a gas-driven device with a stopcock valve to regulate administration of the infusate. I personally prefer the gas-driven type because it provides more even flow.

Tourniquets

Tourniquets can be used to limit blood loss when excising wounds on the extremities. It is very useful if the tourniquet can be sterilized; if the whole limb is burned, the upper portion can be excised before application of the device without contamination of the operative field. When using tourniquets during burn wound excision, areas requiring electrocautery for hemostasis will not bleed until the tourniquet is removed, thus obviating the usefulness of the tourniquet. One way to avoid this bleeding is to deflate the tourniquet briefly while the extremity is wrapped with a moist gauze and elastic bandages. When the tourniquet is reinflated, the outer elastic dressings can be removed and significant bleeding areas will be marked by blood staining. This limits blood loss, identifies bleeding vessels in need of hemostasis, and provides a measure of the adequacy of excision by allowing inspection of the wound. My personal practice is to avoid the use of tourniquets except in reconstructive operations. I rely instead on meticulous attention to hemostasis in a wound bed after a timely excision before moving to another anatomical area requiring excision.

Knives

A variety of knives are used for burn wound excision. Standard #10 and #15 surgical blades are used for sharp excision, incisions into fascial planes, and other procedures. Specialized knives used for tangential excision include the Goulian knife (Weck blade), and the Watson modification of the Braithwaite knife (Picture 2). The Goulian knife is a blade inserted into a handle, over which a guard is placed. The guard can be chosen to regulate the depth of the excision, which ranges from 4 to 16|1000 inch. This blade is generally used for excision of delicate areas such as the face and hands. It is also used to finish the further excision of small areas within wider areas. The Watson knife is much larger, with an 6 inch blade. This knife blade is placed into a handle that has an adjustable guard. It generally used to excise larger areas on the trunk and limbs. Both of these knives can be used to take skin grafts, but it is technically difficult to get consistent grafts of uniform thickness using this technique.

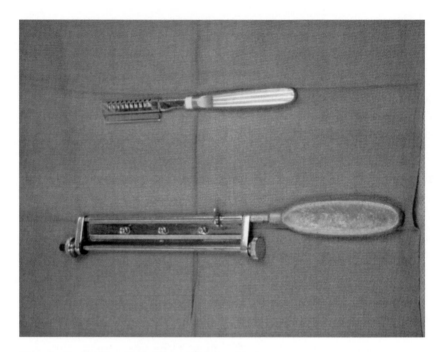

Picture 2   Braithwaite knife and Goulian blade.

Dermatomes

Most surgeons use either electric or gas-driven dermatomes, such as the Zimmer
or Padgett dermatome, to obtain wide, even skin grafts (Picture 3). The depth of
excision is adjustable, and guards from 1 to 4 inches can be placed on the dermatome to regulate width. Some surgeons also use the dermatome for eschar
excision because the depth is very even. I personally prefer the Zimmer gas-
driven type.

Surgical Instruments

The number of typical instruments used in burn surgery is minimal. What is
needed most are scissors of the Mayo type and Metzenbaum type. Straight suture
scissors are also necessary. The Kelly clamp and the tonsil clamp are also commonly used for staple removal and to control bleeding vessels. Forceps are also
very important. I find that the Russian-type forceps are the most useful: they are
versatile and do not have fine ends that can catch the end of grafts and displace
them. Retractors are used rarely but should be available. Instruments used in

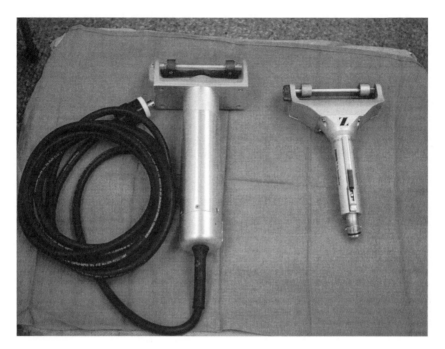

Picture 3   Electric Pagett dermatome and gas-driven Zimmer dermatome.

bone resection are more commonly used, and should also be available but not necessarily opened.

Hemostasis

A number of agents can be used to improve hemostasis during burn operations. The purpose of eschar excision is to remove the dead tissue to viable tissue. This can be reliably achieved by tangentially excising until the tissue bleeds. Once this occurs, the bleeding must be stopped using electrocautery devices or pressure. Even pressure can be obtained on an extremity with the use of wide elastic bandages (4 and 6 inches wide). Irrigants containing epinephrine (1 : 100,000 mixture) or thrombin can be applied directly to the excised bed. Fibrin sealants have recently become available and popular. This mixture of activated thrombin and fibrin is sprayed onto the wound in a thin, even sheet using an aerosol machine available from the fibrin sealant provider (Baxter and Haemocure).

Meshers

Once the skin grafts are taken, it is often best if the grafts are meshed to improve graft take by decreasing the chance of seroma or hematoma formation, and if

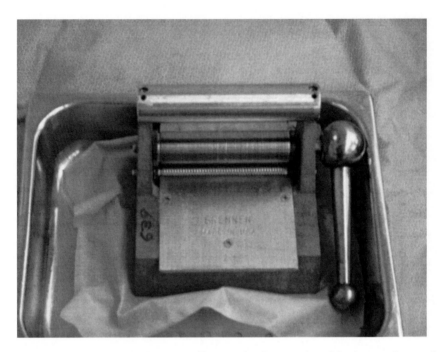

Picture 4 Brennen 2:1 mesher. Sheets of skin are placed in the mesher and advanced with the handle. Other ratios are available.

indicated, to widen the coverage area of the same graft. Three types of meshers are currently available and widely used. The Brennen mesher has a fixed mesh ratio (1:1, 2:1, and 4:1) (Picture 4); if more than one ratio is desired, a different machine must be used. The Zimmer mesher relies on skin carriers to produce different ratios, thus one machine can mesh at several ratios. The Meeks mesher actually cuts the donor skin into 3–4 mm squares, which are then adhered to a expandable template. Once expanded, the skin pieces are then transferred to another carrier to be placed on the wound bed. A 9:1 expansion ratio can be reliably achieved using this technique.

Homografts

Occasionally homografts will be used for wound closure after burn wound excision. A decision should be made pre operatively, as to whether this is likely, and if so, how much will be required. These homografts should be available in the room with the patient, so they will need to be procured preoperatively. The amount of skin required can be estimated from burn diagrams. One square meter of burn surface area requires approximately 10 square feet of homograft skin for closure. The use of homograft skin will be discussed later in this chapter.

Blood Products

Significant amounts of blood are generally lost during burn operations due to the nature of the excision and procurement of autografts. We have found that these losses are best replaced with blood products. To perform timely operations, these blood products must be available in the room before beginning the procedure. In general, 1 cc of reconstituted whole blood will be required for each square centimeter of excised wound. Therefore, if 1000 cm^2 will be excised, approximately 2 units of packed red blood cells and 2 units of fresh frozen plasma should be available. We do not use platelets as a rule unless the platelet count is below 10,000/mm^3 and the patient is actively bleeding.

Sutures and Staplers

Once grafts are harvested, meshed, and applied to the wound bed, they are affixed with either sutures or staples. The use of sutures is generally limited to areas requiring very precise work, such as the face and hands, because of the time and effort involved. Absorbable sutures should be used if possible. In other areas, staples are used because the outcomes are similar to those with sutures, and staples are easy to apply. Some surgeons have recently been using fibrin sealant as a glue for grafted areas without application of sutures or staples. This technique will require some fine-tuning and widespread experience before it will be commonly used.

Donor Site Dressings

A number of types of dressings are available. The first type is a fine-mesh cotton gauze that may or may not be impregnated. Dressings of this type include Scarlet Red and Xeroform, which have the advantage of low cost and familiarity. Other types of dressings that have surfaces engineered to improve coverage, healing, and pain include Biobrane and BCG Matrix. All of these are treated postoperatively with desiccation, and are thus lower in maintenance. Moist dressings of cotton gauze include Kaltostat and Acticoat, which may decrease bacterial colonization and lessen pain. An occlusive dressing such as OpSite can also be used. In discussing the topic of donor site dressing with other burn surgeons. I have found that the type of dressing used is dictated primarily by local standards. Each of the dressings has advantages and disadvantages. In preparation for a burn wound operation, one must ensure that the dressings commonly used at any given institution are available in the operating room.

Burn Wound Dressings

Once the wounds have been treated by debridement and possible grafting, a dressing must be applied. These Dressings should be occlusive and antimicrobial. At our institution, we use fine-mesh gauze impregnated with polymyxin B/neomycin/bacitracin/nystatin ointment, although other topical antibiotic agents could be used. We then apply a thick layer of cotton gauze over this, which is held in place by elastic bandages (Ace bandages). We then place wrapped extremities in plastic bags to keep the dressings from getting soiled and to retain temperature. Sometimes bolster dressings will be applied, which consist of a layer of antibiotic fine mesh gauze and a thick cotton dressing held in place by tie-over sutures placed 2–3 cm apart circumferentially around the grafted area. This type of dressing is generally limited to posterior areas on the trunk and perineum.

Splints

A necessary practice to maximize graft take is immobilization to minimize shear stress. This is best done in the operating room before removal of anesthesia for best patient comfort. To do this, splinting materials will be needed. They should consist of either plaster or fiber glass casting material and elastic bandages. Some centers use Thermoplast splinting material for this purpose. Prefabricated knee and elbow immobilizers can also be used, depending on the size of the patient and the overlying dressings.

Air Beds

To minimize shearing and pressure on posterior areas, air beds have been created that keep the patient elevated on a column of air in a sand base (Picture 5). We have found that the use of these beds improves posterior graft take over that found in regular beds, and decreases (but does not eliminate) development of pressure sores during prolonged treatment for massive burns. The flow of air also improves donor site dressing care over posterior areas. We use these types of beds for patients with posterior wounds and donor sites. If using such a bed postoperatively is considered, it should be procured before the operation so that transfer of the patient from the operating room is not delayed.

BURN WOUND OPERATIONS

The burn wound operation can be conceptually classified into five parts: planning, induction of anesthesia and preparation, excision and hemostasis, grafting, and application of dressings.

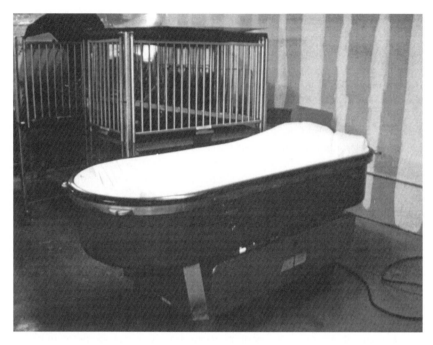

PICTURE 5   Kin-Air air bed with a sand base and air flow through the sand to levitate the patient, thus decreasing pressure and shear forces on the skin.

Planning

Planning begins with an accurate assessment of the area, depth, and location of the wound. From this assessment, plans can be made as to which areas will be excised and which will just be débrided. Once this is decided, plans for wound closure can be made: whether autografts, homografts, or just dressings will be applied. Once this is decided, the operation should be scheduled and the necessary items listed above procured. We believe that once a decision is made to operate, further delay in proceeding to the operating room only increases complications. For this reason, we will schedule the operation for the next available time slot, and will usually perform the operation within 24 h of initial examination. The wisdom of this practice has been borne out in the finding that early operations decrease septic complications.[9] Occasionally, it is reasonable to delay operations for up to 24 h to continue to resuscitate and stabilize the patient. Delays greater than this in patients with burns over 40% of the body surface area requiring operation are not indicated regardless of the physiological condition, because the condition is unlikely to improve without ablation of the wound.

The plan for operation must be discussed beforehand with the patient and his or her family. The discussion should address the typical process of wound healing including those of partial-thickness and full-thickness burns. Deep partial-thickness and full-thickness burns generally will not heal in a timely fashion without operative wound closure, which explains the need for and benefit of the operation. The technical aspects of the procedure should be reviewed, including excision of tissue and planned donor site areas. Risks should also be discussed, including blood loss and the likely use of blood products, risk of infection and development of organ failure, loss of tissue and at times loss of limbs, scarring, pain typically associated with donor site and donor site scarring, and lastly, failure of the operation to achieve its goal (graft loss) generally from technical error. At this time, all questions regarding the procedure and the likely outcomes should be answered. Patients and their families will usually consent to the operation. However, at times the patient and family may refuse an operation. If, after further discussion, this is still the decision of the patient, the time for complete wound closure and the prospect for severe scarring should be made clear, and this should be well documented.

Induction of Anesthesia and Preparation

When the patient arrives at the operating room, several things should be in place. First, the ambient temperature of the room should be at least 30°C (86°F) because the patient will be mostly exposed for the procedure and will not be able to regulate core body temperature. In fact, it may be necessary to increase the temperature further should the patient get cold. Once the patient arrives, anesthesia should be induced with endotracheal intubation. Anesthetic techniques are discussed in another chapter of this book. In our practice, we almost always accomplish intubation by fiberoptic means through the nose. This allows for decreased vulnerability of the airway and for a fiberoptic examination of the upper and lower airways in patients with suspected inhalation injury. Attention then should be turned to placement of intravenous lines and invasive monitors such as arterial lines. We generally, perform operations with a multilumen subclavian venous catheter with one other large-bore venous line. This may not be necessary in patients with smaller burns. We also place a catheter in the femoral artery to measure blood pressure continuously during the operation and to obtain arterial blood for gas analysis; again, this may not be necessary in cases of smaller burns. An oxygen saturation monitor and continuous electrocardiogram leads should also be placed. We have found that alligator clips attached to staples inserted into the skin work well as electrocardiographic leads instead of adhesive pads. A Foley catheter equipped with a temperature probe should be placed.

Once the monitors are in place and anesthesia induced, the patient can be prepared for the operation. While the patient is in the supine position, the head should be shaved if the scalp is burned or if the scalp will be used as a donor site. Other donor site areas then should also be shaved. The skin for the donor site area as well as the burn wound should then be prepared by gentle scrubbing and washing with an antiseptic solution such as Betadine or chlorhexidine solution. For burns over 20% of the body surface area, this will include most of the body; therefore, in these cases we will prepare the skin of the whole body in order to make all the donor sites available. In fact, it is rare for us to prepare and drape specific areas without preparing the whole body. Once the anterior areas are scrubbed, the cleaning solution is irrigated away with warm water (37°C). Then we turn the patient on his or her side to wash and irrigate the back. During the irrigation, the bed should be tilted toward the drain to facilitate removal of the irrigant. Before rolling the patient back to the supine position, a foam pad is placed, which is covered by sterile drapes under the patient. A sterile shoulder roll is then added. The patient is then properly positioned to begin the operation. The last task required before beginning the operation is to ensure that the electrocautery devices are functional, that the dermatome is functional and calibrated properly, and that the table is at the proper height for the surgical team. Consideration should also be given at this point to whether perioperative antibiotics (if to be used) have been given.

Excision and Hemostasis

The operation can then be started. What I will describe in the next few paragraphs are the principles of an operation for a massive burn (>50% TBSA). These principles can be modified to other smaller burns as indicated. In general, excision and donor site procurement should be done anteriorly followed by repositioning of the patient to the prone position. Posterior donor sites procurement and excision can then take place, followed by placement of grafts. The patient is again rolled supine, with placement of grafts anteriorly.

Beginning the operation can be done in one of two ways, depending on the depth of the burn. If most of the wound is of an indeterminate depth, it is not clear whether autograft skin will be necessary at all. In that case, excision of the wound should take place first. I generally do this by passes with a dermatome set at 10/1000 inch. If good punctate bleeding is reached with one or two passes at this depth and dermal elements are still present in the wound bed with no exposed fat, this wound will heal spontaneously and will not require autografting. Once hemostasis is established, appropriate dressings can be applied (discussed later in this chapter). If it is found to be of a depth that will require autografting, these can be obtained after excision. In most cases, what will be found is that some areas will heal spontaneously and others will not. The appropriate amount of donor site skin can then be procured, thus minimizing donor site scarring.

In wounds the majority of which will clearly require autografting, it is best to make an estimate of the amount of donor site skin required, and then to begin the operation by obtaining these. I generally begin by taking anterior donor sites at 10/1000 of an inch with a Zimmer dermatome. If possible, donor sites should be chosen that are conspicuous and will have a good color match for the wound bed. Donor sites on the abdomen, in the groin and perineum, and in the axillae are best harvested after clysis of the sites with a Pitkin's device. I generally avoid taking donor grafts from the dorsum or sole of the foot because of poor healing and improper skin type for most wound beds, respectively. Once the planned donor sites that are accessible anteriorly are taken, the donor site dressings should be applied and secured.

Excision of the wounds is then begun. This can be done with the Braithwaite knife, dermatome, or Weck blade. In general, the large areas such as the chest/abdomen and anterior thighs and legs are attended to first. Excision of the arms and hands can wait until later in the operation. The excision is best accomplished with traction on the eschar coming through the knife. The excision is completed when good bleeding viable tissue is reached. Sometimes, this layer may be in the fat, but the color is red instead of glistening yellow. In this case, the excision should be extended further until good yellow glistening fat is reached (the mnemonic being red is dead).

On occasion, it may be necessary to extend the excision down to the level of the fascia for very deep wounds. It also may be necessary to go to this level should invasive wound infection occur in a previously excised bed. I try to avoid fascial excisions, because this causes problems in the reconstructive phase due to contour difficulties. In addition, if a fascial excision is carried out unnecessarily early in the course of treatment or if invasive infection ensues, options for excisional treatment are very limited (i.e., amputation).

Once it is confirmed that the proper layer has been reached for all the anterior areas, hemostasis can begin. I do this by applying dry laparotomy sponges to the wound beds and applying pressure if possible with elastic bandages (e.g., on the legs). I then make the sponges damp with dilute epinephrine solution (1:400,000 concentration). The sponges are then carefully removed beginning at the edge of the excised area, and the electrocautery pen is used to cauterize large vessels. Capillary bleeding generally stops with observation for 20–30 s. If bleeding persists, fibrin sealant can be used to secure hemostasis. After this is completed, apply gauze sponges again with elastic dressings, if possible, in preparation to move the patient to the prone position.

Before the patient can be moved to the prone position, some monitors must be disconnected so that that they are not lost. I disconnect the arterial line in the groin, the oxygen saturation monitors, and the Foley catheter temperature monitor. Then, I position two members of the surgical team on one side of the table: one at the shoulders and another at the hips. The patient is then rolled prone into the arms of these two surgeons and completely lifted from the table. Another sterile roll is placed where the hips will reside, and then the patient is laid back on the table. All of these maneuvers are done while the anesthesia team has direct control of the airway. A stack of towels is placed under the forehead and another under the ankles. The monitors are then reconnected.

The posterior excision can then begin. It is done similarly to the anterior excision, depending on the estimated depth of burn. I prefer to take scalp donor sites in the prone position, because this gives better access to the entire area. The Pitkin's device should be used for clysis of the scalp, and is also useful in taking buttock donor sites. Excision of the back is followed by completion of leg eschar excision. I still do not excise the arms at this point, as they can be adequately accessed from the supine position. Attempting to excise these in the prone position often leads to inadvisable traction on the brachial plexus, which can lead to nerve injuries. Hemostasis is obtained as previously described.

Grafting

Once the excision has been performed, and the necessary donor sites obtained, a decision must be made as to what will be grafted, and how the grafts will be handled (meshed). In the case of partial-thickness injury, a number of options are available, including placement of antimicrobial dressings, cadaveric homograft to attain wound coverage, or placement of a skin substitute. Antimicrobial dressings consist of Silvadene or Polysporin; antimicrobial soaks of silver nitrate, Dakin's solution, or Sulfamylon, or a silver-impregnated dressing (i.e., Acticoat). These can be applied with the plan for routine dressing changes. I generally avoid this because the consequent dressing changes are painful. This type of treatment is limited in our practice to wounds with adherent pseudoeschar 5–7 days after injury that is very difficult to remove without full-thickness excision.

The option of applying homograft to excised partial-thickness burns is attractive, since the wound has been definitively treated without the need for continued debridement and dressing changes. Usually the homograft will reject after 2–3 weeks. The drawback to this technique is that on occasion some dermal elements of the homograft will incorporate, leaving a meshed pattern in the skin that is cosmetically less acceptable. I generally use this technique if large areas will remain open (>50% TBSA).

The final step is application of a skin substitute such as Biobrane. This substance is elastic, and can be stretched circumferentially around the extremities with excellent adherence rates. It can also be applied as sheets over the trunk and secured by staples. Biobrane is also available in a glove form to facilitate coverage of the hands. If Biobrane is used, the substance should overlap the wound edges to ensure complete coverage and maximize adherence. We have had great success in treating partial-thickness wounds in this way in areas up to 70% of TBSA.

Full-thickness wounds are optimally covered with autograft. In planning autograft coverage, the smaller the mesh ratio, the better the cosmetic outcome (sheets $>$ 1:1 $>$ 2:1 $>$ 4:1 $>$ 9:1). However, this must be weighed against how much autograft is available and how much wound is present. If the amount of autograft is insufficient to close the wound if applied in sheets or 1:1 mesh ratio, a 2:1 ratio should be considered. If even this is insufficient, 4:1 or 9:1 ratios should be considered. I usually try to limit 4:1 or 9:1 ratios to coverage of the trunk, thighs, and upper arms for cosmetic reasons. An estimate can be made of how much autograft skin will be required for 4:1 closure of the trunk, thighs, and upper arms. This amount of autograft is then meshed in that fashion. The rest of the autograft skin is then meshed in a smaller ratio and applied to other areas. If even widely expanded autografts are insufficient to close the wounds, the remaining open areas should be treated with application of homografts. These can be removed at subsequent operations, with application of autograft taken from the available donor sites that have healed. When donor sites have been taken at 10/1,000 of an inch, the donor sites usually heal within a week, and are ready to be reharvested. In truly massive burns ($>$80% TBSA) complete wound closure may require up to eight operations in this fashion.

Application of autografts to excised wound beds assumes that hemostasis has been obtained. As stated previously, one of the reasons for graft loss is development of hematoma under the grafts, thus depriving the transplanted cells of nutrients and the ability to vascularize. If a wide mesh is used (4:1 ratio), this is of less concern. Placement of autografts should be designed so that the lines inherent in the graft from seams and the mesh pattern follow the lines of Langer when possible. In our practice, autograft skin is placed dermal side up on a fine-mesh gauze backing after it is meshed to facilitate placement on the wound bed. Natural curling of the autograft toward the dermal side can be obviated by gentle irrigation with a bulb syringe to expand the graft completely while it is on the mesh. The autograft is then applied to the wound bed and the fine mesh gauze removed. At this point, I usually affix one side of the graft with staples and maximally expand the graft in the other directions. Grafts can then be applied adjacent to this as required for wound closure.

When using 4:1 or 9:1 mesh ratios, the wound will still be mostly open after application of the autograft. At this point, we advise that the wound be completely closed by application of cadaveric homograft over the autograft (Fig. 2). When using this technique, staples are not applied until all layers of the skin are in place. With successful graft take using this technique, the autograft and homograft become adherent and vascularized. With time, the homograft cells reject while the autograft cells expand, thus completing wound healing.

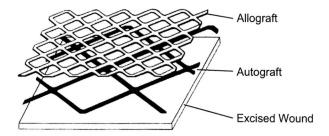

FIGURE 2 Homograft coverage of 4:1 autografts.

Selection of the donor sites, mesh ratio, and placement of the grafts comprise the majority of the art of burn surgery. The wound bed can be viewed as a puzzle, and the autograft as pieces of it. The advantage of this model is that the pieces can be cut to fit the puzzle. However, efforts should be made to keep the pieces whole in order to minimize seams.

Application of Dressings

Once the grafts are in place posteriorly, dressings should be applied. In areas that are dependent such as the back and the buttocks, tie-over bolsters should be placed to minimize shearing. This is done by placing # 0 silk sutures around the wound bed. Sutures should be placed in such a way that a geometric shape results when they are tied (rectangles or squares work best). In the case of a wound bed that goes around to the anterior trunk, it is only necessary to bolster to the posterior axillary line. Once the sutures are in place, a layer of one-half polysporin 1% ointment and one-half nystatin 1% ointment (polymyco)-impregnated fine-mesh gauze should be placed over the wound. Several layers of cotton gauze (5–6 cm) are placed over this, and the sutures are tied over all this firmly so that the dressing does not slide. In the case of the buttocks, polymyco gauze should be wrapped over the cotton gauze to minimize soiling. The legs do not require bolsters, because they can be wrapped circumferentially once the patient is in the supine position. I generally do not apply any dressings at all on the legs until the patient is placed back in the supine position.

At this point, the patient can be returned back to the supine position. This is accomplished by disconnecting the monitors again and covering the patient with a clean drape. The patient is then rolled back into the arms of two members of the surgical team at the shoulders and hips. The patient is lifted completely off the bed, the hip and ankle rolls are removed, and the patient placed back onto the shoulder roll as the monitors are reconnected.

Attention is then given to placement of the grafts anteriorly on the legs, perineum, and trunk. Simultaneous with this, the arms are elevated with hooks (as described above), and the excision carried out on them. After hemostasis is obtained, grafts are placed. Dressings are applied as previously mentioned on the trunk, but bolsters are not necessary. The limbs are dressed with circumferential strips of polymyco gauze followed by layers of cotton gauze and an elastic bandage.

The limbs should be splinted in extension at the elbows and knees. This can be done by the surgeon with plaster or fiber glass placed posteriorly followed by another elastic bandage. As an alternative, splints can be applied with Thermoplast in the recovery room by either the surgeon or experienced occupational and physical therapists.

The Surgical Team

For these operations to be done in a timely manner requires at least two experienced surgeons, and up to four are preferable. Many of the tasks detailed here can be done simultaneously. The senior surgeon makes decisions regarding the adequacy of excision, which donor site areas will be taken, and how the skin will be meshed and where it will be placed. He or she also participates in excision, placement of the grafts, and application of dressings with assistance from the other surgeons.

The anesthesia team and nursing team also play key roles in the actual performance of the operation. At our institution, the anesthesia team not only administers anesthesia, but also participates by holding the airway during position changes, turning on the air pressure for the Pitkin's device, and irrigating the wounds with dilute epinephrine solution. The nursing staff has the responsibility not only for providing instruments and other equipment required to do the operation but also for meshing the grafts. For excision of large burns (>40% TBSA), we have found that two of the nursing staff should be scrubbed, with one providing instruments and another meshing the skin.

TREATMENTS SPECIFIC TO ANATOMICAL LOCATION

Particular anatomical regions require specific treatments. These issues should be considered and incorporated into the operative plan.

Head and Neck

The head and neck have an ample blood supply that enable it to resist invasive infection better than other parts of the body. It is also probably the most important area in terms of cosmesis and function (eyes, mouth). The color of the skin in this area is relatively specific. For these reasons, it is treated differently than other areas. Since the face is so important cosmetically, sharp excision of eschar is not recommended in order to preserve any dermal and epidermal structures

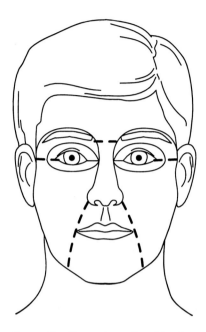

Figure 3 Cosmetic units of the face. Application of sheet grafts should be in this distribution, if possible.

that may survive. This practice is tolerated because of the excellent blood supply to the area that resists infection. Once the eschar separates in 10–14 days, the underlying wound can be grafted. Because of the unique skin coloration in this area, autograft skin should be obtained from donor sites above the clavicles. I generally use donor skin taken from the scalp for this purpose. The autograft skin should be applied in sheets to minimize scarring. Since it is almost always necessary to have seams in the grafts, the autograft skin pieces should be applied in cosmetic units, which are designed to hide the seams in natural lines on the face (Fig. 3).

Nipple/areolar Complex

Because of the nature of the mammary ducts, keratinocytes are often found deep beneath the skin. These will proliferate and affect wound closure in this area if left in place. The coloration of the areola is also very specific, and not easily reconstructed outside of color tattooing. For these reasons, the nipple/areolar complex should not be excised even if it appears to have eschar and all the surrounding skin is lost.

Buttocks and Perineum

The buttocks and perineum are in a very difficult position for skin grafts to take, since the dressings applied are often soiled from excrement, and cleaning the result often shears the grafts. For this reason, I always try to graft this region first, before loose stools occur. If this is unsuccessful, it may be necessary to leave the patient in the prone position at later operations after application of grafts to this area while they adhere.

The penis and scrotum have an excellent blood supply, so they will usually heal in a timely fashion. The skin in this region occupies a highly important function, so, in general, excision is avoided. In the case of a small burn to the shaft of the penis, excision and primary closure akin to a circumcision can suffice. The scrotum is also a very good donor site because it heals well, is relatively hidden, and can be vastly expanded to provide a surprising amount of donor skin.

Hands

The hands are a very important in terms of function and cosmesis. Most burns of the hand are limited to the dorsal surface as the hand is clenched during injury. Unfortunately, sometimes the digits sustain a second injury associated with diminished perfusion during resuscitation. Therefore, it is not uncommon for some parts of the digits to be lost. I usually allow the necrotic part to demarcate clearly prior to amputation in an attempt to preserve as much length as possible; even a few millimeters will contribute greatly to function. Once a viable wound bed is achieved on the hand, grafts should be placed that are either not meshed or meshed tightly at a 1:1 ratio to improve cosmesis. Because of the anatomical structure on the dorsum of the digits, burns through to the extensor tendons can result in boutonniere deformities even with complete wound closure due to sliding of tendons medial and lateral around the proximal interphalangeal joint. Extension contractures at the metacarpophalangeal joint are also common because the burn and subsequent scarring are limited to the dorsal surface. For these two reasons, consideration should be given to fixing the digits in extension at the proximal interphalangeal joint and flexion at the metacarpophalangeal joint by insertion of threaded Kirschner wires which are removed after complete wound healing, and position can be maintained easily with splints. Early mobilization of the hand will also decrease these contractures.

The skin on the palm of the hand is specialized in that it is very thick and highly keratinized to withstand the significant shearing forces. Burns to the palm of the hand are uncommon, but when they occur, should be treated with debridement and spontaneous separation, as they will often heal spontaneously because of the depth of the skin. Allowing this to happen preserves the skin type and thus function. Should the palm of the hand sustain a full-thickness burn, the autograft skin should come from the sole of the foot to match the keratinocyte function.

Feet

The foot has two specialized surfaces; the sole and the dorsum. The sole is very thick with both keratin and layers of keratinocytes, therefore it often will heal spontaneously similarly to the palm of the hand. The dorsum of the foot, however, has a thin layer of skin that has a different pliability than other areas of skin. For this reason, it does not make a good donor site for anything other than the dorsum of the other foot. Great care must also be taken with excision of full-thickness eschar in this area, because the extensor tendons are in very close proximity to the skin. Autograft skin applied to this area should be of a narrow mesh to avoid hypertrophic scarring, which can make it difficult to fit shoes. The toes require the same considerations as the fingers; portions of them can become necrotic both from the burn itself and from the vagaries of resuscitation. I treat all the regions of the foot in a fashion similar to the hand, except for the use of Kirschner wires.

BURN SIZE AND THE STAGING OF OPERATIONS

Small Burns

Burns involving less than 10% of the total body surface area can almost always be managed with a single operation. The most important decision lies in whether some or all of the wound can be closed with local flaps and, if not, where the donor site can be taken that will minimize scarring. The scalp has been shown to be a safe donor site that will provide for minimal donor site scarring and will heal quickly because of its excellent vascularity. For this reason, it is one of my preferred donor sites for small burns. The problem arises with the complication of alopecia resulting from technical error, and the potential for significant donor site scarring with the development of male pattern baldness in some patients. These possibilities should be discussed with the patient and his or her family before a decision is made. Other potential donor sites include the upper anterior thigh or the buttock, which also remain hidden with normal clothing. Selection of the donor site should also consider the color match of the wounded area, which is most significant on the head and neck. Some surgeons also prefer to close these wounds with full-thickness grafts taken from the groin that will provide for better function and cosmesis at the wound site, and minimize donor site morbidity because the donor site can be closed primarily.

Autograft application should be either in sheets or 1:1 meshing. Once excision and grafting have taken place, the wound must be dressed. On occasion, it will be better to apply a bolster-type dressing regardless of the anatomical area, because this will allow for greater patient mobility. In the case of the foot and lower leg, consideration should be given to application of an Unna's paste wrap over an antimicrobial dressing, which will provide for pressure to the wound bed and splinting of the extremity. If the dressings are applied in either of these fashions, this can sometimes be done as outpatient surgery without admission to the hospital. Inspection of the wound and dressing changing can then be done in the outpatient area 5–7 days later.

Medium to Large Burns

Burns involving 10–40% of the TBSA are treated differently. These burns generally will require meshed autograft at a 2:1 ratio, and at times, more than one operation. Staging the closure has the benefit of minimizing donor sites to the conspicuous areas of the scalp and thighs. Those that are cosmetically acceptable are taken twice with closure of the wound with homograft in the interim while the donor sites heal. The drawback to this practice is that the patient will be in the hospital longer as the donor sites heal, with the added risk of two procedures. If this is not desirable, consideration can be given to either taking autograft donor sites from more visible areas such as the abdomen, back, arms, and legs, or meshing the autograft at a 4:1 ratio. This will, however, lead to cosmetic deficits. These possibilities should be discussed with the patient and his or her family, and a decision reached prior to the operation. Otherwise, these operations should proceed as previously described.

Massive Burns

Burns involving more than 40% of the TBSA will almost always require staged operations for closure because of donor site limitations. It is also a race to restore skin continuity as soon as possible to maximize survival. It is our practice to procure all available donor sites in these situations, and use widely expanded autografts. We begin by applying the available autograft to the posterior areas of the back and buttocks first to maximize wound closure. It is our observation that the first excision and grafting procedure is associated with the greatest graft take, thus the posterior areas are addressed first, as these are the most difficult to close in later operations. If some autograft is left over, it can be applied to the posterior thighs or other anterior areas. Remaining open areas are closed with homograft. The patient is then returned to the operating room when the donor sites have healed in about a week, addressing further areas as required. The order in which anatomical areas is addressed in my practice is as follows: back and buttocks, posterior thighs and legs, anterior trunk, anterior thighs and legs, arms and hands, and finally, the head and neck. As these staged procedures proceed, consideration can be given to tightening the mesh ratio to improve cosmesis and function particularly in the hands, arms, and face after the majority of the wounds are closed with a larger mesh ratio.

Burns upwards of 85% of the total body surface area might be best treated with cultured epithelial autografts because of the extreme donor site limitation.

If this is a consideration, a full-thickness skin biopsy should be sent for study at the first operation. The resulting grafts can be applied 3–4 weeks later. In the meantime, staged operations with autograft obtained from the available donor sites should continue to affect wound closure. Even after application and adherence of the cultured skin, it is our observation that the resulting skin is very fragile. It will require repeated operations to replace the skin with autograft taken from the available donor sites to gain durable wound closure.[10]

DERMAL EQUIVALENTS

Scarring can be minimized with the use of full-thickness grafts that have a complete layer of epidermis and dermis. Most of the techniques described above with partial-thickness skin grafts provide for epidermal coverage, but do not address the loss of dermis, leading to significant scarring. An extrapolation of the finding of decreased scarring with full-thickness grafts has led to the search for a dermal replacement to be used with partial-thickness skin grafts. Two products are currently available that hold this promise: Integra and AlloDerm. These two products have different properties and are thus used differently. These products are currently being widely used in many centers based on the hope that they will improve outcomes. These improvements, however, have not yet been firmly established. Their use is also associated with significant increases in cost.

Integra

This is a skin substitute with a dermal equivalent layer consisting of collagen and other matrix proteins that vascularizes and functions as a neodermis. With good take, this neodermis is reported to improve the pliability and appearance of the scar. Integra also has an epidermal component of a silicone layer that functions as a barrier while the underlying neodermal layer vascularizes. After this takes place over 10–14 days after application, the silicone layer can be removed and replaced with thin split-thickness autografts. In the interim, the wound is completely closed.

Integra is applied and treated postoperatively similarly to autograft or homograft skin. Some practitioners apply it in sheets, while others will mesh it at a 1:1 ratio to minimize underlying fluid accumulations. Securing staples are generally not placed between sheets of Integra. Instead the staples are applied to single sheets to minimize losses due to shearing, because the sheets of Integra are not as pliable as skin because of the silicone layer. The Integra will progressively vascularize over 10–21 days, which is signified by increasing redness upon inspection. When the silicone layer begins to separate spontaneously, it must be replaced with autograft in a staged procedure. This is one of the drawbacks of this product; it requires more than one procedure.

AlloDerm

AlloDerm is obtained from cadaveric homograft skin treated to remove all the cells, leaving only the dermal matrix. This process removes all the allogenic properties from the dermis, so that it does not induce rejection. This product is a dermal replacement that does not have an epidermal component, which must be provided with autograft. Its use, therefore, is predicated on the availability of autograft skin to close the wound. It is generally applied to the wound bed directly followed by application of autograft on top of this in a sandwich fashion. All of this then vascularizes, leaving wound coverage with both a dermal layer and epidermal layer in one procedure.

REFERENCES

1. Pruitt BA, Goodwin CW, Mason ADEpidemiologic, demographic, and outcome characteristics of burn injury. In Herndon DN, Ed Total Burn Care. London: W.B. Saunders, 2002:16–30.
2. Brigham PA, McLoughlin E. Burn incidence and medical care use in the United States: estimates, trends, and data sources. J Burn Care Rehab 1996; 17:95–107.
3. Bull JP, Fisher AJ. A study in mortality in a burn unit: standards for the evaluation for alternative methods of treatment. Ann Surg 1949; 130:160–173.
4. Herndon DN, Gore D, Cole M, Desai MH, Linares H, Abston S, Rutan T, Van O, sten T, Barrow RE. Determinants of mortality in pediatric patients with greater than 70% full-thickness total body surface area thermal injury treated by early total excision and grafting. J Trauma 1987; 27:208–212.
5. McDonald WS, Sharp CW, Deitch EA. Immediate enteral feeding in burn patients is safe and effective. Ann Surg 1991; 213:177–183.
6. Sheridan RL, Remensnyder JP, Schnitzer JJ, Schulz JT, Ryan CM, Tompkins RG. Current expectations for survival in pediatric burns. Arch Pediatr Adolesc Med 2000; 154:245–249.
7. Stassen NA, Lukan JK, Mizuguchi NN, Spain DA, Carrillo EH, Polk HC. Thermal injury in the elderly: when is comfort care the right choice. Am Surg 2001; 67: 704–708.
8. Yeong EK, Mann R, Goldberg M, Engrav L, Heimbach D. Improved accuracy of burn wound assessment using laser Doppler. J Trauma 1996; 40:956–962.
9. Wu XW, Herndon DN, Spies M, Sanford AP, Wolf SE. Effects of delayed wound excision and grafting in severely burned children. Arch Surg 2002:1049–1054.
10. Barret JP, Wolf SE, Desai MH, Herndon DN. Cost-efficacy of cultured epidermal autografts in massive pediatric burns. Ann Surg 2000; 231:869–876.

10

Surgical Approaches to the Major Burn

Juan P. Barret
Broomfield Hospital, Chelmsford, Essex, United Kingdom

The treatment of major burn injuries with immediate (within 24 h from the injury) total burn wound excision (all full-thickness and deep dermal injuries are excised and homografted) has been described in chapter 9. Two main approaches have proven effective for the treatment of massive burn wounds:

Immediate burn wound excision
Serial or sequential early burn wound excision

They differ significantly in terms of timing of surgery (first 24 h vs. first 72 h) and extent of the excision (total or near total vs. sequential). They represent an alternative for each other, and there is still great debate regarding the timing and extent of excision, especially in patients whose survival is questionable. The general philosophy of the major burn excision reviewed in Chapter 9 is entirely valid for both approaches. However, intraoperative and postoperative care issues differ as to the extent of the surface to be excised and the number of times the patients has to return to for further skin autografting procedures.

A third therapeutic approach used in some burn centers throughout Europe is the treatment of massive burn injuries with daily or twice-daily application of cerium nitrate–silver sulfadiazine (Flammacerium) and delayed excision and autografting. Some reports suggest that patients present with improved and recovered inmunological function and good protection against invasive burn wound infection. All three therapeutic approaches are summarized and compared in the following sections.

IMMEDIATE TOTAL BURN WOUND EXCISION

In this therapeutic approach, all deep dermal and full-thickness burns are excised after admission, ideally within 24 h of injury. Resuscitation is started and carried on during surgery, and urine output and other hemodynamic parameters govern it. Operative losses are replaced with reconstituted whole blood (one unit of fresh frozen plasma + one unit of packed red cells) calculated to replace a blood loss of 0.5 ml/cm^2 excised. Blood gas analysis and measurement of blood count and electrolytes are repeated every 30 min during surgery to determine the adequacy of fluid resuscitation and operative blood loss replacement. Patients receive perioperative antibiotics to prevent postoperative sepsis due to bacterial translocation from the gut.

Donor sites are harvested first, unless paucity of donor sites necessitates the use of culture keratinocyte techniques, in which case a skin biopsy is obtained to perform such techniques. If planned wound closure includes the use of Integra, donor sites are not harvested at this time.

The patient is placed in the supine position and any deep dermal and full-thickness burns on the anterior torso and abdomen are excised. Active arterial and large venous bleeder points are controlled with diathermy and bipolar cautery. Epinephrine-soaked (1:10.000) Telfa dressings and laparotomy pads soaked in epinephrine solution are applied and secured with sterile drapes. A second operative table is placed parallel to the main operative table and the patient is turned prone. The back is then excised and hemostasis is obtained in the standard fashion. When complete hemostasis has been obtained, the wound is closed. Wound closure may proceed by three different but complementary approaches:

1. Integra
2. Split-thickness autografts meshed 4:1 with an overlay of nonmeshed allografts (sandwich technique)
3. Split thickness autografts meshed 2:1

The meshing pattern used for wound closure depends on burn surface area and donor site availability.

Following wound closure, the grafts or skin substitutes are secured with a bolster (should include the whole back), or Biobrane. After completion, the patient is returned to the main operative table. This order is advised to prevent any blood loss pouring onto the dressing applied on the back. If the back is excised first and the excision proceeds on the anterior trunk, the bolsters will inevitably become soaked with blood, saline, and debris.

The anterior trunk is checked for appropriate hemostasis and the wound is covered with Integra or sheet homografts (usually all available autografts have been already used to autograft the back). If some areas can still be autografted, meshing expansions no bigger than 3:1 are used.

Attention is then turned to the upper and lower limbs. Excision should proceed in an orderly fashion. Excision under tourniquet is strongly advised. If tourniquets are not used, no more than one team should operate at the same time. The simultaneous excision of two limbs without tourniquet control can lead to patient exsanguination and cardiac arrest. If tourniquets are used, no more than two teams should operate at the same time. In general, tourniquets are inflated and excision proceeds from top to bottom and medial to lateral until all burned tissue has been removed. Hemostasis proceeds in the standard fashion and the wounds are closed with either Integra or homografts (not meshed). If the axillary area is excised, the grafts or skin substitutes are secured with bolsters.

Wounds are dressed with petrolatum-impregnated fine-mesh gauze and burn dressings (large padded cotton-based dressings). Topical antimicrobial solutions may be used (i.e., silver nitrate, Sulfamylon). As an alternative, the wounds may be covered with Acticoat, a nanocrystalline silver nitrate dressing (petrolatum-impregnated fine-mesh gauze should then not be applied directly to the wound). It is normally necessary to change the outer burn dressings at 48–72 h because of oozing and exudates from the wound (burn wound edema). Splints are fabricated in the operating room before the patient is fully dressed. Patient may benefit from an air-fluidized bed if their back has been grafted or harvested.

The postoperative surgical plan differs depending on the wound closure strategy utilized:

Integra: Patients return 2–3 weeks following the first operation to start Integra grafting with super-thin (6/1000 inch) split-thickness skin autografts.

Autografts: Patients return at weekly intervals (for further autografting and change of homografts) until complete wound closure has been achieved. When patients' wounds are fully covered, an aggressive rehabilitation program is started (in the meantime, patients benefit from active and passive therapy between operations).

SERIAL OR SEQUENTIAL EARLY BURN WOUND EXCISION

Serial or sequential excision is less aggressive but its goal is to excise the whole burn wound within a week before colonization of burn wound by gram-negative bacteria has occurred.

Burn patients are resuscitated and burn wounds are treated with the application of silver sulfadiazine or cerium nitrate–silver sulfadiazine dressings for

48–72 h. Two to three days after the injury, patients–undergo surgical excision and closure of the wound. The burn wound is serially excised in sessions of up to 20–25% total body surface area burned. The patient returns then at 48 h intervals for further surgery until the whole burn has been excised.

Excision starts with large burned areas. The back is excised first in the first operation. If the back has not been burned, the excision starts with the anterior trunk and proceeds from major to minor areas until all burns are excised. The following is the orderly fashion of sequential or serial early burn wound excision. If one of the areas has not been burned, excision proceeds to the next area awaiting excision:

1. Back
2. Chest and abdomen
3. Lower limbs
4. Upper limbs
5. Face and neck (day 10)

After excision of one of the burned areas is completed, patients return to the burn intensive care unit where general treatment as per unit protocols is continued. Patients are stabilized and prepared for the next operative session. Nonexcised burns are treated with daily or twice-daily application of silver sulfadiazine or cerium nitrate–silver sulfadiazine creams. Patients should receive peroperative antibiotics based on burn unit sensitivities to prevent sepsis from bacterial translocation.

Massive burns are generally closed with Integra. If Integra is not to be used, the sandwich technique may be utilized, although mesh expansion of 2:1 up to 3:1 should be used in an attempt to minimize scarring. If Integra is not used, excised areas are closed with nonmeshed homografts, which are changed 7–15 days posthomografting.

Patients whose wounds have been closed with Integra, return generally between day 15 and 18 to undergo skin autografting (or day 21 or later if Integra viability is in doubt). If, on the other hand, the patient has been treated with sandwich technique or skin autografts and homografts, he or she returns weekly for further autografting and change of homografts.

As with patients treated with immediate burn wound excision, patients benefit from air-fluidized beds, splints, early physiotherapy, and aggressive rehabilitation following completion of wound closure.

CERIUM NITRATE–SILVER SULFADIAZINE (FLAMMACERIUM) AND DELAYED EXCISION AND AUTOGRAFTING

Excellent reports of patients with massive burns treated with cerium nitrate–silver sulfadiazine have been published by groups in France, Belgium, and the Netherlands.

The rationale for this regimen is based on preservation of cell-mediated immunity, a broad antimicrobial spectrum, and a calcification of the burn eschar, which, all together, have led to highly favorable mortality data in burn patients with very large, ostensibly lethal injuries.

Upon admission, patients are resuscitated and general treatment is started according to burn unit protocols. Burn wounds are debrided of blisters and loose debris, and cerium nitrate–silver sulfadiazine (Flammacerium) is applied. A generous application of the cream is necessary to cover the entire wound and allow penetration of the cerium nitrate in the wound. It is the author's experience that either silver sulfadiazine or cerium nitrate–silver sulfadiazine provides the best antimicrobial properties and eschar saturation if the antimicrobial creams are applied twice daily. During the first week after injury, patients undergo surgical donor site harvesting and areas of 10–15% total body surface area (TBSA) burn are excised and grafted. Patients are returned to the operating room when donor sites are healed for further autografting of limited burn areas. Unexcised burns continue to be treated with cerium nitrate–silver sulfadiazine.

GENERAL DISCUSSION

The burn wound is the source of almost all ill effects, local and systemic, seen in a burned patient. Surgical removal of the burn wound results in a much improved patient and, when done early, improvements in survival as well as in a decline in morbidity. Burn patients were treated conservatively for many decades, allowing the burn eschar to separate by the action of human and bacterial collagenases. Patients were admitted to the most isolated wards in the hospital, where pain, odor, and human misery were hidden. Those who survived their injuries were condemned to disfigurement and disability.

Although burn injuries are frequent in our society, many surgeons are uncomfortable in managing patients with major thermal trauma. With an overall incidence of more than 800 burn cases per 100,000 person/year, only motor vehicle accidents cause more accidental deaths than burns. During the past century, many lessons were learnt regarding the initial management, resuscitation, infection control, and local treatment of burns. Early in the 1960s, it was becoming plain that burn care is a complex enterprise involving many professional disciplines. From a logistical point of view, it was sensible to concentrate severely burned patients in the same ward so that an experienced team could be trained to provide Continuing care, both medical and psychosocial. Soon after, the development of new and more effective resuscitation formulas and the synthesis of silver sulfadiazine opened a new era in burn treatment. Severely burned patients were no longer doomed to death from burn shock or burn wound sepsis.

A new challenge, however, appeared on the horizon of burn care. Surgeons were faced with patients who survived beyond the initial phase of their injury, and definitive care of the burn wound began to be the main focus of all clinical and research efforts. Previously, nearly all large, deep burns had been treated expectantly: eschar was permitted to slough spontaneously, and open wounds were left to granulate. Split-thickness skin grafts were then applied, in a process that lasted weeks or, frequently, months before permanent wound closure could be achieved. Conservative treatment was recognized as being contrary to the fundamental principle in the treatment of other traumatic wounds learned during the two world wars: the prompt excision of all devitalized tissue. The debate remained hypothetical because of numerous practical clinical constraints. Then advances were made that changed the clinical environment: the availability of new powered dermatomes and mesh-expanding techniques, and sophisticated intraoperative and critical care monitoring. Pediatric burn patients have benefited most from this new era of early excision and grafting. Children present with the best survival rate among burn patients, with an excellent psychosocial adaptation to normal living.

The approach most used often in burn centers today throughout the world is the staged surgical wound closure. In this approach, unequivocally deep burns are excised at intervals of approximately 7 days, with immediate coverage of all exposed areas by autologous skin grafts. The timing of the first surgical procedure is dependent on the patient's physiological status and on the clinical estimate of burn depth. Burns that are left non-excised are usually treated with silver sulfadiazine or cerium nitrate–silver sulfadiazine. Early or immediate total excision has emerged as an alternative to staged surgical wound closure. This approach requires an experienced team and is logistically demanding of both personnel and resources. It has been claimed that this aggressive approach may increase catabolism and the inflammatory response, without real gains in patient survival. Moreover, it is generally believed that a short delay in surgical therapy is not harmful.

Early excision of the burn wound gained popularity in the early 1980s, when excising the entire wound within the first 2 weeks postinjury began to be feasible. The exact timing for wound excision, however, is still debatable. Many kinds of local wound treatments have been described, but the two main approaches described above are in use in most institutions.

Conservative treatment of burn wounds with 1% silver sulfadiazine or cerium nitrate sulfadiazine followed by serial excision of full-thickness burns is currently the standard of care in many burn centers throughout the world. Burns are excised in areas of as much as 20% total body surface area (TBSA) in one operative setting, and patients return to the operating room when donor sites are fully healed and ready to be harvested again. All full-thickness burns can be excised first. Deep dermal and indeterminate-depth wounds are addressed later, preventing excision of potentially viable tissue. Intraoperative and postoperative management of patients is easier, but the patient needs to return many times to the operation room. Episodes of bacterial translocation, bacteremia, and cardio-

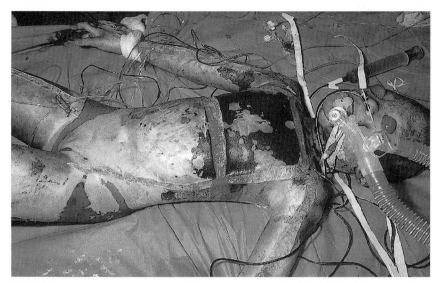

A

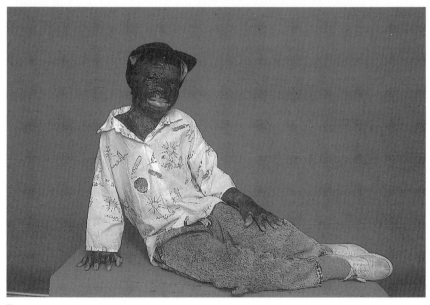

B

FIGURE 1 A patient with 95% TBSA burns (A) treated with immediate burn wound excision and grafting. Currently, all children and young adults are candidates for survival. No matter what surgical approach is utilized, the aim should be to obtain LD50 over 90% TBSA burned (B).

vascular instability are therefore repeated. Other disadvantages include exaggerated blood losses, prolongation of the hypermetabolic response, and increased risk of infection and sepsis from remaining eschar in which bacteria proliferate.

Immediate near-total wound excision has been advocated as an excellent alternative to serial debridement in patients with massive burns. All full-thickness and deep partial-thickness burns are excised within 24 h of admission, and the excised wounds are covered with autografts when feasible and homologous skin grafts or skin substitutes to other areas if the burn exceeds the donor-site supply. Infection control is easier. Burn eschars are excised completely so that burn wound sepsis is no longer the major cause of death in these patients. Potentially viable tissue, however, may be sacrificed with this technique. It has been postulated that the surgical trauma of immediate burn wound excision may aggravate the inflammatory and catabolic response, leading to potentially fatal complications. Furthermore, it is believed that the hemodynamic instability of burn patients during the first 72 h after the injury makes their surgical management more likely to lead to postoperative complications. Therefore, many authors still question the safety and efficacy of immediate burn-wound excision in patients with massive burns, preventing the spread of this technique.

Survival has increased dramatically during the past two decades. Reports from institutions that carry out programs of immediate burn wound excision and sequential burn wound excision have produced LD50 over 90% TBSA burned in children and young adults and over 40% in patients older than 60 years old.

No matter the approach used to manage the burn wound, the program should aim for these results. Currently, all young adults and children are candidates for survival (Fig. 1)

BIBLIOGRAPHY

1. Barret Juan P. Surgical management and hypermetabolic modulation of pediatric burns. Groningen. The Netherlands: University of Groningen, 2002.
2. Herndon David N. Total Burn Care. Second Edition. London. UK: W. B. Saunders, 2002.
3. Luce Edward A. Burn Care and Management. Clin Plast Surg 2000; 27(1).
4. Barret Juan P, Herndon David N. Color Atlas of Burn Care. London. UK: W. B. Saunders, 2001.
5. Wasserman D et al. Use of topically applied silver sulfadiazine plus cerium nitrate in major burns. Burns 1989; 15:257–260.
6. Boeckx W et al. Effect of cerium nitrate-silver sulphadiazine on deep dermal burns: a histological hypothesis. Burns 1992; 18:456–462.
7. Hermans RP. Topical treatment of serious infections with special reference to the use of a mixture of silver sulphadiazine and cerium nitrate: two clinical studies. Burns 1984; 11:59–62.

11

The Hand

Tomás Gómez-Cía and José I. Ortega-Martínez
Hospital Universitario Virgen del Rocío, Seville, Spain

INTRODUCTION

Resuscitation therapy in burn patients, early nutrition, topical treatment, and prophylaxis against burn wound infection and its complications, as performed by a multidisciplinary team of specialists in the burn units, have increased survival of burn patients [1,2]. Psychological support and pain therapy have improved adaptation to the accident, thus decreasing emotional sequelae.

The hands and the face are frequently involved in burn accidents. The functional repercussions of severe burns on the hands are obvious, and for this reason we believe that their correct treatment is very important. Thermal damage to the hands, patient's age, and percentage of burned body area requiring grafts are the determining factors of the patient's ability to return to his or her working situation [3].

Factors that increase the severity of burns of the upper limbs include bilateral involvement of hands, from causes such as flames, chemicals, or high-voltage electricity (greater than 1000 V), deep burns involving the dorsum of the fingers, and burns that are circumferential and/or causing inelastic wounds.

The primary objective of surgical treatment of burn patients is to increase survival. However, surgery is also necessary to achieve a greater degree of functionality of the burned areas, which has a considerable effect on the patient's life

[4]. Furthermore, burn surgery reduces treatment costs by reducing patients' length of hospital stay and the number of complications and sequelae.

TOPICAL TREATMENT

After stabilizing the patient correctly and diagnosing the extent and depth of the wounds and associated lesions, trauma, smoke inhalation, and other factors, we begin treatment with intravenous fluids. Our overall objective is to achieve permanent coverage of the burns as quickly as possible.

Topical treatment of burned hands is similar to that of the the rest of the body. The first step is to eliminate the causative agent, dissipate the heat, and reduce the temperature of the tissues in the first moments after the accident (cooling also reduces inflammation and relieves pain). This can be done by profusely flushing the burns (which is especially important with chemical burns), or removing the patient from contact with an electrical source. Local treatment of burns continues with the elimination of devitalized superficial tissue, such as blisters on the hands that have ruptured. Although there is controversy over the subject, we closely evaluate the evolution of blisters that have not ruptured, watching for secondary ruptures, symptoms of a secondary infection, or a delay in epithelialization, which would indicate a deep full-thickness burn. Once the patient is under analgesia, the wounds are profusely washed with a chlorhexidine gluconate soap. When there is a loss of epithelium, they are covered with a petrolatum-impregnated gauze and absorbent dressing. Each injured finger is bandaged individually, to allow greater mobility. When a topical antiseptic is necessary we prefer 1% silver sulfadiazine, which is effective against gram-positive and gram-negative bacteria, including *Pseudomonas spp*. Mafenide acetate is not available for clinical use in Spain, nor are silver nitrate solutions used commonly.

Full-thickness circumferential burns, especially those on the upper limbs, can cause compartment syndrome, which should be actively watched for in the initial hours following the accident with every change of dressing. When it is suspected, a decompresssion escharotomy should be performed (see below).

We emphasize to the patient the importance of postural drainage using early elevation and active mobilization of the affected extremity. If patients are unable to assist in their care due to their clinical condition, we place elastic traction at the zenith to hold the injured upper limb upwards [5].

Bandages are changed at least once a day in the first days, and more frequently if necessary. For outpatients with less severe burns, if there are no signs of infection or pain, dressings can be changed after up to 48 h.

SURGICAL TREATMENT

General principles

The scientific foundations of current surgical treatment of burn patients, early escharotomy, and wound coverage, were introduced in the late 1960s and early

1970s by various authors [6]. They became widespread during the 1980s and today are standard procedure in most burn units. Burns of the face and hands are considered to be areas of high priority for treatment.

Surgical treatment of burned hands is limited to deep dermal burns and full-thickness burns. It consists of surgical removal of the burned tissue and coverage of the wound. Depending upon the location of the burn, depth, and deep structures exposed after debriding, coverage of the burn will take the place of secondary epithelialization. A partial or full-thickness cutaneous graft and local or distant flaps are used; it will occasionally be necessary to use free flaps.

The objective is to provide cutaneous coverage within a maximum of 3 to prevent the appearance of inelastic and/or retractile scars, joint rigidity, pain, and functional weakness in the affected extremity [7]. There is controversy over the optimal time for surgical treatment of burned hands. Although there is consensus that early excision and grafting of the hands lead to better functional outcomes, some authors suggest that expectant treatment of burns of undetermined thickness followed by selective surgical debridement and coverage will reduce blood loss. This method avoids the removal of vital tissues and preserves donor areas, with acceptable functional results in the long term [8].

The main components of rehabilitative treatment in these patients are postural drainage of burned hands and splinting in the intrinsic plus position. The thumb is splinted in flexion and abducted when active or passive mobilization supervised by a physical therapist is not being performed [9].

As Robson advocated, the basic objectives of surgical treatment of the burned hand in the acute phase include [10,11] the following:

1. Do not cause damage.
2. Maintain circulation, avoiding edema if possible, performing the necessary escharotomies, especially in the case of high-voltage electrical burns, including fasciotomies in those cases.
3. Prevent infection by using adequate topical wound treatment and then proceed to early escharotomy of full-thickness burns.
4. Provide adequate coverage.
5. Preserve/recover mobility by appropriate splinting of the hands when active or passive mobilization is not being performed.
6. Rehabilitate function.

Strategies

In our burn unit, we follow the flow charts documented in Figure 1 for surgical treatment of hand burns.

Surgical treatment of hand burns depends on the depth and location of the wounds. Burns rarely require surgical treatment on the palm of the hand, except with very severe burns or electrical burns. However, the dorsum of the hand and

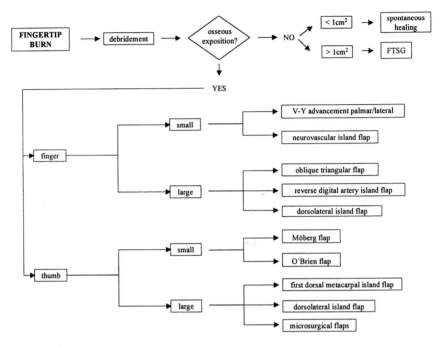

FIGURE 1   Flow chart for coverage of hand burns.

digits frequently require surgical debridement and appropriate cutaneous coverage.

Escharotomies

Compartment syndrome following burns

Compartment syndrome occurs when interstitial tissue pressure becomes greater than the perfusion pressure of the tissue as a result of inflammation and edema in a space that has reached its maximum distensibility (30 mmHg is considered the highest tolerable pressure). The upper limbs in general, and particularly the hands, are especially prone to this syndrome following a burn. This is because they are approximately tubular structures with a small diameter and are frequently affected with circumferential burns.

Various methods have been used to diagnose compartment syndrome. Intense, hard edema in the area of a full-thickness circumferential burn is highly suggestive of this complication. Surgical treatment, which involves decompression escharotomy with or without decompression of the carpal tunnel at the level of the wrist, should be performed urgently. In our unit, we do not perform invasive monitoring of this complication.

Surgical technique

Escharotomy of the burned hand is, in our opinion, an urgent and major surgical procedure. In our burn unit it is performed in the unit's surgery room with the collaboration of an anaesthetist and the necessary nursing staff.

The technique involves making longitudinal incisions in segments with inelastic circumferential burns, usually of full thickness. The areas of skin that are not burned are preserved. The incisions, all of which are interconnected, are made on the lateral aspect of the digits, the dorsum of the hand, and at the level of the forearm and the arm on their dorsal and volar aspects. With escharotomies at the level of the articular folds, the incisions should follow a sinuous path, which avoids later scars perpendicular to the folds and retraction.

In the case of high-voltage electrical burns with suspected compartment syndrome, the incisions should include the eschar and the deep fascia of each of the affected muscle compartments, beyond the cutaneous burn lesion.

With circumferential burns of the wrist and with severe electrical burns, we suggest performing a carpal retinaculotomy to release the median nerve at the level of this anatomical gap.

It is vital to maintain careful hemostasis using ligatures and/or an electroscalpel after making the drainage incisions. Otherwise, it will often be necessary to establish hemostasis again later on in the treatment of the wound.

After performing the escharotomy of the upper extremity, we then generally use a loose elastic suture with a vessel-loop in a fixed zigzag pattern, using clips at the borders of the incision. Several days after the decompression escharotomy, when the danger of compartment syndrome has passed, the ends of the elastic sutures are subjected to progressive traction, which will approximate the edges of the escharotomy. This favors a progressive closure of the exposed surface and decreases subsequent scarring as a result of decompression.

Justification

The clinical justifications for an early escharectomy have been described in other chapters.

The hands constitute approximately 4% of the adult body surface. Therefore, early escharectomy of burned hands on a patient with extensive, life-threatening burns may not be a priority from a systemic point of view. However, from a functional standpoint, the hands, as well as the face, are of high priority since they help determine the quality of life for patients who survive.

We, therefore, believe that surgical treatment in the form of an escharectomy of deep partial-thickness burns and full-thickness burns of the hands should be undertaken as soon as possible.

Surgical techniques

Methodology. The escharectomy of the burned hand is considered a major surgical procedure. It is performed under general anesthesia or with an axillary block when feasible, alone, or in association with other surgical procedures to remove devitalized tissue. It is, therefore, indicated for patients with deep partial-thickness and full-thickness burns. This should take place early: after the third day in patients with hemodynamic instability following the accident, and before that in patients with isolated burns of the hands [12,13].

Two methodologies have been identified: tangential escharectomy, which is more commonly used, and escharectomy, at the fascial level.

Tangential escharectomy. This method, which is described in detail in other chapters in this book, is also the method of choice for burned hands. Aspects of this anatomical zone that differ from other areas of the body are the possibility of performing the procedure under ischemic conditions using a pneumatic tourniquet. This procedure requires a modification of the criteria for a sufficient escharectomy since we eliminate bleeding as an indicator of having reached the level of healthy tissue. We are also faced with the difficulty of performing the procedure in the interdigital spaces and on the dorsal aspect of the digits, which makes it appropriate to use smaller dermatomes (such as the Goulian dermatome). If it has not been affected, it is essential to preserve the areolar connective tissue covering the deep structures of the dorsum of the hand and digits. This is essential for recovery of the wounded area with the use of cutaneous grafts.

To promote hemostasis, we use electrocoagulation or sutures, elevation of the extremity being operated on, and compression bandages soaked in a 1:250,000 solution of epinephrine in crystaloid solution as a hemostatic agent. We do not have experience in the use of topical clotting factors. Careful maintenance of hemostasis is particularly important on the dorsum of the hand and digits, which are anatomical areas where venous drainage occurs and may bleed profusely during a tangential escharectomy.

Tangential escharectomy of the dorsum of the hand and digits has clear advantages over escharectomy at the fascial level, especially with deep partial-thickness burns. Preserving tissues that remain viable beneath the eschar promotes faster wound healing. This will lead to reduced hospital stays and associated costs and, most importantly, reduced incidence of secondary and hypertrophic scarring, providing good functional results after coverage with cutaneous grafts.

Escharectomy at the fascial level. Escharectomy at the fascial level can be used for full-thickness hand burns that have defined limits. This method is sometimes associated with digital amputation. The surgical technique, which has been described in other chapters, does not differ with the hands. We again wish to emphasize the importance of maintaining very careful hemostasis. Following this kind of escharectomy, deep structures of the hands and digits, such as extensor tendons lacking tendon sheaths or interdigital joints, are often exposed, and this determines wound coverage. In this circumstance, cutaneous grafts would not be indicated, which makes it necessary to use flaps of some type.

Coverage

Temporary coverage

Once the escharectomy is complete, it is important to provide coverage for the wound to prevent desiccation and the resulting increase in depth of the wound with the appearance of new eschars. The treatment of choice for coverage of hand burns after an escharectomy is usually a cutaneous graft taken from the patient. When the condition of the patient or the wound requires it, or when cutaneous graft donor areas are very scarce, we cover the wound with temporary dressings. However, we consider the face and hands to be priorities in the surgical treatment of burn patients, and are therefore less limited by these conditions.

Some of the materials used, in order of preference, include the following:

Biological substitutes
  Cadaveric skin: fresh, cryopreserved, or preserved in glycerol
  Cryopreserved amniotic membrane
  Porcine xenografts
Biosynthetic wound dressing: Biobrane (Woodruff Labs, Santa Ana, CA, USA).
Bioengineered skin substitutes
  Epidermal substitutes: Autologous keratinocyte cultures, such as Epicel (Genzyme, Cambridge, MA, USA)
Dermal substitutes
  Transcyte (Smith and Nephew, Largo, FL)
  Integra Artificial Skin (Integra Life Sciences, Plainsboro, NJ, USA)
  Alloderm (Lifecell, Woodland, TX, USA)
  Oasis (Cook, Spencer, IN, USA)
  Dermal–epidermal substitutes: Apligraf (Organogenesis, Canton, MA, USA)

For a more complete description of these substitutes, which are rarely used on hand burns in our unit, we refer the reader to other chapters in this volume.

Definitive coverage

Deep, partial-thickness burns and full-thickness burns require permanent coverage of the wound.

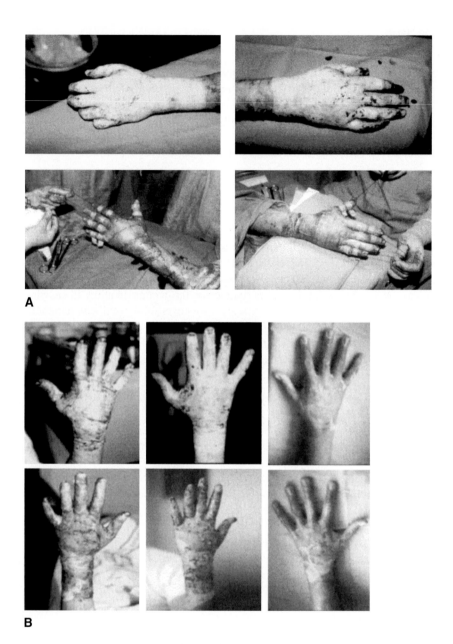

A

B

FIGURE 2 Partial-thickness, intermediate-width laminar cutaneous grafts are the most frequent indication for coverage of the burned hand after a tangential eschare-ctomy. We have found adhesive sutures to be useful for securing the graft on the digits. The definitive results should be evaluated once the phase of secondary scarring has been completed, between 6 and 12 months after the burn in cases in which hypertrophic scarring does not occur.

264

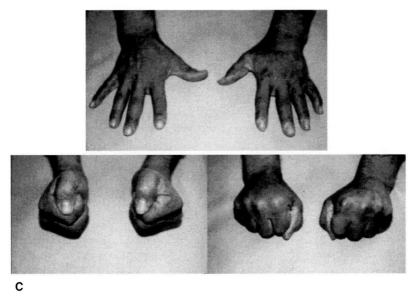

C

FIGURE 2 (Cont.)

Cutaneous grafts. The recovery method of choice for deep burns of the hands following an early escharectomy includes cutaneous grafts taken from the same patient [19]. Limitations in the amount of available cutaneous graft donor areas should not be, in our opinion, a restriction against using them on the hand.

The surgical technique for collecting and placing cutaneous grafts has been described in detail in other chapters.

A thinner cutaneous graft will be better accepted. However, a thicker graft will cause less secondary scar retraction, which is especially relevant when treating burned hands on children [14]. Full-thickness cutaneous grafts may be indicated for hand burns in areas that are sensitive to secondary contraction, especially with pediatric patients. There does not appear to be any significant difference in the functional results of treatment by cutaneous coverage of burned hands based on the thickness of the grafts used on adults. The recommended graft thickness is at least 0.015 inches, with no apparent advantage in using very thick grafts of up to 0.025 inches [11]. Graft expansion methods are generally not indicated for burned hand coverage, since the area to be covered is not extensive. This ensures the quality of the resulting scar.

When placing these cutaneous grafts, we have found that adhesive sutures for coverage of the digits of the burned hand are especially useful (Fig. 2), together with individual bandaging of each digit using well-fitted petrolatum-impregnated gauze. It is very important to splint the hand and digits in the intrinsic plus position, with the thumb in flexion, opposition, and abduction. Some authors suggest placing the hand in fist position when placing the graft because they believe that the amount of graft material needed can be better estimated [15,16].

When the digital extensors, ligamentous apparatus, or joints have been damaged, we use internal splinting of the affected segment using K-wires until the wound has healed.

We examine laminar grafts of the hands 24 hours after surgery to eliminate seromas and hematomas, which may accumulate beneath the graft, and to apply a new nonadherent bandage.

Grafted hands should be elevated with respect to the position of the patient's body by placing them on a pillow or by elastic traction above the patient, and splinted in the position described previously. Occasionally, skeletal traction may be useful alone or in association with devices such as the ukelele, horseshoe, or others.

Once the graft is secure, the patient should then begin active and passive mobilization of the joints of the digits, hand, and wrist. A splint is used to maintain the correct position of the hand while the patient is resting.

Flaps. If deep structures are exposed, such as tendon lacking a peritenon, bone lacking periosteum, joints, or nerves, after burn debridement, cutaneous grafts are not indicated. In such cases, it is necessary to use local flaps, distal flaps, or occasionally free flaps [17].

LOCAL FLAPS. Local flaps are primarily indicated for the treatment of burned digits. In addition to the classic flaps, based on a proximal, random, or axial vascular pedicle, proximal cutaneous regions based on distal vascular pedicles using inverse flow are also useful.

Cutaneous losses in the pulp of the long digits occurs frequently with low-voltage electrical burns in children. When bone is not exposed and the injury is less than 1 cm^2, it is justifiable, in our opinion, to take a conservative approach and allow the wound to close by spontaneous scarring. If the injury is greater than 1 cm^2, it may be covered with full-thickness skin graft.

If bone is exposed, and if the injury is small, we identify two distinct approaches: If the injury is perpendicular or bevelled dorsally, we can use the V-Y advancement palmar flap [18,19], which is based on the ascending arteries that branch off of the distal central artery of the pulp. If the injury is bevelled obliquely on the palmar surface, we do not use tissue from the part distal to the pulp and proximal to the injury. We use tissue lateral to the pulp by means of the V-Y advancement lateral flap [20]. The advancement–rotation quadrangular flap [21] may also be used to close such small injuries. The difficulty with this technique is that the area that is most damaged, which is the part that must cover the end distal to the pulp, is the least sensitive part of the flap.

These three flaps have the advantage of being simple, but they provide less sensation than the neurovascular island flap [22]. This flap involves V-Y displacement of the side of the digit that includes the complete collateral pedicle from the side of the injury. For this reason, most authors consider this the method of choice for such injuries. This type of flap is indicated especially for perpendicular injuries. However, even if the injury is oblique, it is preferable to use a modification of this method: the so-called modified triangular flap [23]. This type of flap is very similar to that just described: it differs in that it involves a more oblique palmar incision, which provides more skin from the palmar aspect of the middle phalanx. An alternative to the previous method is the dorsolateral island flap [24], which is based on small arteries that exit the collateral artery distally to supply the dorsum of the distal phalanx and allow that skin area to be included in the flap. The difficulty with this flap is that skin on the dorsum of the hand is of poor quality for reconstruction of the pulp compared to the skin of the palm or the lateral aspect of the digit. For this reason, another possibility in such cases is to cut a flap in the skin on the lateral aspect of the proximal phalanx, based distally on the collateral pedicle of that side, and invert it distally toward the pulp. This is the reverse digital artery island flap [25]. Blood reaches the flap from the collateral artery of the other side via the distal arcades that connect both collateral arteries near the ends of the phalanges. The proximal end of the collateral nerve in the flap is sutured, if possible, to the sectioned distal end of the collateral nerve of the other side of the digit, thus increasing its sensitivity.

When none of these flaps can be used because the skin of the affected digit has also been burned, we use an adjacent digit by means of a heterodigital reversed-flow neurovascular island flap [26] or a ''boomerang'' flap [27]. Both flaps are based on an anastomosis between the palmar collateral system and the dorsal arterial network of the finger. In the rare case in which none of these flaps is available, we use a cross-finger flap to provide coverage of the pulp of a long digit.

If an injury of the pulp of the thumb is not more than 2 cm^2, we have the choice of two different neurovascular palmar advancement flaps [28,29]. Unlike on the long digits, the dorsal skin of the thumb is supplied by two dorsal collateral arteries. This allows us to separate the skin on the palmar surface of the thumb completely from that of the dorsum and advance it distally to cover injuries of the pulp without fear of causing necrosis of the skin on the dorsal surface. The Möberg flap uses flexion of the metacarpal–phalangeal joint to advance all the skin of the palmar surface towards the pulp. O'Brien [29] cuts a proximal flap based on both palmar pedicles and covers the secondary injury with a skin graft. If the burn is large, we can use the dorsolateral island flap [30], which has an identical vascular base and design to Joshi's flap for the long digits [24], or we can use the first dorsal metacarpal artery island flap [31] if the injury is even larger, since the latter can cover almost the entire palmar surface of the thumb. More complicated flaps for thumb pulp reconstruction are described in the literature. These methods require microsurgical technique and include the wraparound flap [32], the great toe pulpfree flap, the sensate medial plantar free flap [33], and the free palmaris brevis musculocutaneous flap [34], among others.

To provide coverage for injuries to the palmar surface of the proximal phalanges, we use tissues that provide stability. Sensitivity is less crucial in this area. When possible, while performing reconstruction, we preserve functional units and keep in mind the main arterial supplies of each digit (the collateral cubital artery for the first three digits, and the radial for the fourth and fifth). For deep burns that are small, the advancement–rotation quadrangular flap may be used. For larger burns of the long digits, the injury can be covered with a laterodigital island flap or with a cross-finger flap. For coverage of the proximal phalanx of the thumb, the flap of choice is the first dorsal metacarpal artery island flap (Fig. 3). It is also possible to use the second dorsal metacarpal artery island flap or a pulp finger heterodigital island flap, usually from the fourth finger, when the two previous ones are not available.

For injuries of the dorsal surface of the digits of limited size, we can use the advancement–rotation quadrangular flap or the bipedicle strap flap [35] (longitudinal or transverse). If the injury is distal to the proximal interphalangeal (PIP) joint, we can also use the adipofascial turnover flap [35a]. When we do not have healthy tissue located proximally on the same digit to cut this flap, we must use skin from the dorsal surface of an adjacent digit by means of a heterodigi-

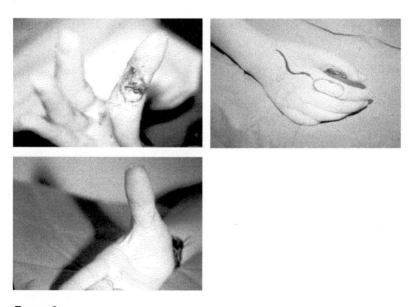

FIGURE 3

tal reverse-flow neurovascular island flap, a so-called boomerang flap, or a de-epithelialized cross-finger flap.

For injuries distal to the PIP joint, the available options are the reverse dorsal digital flap [36,37] and the de-epithelialized cross-finger flap. If the injury is very large, we must mobilize healthy tissue from the skin on the dorsal surface of the hand. The existence of communicating arteries between the palmar and dorsal vascular systems of the hand at the level of the commissures or near the ends of the metacarpal bones allows us to cut reverse-flow flaps in the dorsum of the hand and cover cutaneous injuries of the dorsal surface of the digits. These are the commisural perforators flap [38] and the dorsal metacarpal reverse-flow flaps [39]. These flaps are indicated for proximal injuries since their coverage area does not reach beyond the PIP joint. For injuries distal to the PIP joint that cannot be covered with an adipofascial turnover flap due to the size of the injury, we can use the dorsal digitometacarpal flap [40], based on the proximal dorsal cutaneous branches of the digital collateral arteries through the anastomotic arterial network of the webspace.

For large injuries covering nearly the entire dorsal surface of a digit, we can use a U-I flap [41]. This flap uses skin from the dorsal surface of the hand and is based on the existing communicating branches between the second dorsal intermetacarpal artery and the palmar system. Its vascular axis is the second dorsal intermetacarpal artery, the dorsal arch of the carpus, the dorsal branch of the radial artery, and the first dorsal intermetacarpal artery.

To cover injuries on the dorsal surface of the thumb, we use the first dorsal metacarpal artery island flap, although we can also use the second dorsal metacarpal artery island flap when the second digit is also burned.

The lack of mobility allowed by the skin of the palm of the hand makes it impossible to cut local flaps from this area. This changes in the case of the dorsal surface of the hand due to the elasticity of the skin in this area. Random flaps, such as the rotation flap, the bipedicle flap, or the rhomboidal flap, can be used to close small and moderately sized injuries.

If none of these flaps will work for the injury being treated, we use an axial flap. The most frequently used in this area are those based on anastomoses between the dorsal and palmar intermetacarpal systems [38,39], the commisural perforator flap and the dorsal metacarpal flaps, and the first dorsal metacarpal artery island flap.

DISTANT FLAPS.   For more extensive full-thickness burns where a cutaneous graft is not indicated, we use distant flaps. Burns occasionally cause so much tissue destruction that burn coverage using local flaps is not a viable option.

The groin flap, as described by McGregor and Jackson in 1972, based on the pedicle of the superficial circumflex iliac artery, has frequently been used to treat soft tissue injuries of the dorsum of the hand and digits [42]. Syndactylization usually results, which necessitates a subsequent surgical procedure to separate the reconstructed digits. The lateral thoracic wall, and even the contralateral arm, have also been used as donor areas for this type of flap. The need to wait at least 3 weeks until the second surgery and the separation of the flap from its donor tissue make it very difficult to care for the burned limbs and prevent proper mobilization therapy and splinting. This tends to result in chronic edema of the burned hand. For these reasons these flaps are increasingly being replaced by regional fasciosubcutaneous flaps, or free flaps, for coverage of complex injuries of the limbs.

Some very useful examples are fascial axial flaps, fasciosubcutaneous flaps, or reverse-flow fasciocutaneous flaps based on the radial, cubital [43], or posterior interosseous arteries for hand coverage. These flaps also allow the transfer of segments of tendon, muscle, or bone, which adds great versatility to reconstruction methods. Its zone of coverage may even reach the ends of the digits.

The reverse-flow radial flap, as described by Lu in 1982, is a modification of the free antebrachial fasciocutaneous flap described by Yang in 1978 [44]. It is a flap based on the septal perforating branches of the vascular system of the radial artery, perfused in a retrograde direction from the palmar arch, whose permeability is tested preoperatively using the Allen test. Venous drainage occurs in a retrograde fashion through the concomitant radial veins, which occasionally creates initial signs of venous congestion that later disappear. It is very important to exercise maximum caution while dissecting the fascial wall to avoid damaging the superficial branches of the radial nerve in the distal third of the forearm. Figure 4 shows an example of the placement of this flap in the treatment of a severe hand burn.

The reverse-flow cubital flap, described by Jin in 1985, is very similar to the one just described and is used less frequently since it is considered the main vascular supply to the hand. The feasible cutaneous territory of this flap is less than the flap based on the pedicle of the radial artery.

The reverse-flow fasciocutaneous flap based on the posterior interosseous artery was described by Zancolli and Angriniani in 1985. Blood flow arrives in a retrograde fashion to the septocutaneous perforating branches from the posterior interosseous artery via the communicating branch, with the anterior interosseous artery located distally in the forearm. This is indicated specifically for treatment of deep burns of the thumb, the first commissure, and the dorsum of the hand (Fig. 5).

In 1988, Ching described the anatomical basis for the antebrachial fascio-subcutaneous flap distally based on septocutaneous perforating branches of the radial and cubital arteries the level of the distal third of the forearm, with the preservation of the integrity of these vascular axes. These flaps are useful for coverage of complex distal injuries of the forearm and hand. The inverted flap is covered with a cutaneous graft.

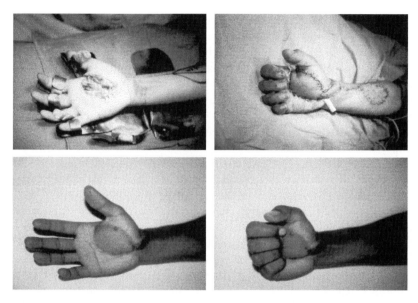

FIGURE 4   Reverse-flow radial flap for treatment of a hand burn.

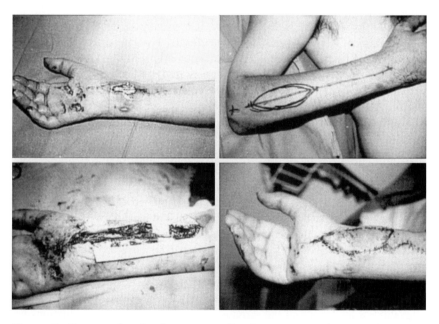

FIGURE 5   Reverse-flow fasciocutaneous flap for coverage of a burned hand.

FREE FLAPS. When tissue destruction prevents the use of local or distant flaps and when, necessary for reconstruction, free flaps are indicated for treatment of burned hands. Using microsurgical techniques, it is possible to transfer in a single surgical procedure the tissue necessary for optimal coverage of the exposed blood vessels, nerves, tendons, joints, or bones. This helps reduce the risk of deep infection and necrosis of the exposed soft tissue structures and facilitates early movement of the burned extremity [45]. This is especially relevant for the treatment of patients who have suffered high-voltage electrical burns of the upper limbs [46].

Coverage of the burned hand requires the use of tissues that are not very thick. The existence of this with a fascial component in the flap that allows sliding of the exposed deep structures is another advantage of free flaps.

The free radial fasciocutaneous flap, described by Yang in 1981, provides excellent coverage with a thin, pliable tissue with a fascial component on its deep surface. It can be reinervated from the antebrachial nerves. Its vascular pedicle is constant, of large caliber, and has supplementary drainage through the superficial veins of the forearm. This type of flap is contraindicated when the Allen test shows insufficient vascular supply from the cubital system and the posterior interosseous of the hand [26,47] or when the skin of the donor region of the forearm has been burned. We do not reconstruct the radial artery after extracting the flap, and we have not observed any case of poor perfusion of the hand of the donor extremity. In occasional cases, scarring of the flap donor area is delayed, with partial losses of the cutaneous graft; it is usually sufficient to administer topical treatment alone to promote wound closure. For a detailed description of the anatomy and steps of operation for extraction of this flap and those to follow, we refer the reader to the text on microsurgery by Dr. Buncke [48]. In Figure 6, we present an example of the use of the free radial fasciocutaneous flap for coverage using a single surgical procedure of a deep burn on the palm of the hand. The functional results in the long term were excellent, with stable and sensitive coverage.

Of the free muscular flaps, the free flap of the anterior serratus muscle, described simultaneously in 1982 by Buncke [48] and by Takayanagi, provides great plasticity and a constant vascular pedicle of good size and length. When covered with a cutaneous graft, stable and long-lasting coverage is achieved. We use the last three muscular digitations for coverage of hand burn injuries that are not very extensive and that require coverage with high vascular density per gram of tissue supplied. They are especially indicated for coverage of high-voltage electrical burn wounds of the wrist, which may sometimes be corrected in association with nerve grafts in the same procedure (Fig. 7). We emphasize the technical difficulties we often encounter when dissecting out the vascular pedicle from the bifurcation of the branch of the serratus and its entrance into the digitations we are going to transfer.

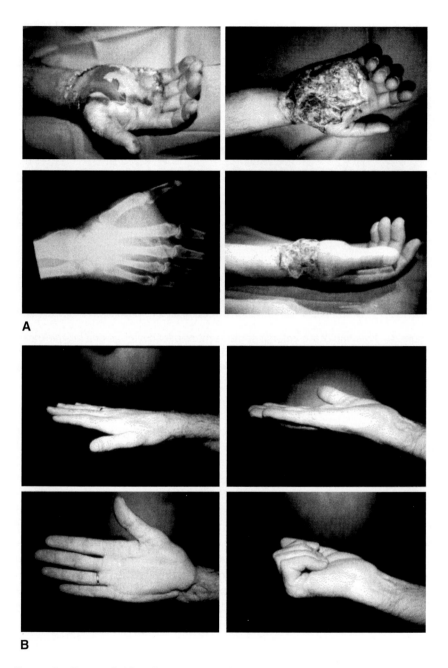

FIGURE 6 Free radial flap for coverage of a hand with a full-thickness burn from contact with a hot solid. There are osseous lesions at the second metacarpal bone and affecting the palmar arch. Excellent functional results: stable and sensitive coverage 2 years after the accident following only one surgical procedure (A, B).

273

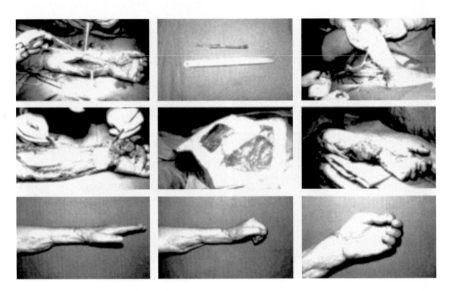

Figure 7 Free flap of the anterior serratus muscle for coverage of a full-thickness injury of the wrist from high-voltage limited electrical burn. A segment of the median nerve has been excised, and a sural nerve graft placed. Excellent functional results 2 years after the accident.

To cover large burn injuries of the upper extremity, we use a free flap of the latissimus dorsi muscle covered by a cutaneous graft. Described by Maxwell in 1978, this flap is still in common use today due to its versatility, accessibility, and ability to provide filling and coverage for large injuries. The vascular system of the donor area is also from the subscapular–thoracodorsal artery (Fig. 8).

The free temporal fascia flap, first described by Smith in 1979, is based on the axis of the superficial temporal arteries and veins and allows coverage of burn injuries on the dorsal surface of the digits and hand. It provides well-vascularized coverage that is extremely thin and flexible and leaves a barely visible cosmetic defect on the scalp. The transferred temporal fascia, which easily allows a partial-thickness cutaneous graft, permits sliding of the deep structures of the digits and hand. A second surgical procedure is occasionally necessary to separate the syndactylized digits (Fig. 9).

OTHER PROCEDURES

Placing the affected extremity in an elevated position, avoiding articular contractures with proper splinting, and limiting movement with proper therapy are crucial for the prevention of hand burn sequelae. In our opinion, it is essential

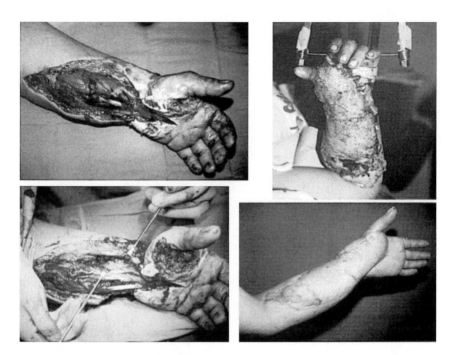

FIGURE 8   Free flap of the latissimus dorsi muscle for reconstruction of a large injury on the volar surface of the forearm from a high-voltage electrical burn. The functional results were poor due to severe tissue destruction.

to have collaboration with the physical medicine and rehabilitation services. Only a multidisciplinary group effort will be able to prevent the occurrence of sequelae and the need for secondary reconstruction of the hands of these patients.

The ideal position for the burned hand depends on the location and depth of the burns. With dorsal and/or circumferential burns, the correct position is in the intrinsic plus (metacarpophalangeal [MCP] joints 50–70 degrees of flexion, interphalangeal [IP] joints in extension), with the thumb in opposition and abducted. The wrist should remain in slight extension. With deep burns of the palm of the hand, it is preferable to place the MCP and IP joints in extension, with the thumb and all the other digits in abduction. The position can be maintained using the appropriate splints. If that does not work, internal fixation using K-wires may be used.

Prevention of hypertrophic scarring requires a correct initial diagnosis that makes possible coverage of the burned hands as soon as possible: within 2 or 3 weeks at the most. With deep burns on the hands, it is important to begin treatment as soon as possible with pressotherapy, especially if the healing process has been

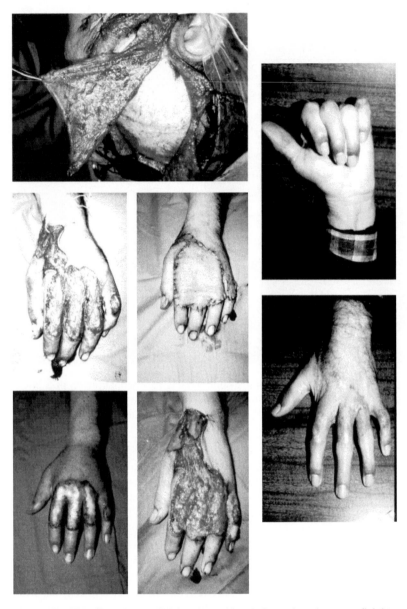

Figure 9 Free flap of superficial temporal fascia based on the superficial temporal arteries and veins for coverage of a burn from contact with a hot solid on the dorsal surface of digits II, III, and IV of the hand. A second surgical procedure was necessary to correct the surgical syndactyly produced by the fascial flap and the graft. The functional results were better than those of the fifth digit, where the burn over the joint was grafted with a thick graft because the burn was more superficial than those of the other digits.

276

delayed or when there is a personal or family history of hypertrophic scarring. In the acute phase, in addition to postural treatment and mobilization, elastic bandaging in strips or tubular forms may be used to decrease edema. Compressive bandages made to fit are the treatment of choice. They should be used for at least 6 months after the burn, and often for longer, until we observe flattening of the scars, which will progressively lose their bright red color and will become softer and more pliable.

REFERENCES

1. Gómez-Cía T, Mallén L, Marquez T, Portela C, Lopez I. Mortality according to age and burned body surface in the Hospital Universitario Virgen del Rocío. Burns 1999; 25:317–323.
2. Gómez Cía T, Franco A, Gimeno M, Fernández-Mota A, et al. Mortality of the pediatric burn population treated at the Virgen del Rocío University Hospital, Seville, Spain in the period 1968 1999. Ann Burns Fire Dis 2000; 13(2).
3. Wrigley M, Trofman K, Dimick A, et al. Factors relating to the return to work after burn injury. J Burn Care Rehab 1995; 16:445–450.
4. Sheridan RL, Baryza MJ, Pessina MA, O'Neill KM, Cipullo HM, Donelan MB, Ryan CM, Schulz JT, Schnitzer JJ, Tompkins RG. Acute hand burns in children: management and long-term outcome based on a 10-year experience with 698 injured hands. Ann Surg 1999; 229(4):558–64.
5. McCauley RL. Reconstruction of the pediatric burned hand. Hand Clin 2000; 16(2): 249–259.
6. Janzekovic Z. A new concept in the early excision and immediate grafting of large burns. J Trauma 1970; 10:1103–1108.
7. Barret JP, Desai MH, Herndon DN. The isolated burned palm in children: epidemiology and long-term sequelae. Plast Reconstr Surg 2000; 105(3):949–952.
8. Zuijlen PP, Kreis RW, Vloemans AF, Groenevelt F, Mackie DP. The prognostic factors regarding long-term functional outcome of full-thickness hand burns. Burns 1999; 25(8):709–714.
9. Barillo DJ, Harvey KD, Hobbs CL, Mozingo DW, Cioffi WG, Pruitt BA. Prospective outcome analysis of a protocol for the surgical and rehabilitative management of burns to the hands. Plast Reconstr Surg 1997; 100(6):1442–1451.
10. Robson MC, Smith DJ, VanderZee AJ. Making the burned hand functional. Clin Plast Surg 1992; 19(3):663–771.
11. Robson MC. Plastic Surgery: Principles and Practice. St. Louis: Mosby-Year Book, 1990.
12. Heimback D. Early burn excision and grafting. Surg Clin North Am 1987; 67: 93–107.
13. Herndon D, Barrow R, Rutan R, et al. A comparison of conservative versus early excision: therapies in severely burned patients. Ann Surg 1989; 209:547–552.
14. Pham TN, Hanley C, Palmieri T, Greenhalgh DG. Results of early excision and full-thickness grafting of deep palm burns in children. J Burn Care Rehabil 2001; 22(1): 54–57.

15. Burm JS, Chung CH, Oh SJ. Fist position for skin grafting on the dorsal hand: I. Analysis of length of the dorsal hand surgery in hand positions. Plast Reconstr Surg 1999; 104(5):1350–1355.

16. Burm JS, Oh SJ. Fist position for skin grafting on the dorsal hand: II. Clinical use in deep burns and burn scar contractures. Plast Reconstr Surg 2000; 105(2):581–588.

17. Barillo DJ, Arabitg R, Cancio LC, Goodwin CW. Distant pedicle flaps for soft tissue coverage of severely burned hands: an old idea revisited. Burns 2001; 27(6):613–619.

18. Atasoy E, Iokamidis E, Kasdan M, Kutz JE, Kleinert HE. Reconstruction of the amputated fingertip with a triangular volar flap. J Bone Jt Surg 1970; 52(A):921–926.

19. Logsetty S, Heimbach DM. Modern techniques for wound coverage of the thermally injured upper extremity. Hand Clin 2000; 16(2):205–214.

19a. Tranquilli-Leali E. Reconstruzione dell'apice delle falangi vaguali mediante autoplastica volare pedunculata per scorimento. Infort Traum Lavoro 1935; 1:186–193.

20. Kutler W. A new method for fingertip amputation. JAMA 1947; 13:29–30.

21. Hueston JT. Local flap repair of fingertip injuries. Plast Reconstr Surg 1966; 37(4): 135–139.

22. Littler JW. The neurovascular pedicle method of digital transposition for reconstruction of the hand. Plast Reconstr Surg 1953; 12:303–319.

23. Venkataswami DR, Subramanian N. Oblique triangular flap: a new method for repair oblique amputations of the fingertip and thumb. Plast Reconstr Surg 1980; 66(2): 296–230.

24. Joshi BB. A local dorsolateral island flap for restoration of sensation after avulsion injury of the fingertip pulp. Plast Reconstr Surg 1974; 54(2):175–182.

25. Garcia-Sanchez V, Gomez Morell P. Electric burns: high- and low-tension injuries. Burns 1999; 25(4):357–360.

25a. Han SK, Lee BI, Kim WK. The reverse digital artery island flap: clinical experience in 120 fingers. Plast Reconstr Surg 1999; 103(3):1095–1096.

26. Adani R, Busa R, Scagni R, Mingione A. The heterodigital reversed flow neurovasclar island flap for fingertip injuries. J Hand Surg (Br) 1999; 24(4):431–436.

27. Legaillard P, Grangier Y, Casoli V, Martin D, Baudet J. Boomerang flap. A true single-stage pedicled cross finger flap. Ann Chir Plast Esthet 1996; 41(3):251–258.

28. Macht SD, Watson HK. The Möberg volar advancement flap for digital reconstruction. J Hand Surg 1980; 5(4):373–376.

29. O'Brien B. Neurovascular island flaps for terminal amputations and digital scars. Br J Plast Surg 1968; 21:258–61.

30. Pho RW. Local composite neurovascular island flap for skin cover in pulp loss of the thumb. J Hand Surg 1979; 4(A):11–15.

31. Foucher G, Braun JB. A new island flap in the surgery of the hand. Plast Reconstr Surg 1979; 63:28–31.

32. Lee KS, Park JW, Chung WK. Thumb reconstruction with a wrap-around free flap according to the level of amputation. J Hand Surg 2000(A); 25(4):644–50.

33. Lee HB, Tark KC, Rah DK, Shin KS. Pulp reconstruction of fingers with very small sensate medial plantar free flap. Plast Reconstr Surg 1998; 101(4):999–1005.

34. Xu Y, Li Z, Li Q. Repair of pulp defect of thumb by free palmaris brevis musculocutaneous flap. Zhong Xiu Fu 1997; 11(5):293–295.

35. Yii NW, Elliot D. Bipedicle strap flaps in reconstruction of longitudinal dorsal skin defects of the digits. Plast Reconstr Surg 1999; 103(4):1205–1211.

35a. Lai CS, Lin SD, Yang CC, Chou CK. The adipofascial turn-over flap for complicated dorsal skin defects of the hand and finger. Br J Plast Surg 1991; 44(3):165–169.

36. Yang D, Morris SF. Reversed dorsal digital and metacarpal island flaps supplied by the dorsal cutaneous branches of the palmar digital artery. Ann Plast Surg 2001; 46(4):444–449.

37. Pelissier P, Casoli V, Bakhach J, Martin D, Baudet J. Reverse dorsal digital and metacarpal flaps: a review of 27 cases. Plast Reconstr Surg 1999; 103(1):159–65.

38. Quaba AA, Davidson PM. The distally based dorsal hand flap. Br J Plast Surg 1990; 43:28–39.

39. Early MJ. The arterial supply of the thumb, first web and index finger and its surgical application. J Hand Surg 1986; 11(B):2.

39a. Early MJ, Millner RH. Dorsal metacarpal flaps. Br J Plast Surg 1987; 40:333–341.

40. Bakhach J, Demiri E, Conde A, Baudet J. Dorsal metacarpal flap with a retrograde pedicle. Anatomic study and 22 clinical cases. Ann Chir Plast Esthet 1999; 44(2): 185–193.

41. Karacalar A, Ozcan M. U-I flap. Plast Reconstr Surg 1998; 102(3):741–747.

42. Rasheed T, Hill C, Riaz M. Innovations in flap design: modified groin flap for closure of multiple finger defects. Burns 2000; 26(2):186–189.

43. Grobbelaar AO, Harrison DH. The distally based ulnar artery island flap in hand reconstruction. J Hand Surg [Br] 1997; 22(2):204–211.

44. Yang D, Morris SF. Reversed dorsal digital and metacarpal island flaps supplied by the dorsal cutaneous branches of the palmar digital artery. Ann Plast Surg 2001; 46(4):444–449.

45. Takeuchi M, Nozaki M, Sasaki K, Nakazawa H, Sakurai H. Microsurgical reconstruction of the thermally injured upper extremity. Hand Clin. 2000; 16(2):261–269 IX.

46. Tredget EE, Shankowsky HA, Tilley WA. Electrical injuries in Canadian burn care. Identification of unsolved problems. Ann NY Acad Sci 1999; 888:75–87.

47. Ciria G, Gómez Cía T. Hand blood supply in radial forearm flap donor extremities: a qualitative analysis using doppler examination. J Hand Surg 2001; 26B(2):125–128.

48. Buncke HJ. Microsurgery: Transplantation–replantation. An Atlas Text. Philadelphia: Lea & Febiger, 1991.

12

The Face

Juan P. Barret
Broomfield Hospital, Chelmsford, Essex, United Kingdom

The goals of acute management of the burned face are similar to those of burns in other parts of the body. However, the outcome of facial burns and hands burns has a significant social and functional implication. Patients whose face and hands have been spared present with excellent rates of social reintegration. Deep burns of the face, and hands however, are devastating, requiring long-term physiotherapy, psychological intervention, and reconstruction.

In general, unless gross destruction of skin and soft tissues is obvious (Fig. 1), a delay in the excision of acute facial burns until day 10 allows better determination of tissue that will not heal within a 3 week period. Subsequent excision of deep partial- and full-thickness burns must be carefully planned and performed in a precise manner following strict principles:

Respect for esthetic units
Sacrifice of less injured tissue to preserve aesthetic units
Minimization of blood loss
Delayed coverage with autografts to minimize postoperative hematomas
Early intervention of rehabilitation services

GENERAL PRINCIPLES

In general, a conservative approach with daily hydrotherapy and topical antimicrobial cream application for 10 days is advised in face burns. This allows for

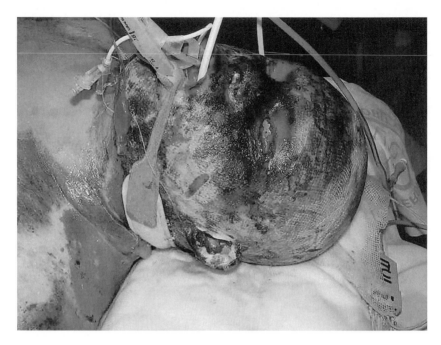

FIGURE 1   Full-thickness burns to the face. Skin and soft tissues have been severely damaged by thermal injury. Early escharectomy is indicated. Patients with
a mixture of deep dermal and indeterminate-depth burns benefit from conservative
treatment for 10 days followed by excision of true full-thickness areas.

viable tissue to heal, and helps to determine which areas will not be healed within
3 weeks of the injury. On admission face burns are debrided of loose blisters
and dead skin. Burns are then treated conservatively with one of the following
regimens:

> Polysporin cream + nystatin
> Silver sulfadiazine
> Cerium nitrate–silver sulfadiazine
> Xenografts

Conservative treatment is then carried out until a definitive diagnosis and treatment plan are outlined.

SURGICAL PROCEDURE

The operation is performed with the patient supine in the reverse Trendelemburg
position under general anesthesia. Extensive bleeding must be expected and blood

products should be available before the beginning of the operation. The endotracheal tube (ET) is suspended from overhead hooks together with feeding tubes. The ET tube is wired to the teeth or secured in similar fashion. The eyes should be protected with either protective contact lens or temporary tarsorraphy stitches. Face burns are normally operated on in a two-stage procedure. Burns are excised in the first operation and the wounds are closed with homografts or skin substitutes. A second-look operation is then performed within 4–7 days and wounds are closed with autografts. This allows for perfect hemostasis, preventing graft loss due to hematomas. It also permits re-excision of nonviable tissue. The operating team staff should be informed of the nature of the operation and to make the necessary arrangements for procurement of homografts and skin substitutes.

Patients are fed via an enteral tube that should be let in place until all grafts are stable, usually by day 7 postgrafting. Nonventilated patients should be left intubated and ventilated for 48 h to preserve integrity of the grafted areas.

The esthetic units that will not heal within 3 weeks of the injury are outlined with markers (Fig. 2). The excision must incorporate the whole aesthetic unit to render perfect outcomes. It is not uncommon to excise minor areas of normal skin or superficial wounds to comply with the aesthetic unit philosophy. When only a small area of an aesthetic unit is burned, it is either left unexcised or grafted, preserving the rest of normal tissue. It is reconstructed at a later stage if the outcome is deemed unacceptable. It is not uncommon that face burns present

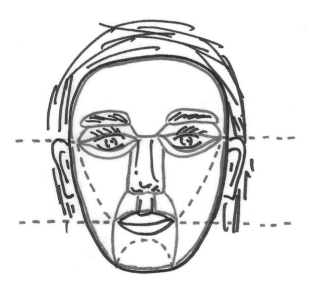

FIGURE 2 Excision of face burns must adapt to esthetic units. The areas included in any given esthetic unit are excised as a whole to provide optimal outcomes.

with different depth of damaged tissue. The excision in these circumstances must be deep enough to excise all skin appendages. This avoids healing underneath the graft with resultant graft loss and bad cosmetic outcomes.

Hemostasis is achieved with epinephrine-soaked Telfa dressings. The excision proceeds in a stepwise manner. Therefore Telfa dressings must be applied meticulously to avoid soaking nonexcised areas. If wounds are impregnated with epinephrine prior to excision, this can lead to inadvertent vasoconstriction and overexcision of living tissue. The infiltration of soft tissues with epinephrine-containing solution should likewise be condemned. They provide good blood loss control, but overexcision of living tissue may result.

Stage One: Excision and Homografting

Face burn excision proceeds in a stepwise manner. The order of excision outlined in here is only a suggestion. Surgeons should find the order that best serves their individual skills and purpose. In general, the center of the face is excised first, followed by excision of larger areas (cheeks and forehead). The following is a description of a full-face excision.

Center of the face

The so-called T area of the face is normally excised first. Extreme care must be exercised to preserve muscles and soft tissues providing the contour of the anatomical areas that allow for preservation of facial features. If the vitality of tissues is in question, they should be homografted and excised further during the second stage. This allows for preservation of vital structures. Soft tissues around canthal areas, tip of the nose, filtrum, and chin should be excised carefully to preserve fibrofatty tissue in an attempt to prevent flat structures that will be difficult to reconstruct at a later stage.

Traction should be applied during excision of eyelids. If temporary tarsorraphy stitches have been placed, they should be left long to allow for countertraction. If corneal protectors are used instead, three traction stitches should be placed on the lid margin. The Goulian dermatome is used with an 8/1000 inch guard. When the excision is complete, the canthal regions are excised next. Fine trip curved scissors or a #ns15 blade is commonly used. Hemostasis is carefully performed before moving to the next area (see next section on Hemostasis).

The Goulian dermatome with the 8/1000 guard is used on the nasal pyramid. The nasal pyramid is well supported and the excision proceeds in the standard fashion. Extreme care must be exercised on the tip of the nose and nares. Counterpressure must be obtained while excising these structures. Soft tissues must be preserved to allow for a good contour. When normal tissue is observed, the excision must be stopped even if vitality is in question.

Countertraction is necessary for the lips in a similar fashion to the excision of eyelids. Three traction stitches are placed on each lip. The Goulian dermatome with an 8:1000 guard is used. The tissue of the philtrum and philtral columns should be managed similarly to the tip of the nose and nares. Soft tissues must be preserved, although vitality is again in question. This allows for a good contour of the philtral area when skin grafts are applied. The areas that are left behind can be excised anew during the second-stage procedure, which permits a better outcome. If they are overexcised until brisk pulsatile bleeding is observed, a flat lip may result, requiring difficult reconstructive procedures in the future to provide anatomical reconstruction.

The Goulian dermatome with the 8/1000 guard is used again to excise the chin. This must be excised as a complete aesthetic unit. It is imperative to preserve as much tissue as possible on the mental prominence to avoid a flat chin that would require future reconstruction. The mental prominence is excised until normal tissue is observed. Even though vitality of the tissue might be in question, it should be preserved and excised at the second-stage procedure if deemed necessary. Hemostasis is performed in the standard fashion.

Excision of periphery (Large flat areas)

Following the excision of the delicate structures of the centre of the face, attention must be turned to the large flat areas on the periphery: both cheeks, forehead, and neck. The excision of these areas must proceed in an orderly manner. They should be excised one at a time to prevent massive blood loss, and excision should proceed from top to bottom and from medial to lateral. Burns are excised with the Goulian dermatome with the 10 or 12:1000 inch guards. Serial passes of the dermatome are performed until living tissues are reached and all skin appendages have been removed. This is assessed by excising all hair follicles. If they are left behind, some re-epithelialization may occur underneath the skin graft, leading to graft loss and poor esthetic outcome. The eyebrows constitute an exception to this general rule. When excision of forehead burns is considered, the eyebrows should be spared to allow conservative healing and regrowth of hair follicles. Hemostasis proceeds as described in the following section (Fig. 3).

Hemostasis

Blood loss can be extensive during excision of facial burns. Serial excision performed in an orderly fashion helps to prevent massive blood loss. Simultaneous excision of two or more areas at any given time should be avoided and condemned. This leads to massive bleeding, poor control of plane of excision, and hemodynamic instability.

Hemostasis is carried out with bipolar cautery and topical epinephrine. Active bleeders are controlled with bipolar cautery, followed by the application of epinephrine-soaked (1:10,000) Telfa dressings. Excision proceeds in an orderly fashion. Therefore extreme care must be taken to keep the epinephrine from running onto unexcised areas, which would lead to spasm, congestion, and overex-

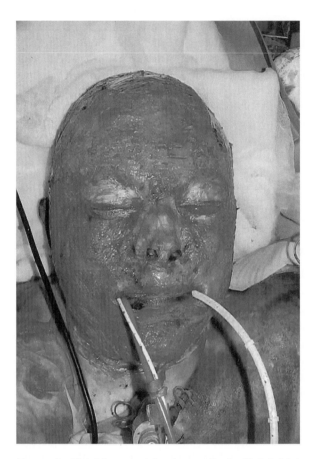

FIGURE 3   Total face excision in a patient with full-thickness burn.

cision of living tissue. Telfa dressings are left in place for 10 min to allow enough vasoconstriction. The blood clot is then wiped out with the same dressing and the zone is inspected for acute bleeders, which are controlled with bipolar cautery. Any remaining capillary bleeding is controlled with serial applications of epinephrine-soaked Telfa dressings left in place for another 7 min. The area can also be sprayed with topical fibrin glue, which provides excellent hemostasis and good graft take.

Wound closure

Following excision and appropriate hemostasis, each area is covered with homografts, placed in similar fashion to autografts. The grafts are tailored to match esthetic units, with graft seams placed in the boundaries of units. Homografts can be secured with staples in the large flat areas, whereas sutures should be used for the eyelids, nose, and lips. Homografts are a good test of wound bed viability. They do vascularize in the presence of viable tissue, and this unique property makes them the temporary cover of choice. Xenografts and Biobrane can be used in a similar fashion, but they do not integrate in the wound and therefore tissue viability is not tested. Graft seams are moistened with bacitracin or chloramphenicol ointments and graft surfaces kept moist with petroleum jelly or polysporin ointment.

Patients are fed with tube feeding. Oral intake is allowed, but wounds should be kept clean to avoid any graft shearing and infection. Speech is allowed with restriction. The head of the bed should be elevated to avoid postoperative edema.

Stage Two: Second Look and Autografting

Approximately 1 week later (between 4 and 7 days after excision and homografting), the patient returns to the operating room for definitive wound closure. Homografts are carefully inspected. It is determined whether they are viable. If homografts are well adherent to the wound bed and there are signs of revasularization, the wound is ready for skin autografting. When the homografts are found to be loose and nonadherent, facial wounds need to be excised and homografted again. In this case, patients return 4 days following the second stage for a further inspection. If homografts are well adherent, surgery proceeds as follows.

Homografts are removed and the wound is inspected. If the wound bed is vital, epinephrine-soaked (1:10,000) Telfa dressings are applied. Split-thickness skin grafts are then obtained. When grafts need to match nonburned or healed face areas, the scalp should be used. When the entire face must be grafted, the scalp does not provide enough quantity of skin graft. Larger donor sites should be used in this circumstance. The skin grafts must be obtained from the same donor site to graft the entire face with the same quality of skin to render a good color match all over the face. It is not acceptable to obtain skin from the scalp and elsewhere at the same time. This will inevitably leave an area of color mismatch that will be not accepted by the patient. When the scalp is used, the size and form of the skin grafts should be drawn on the surface before any subcutaneous infusion is applied. Four good-sized pieces of skin autografts can usually be obtained from the scalp:

> One anterior piece from ear to ear posterior to the hair line
> One posterior piece from vertex to the occipital region
> Two lateral pieces from the retroauricular region to the neck

The scalp is infiltrated with epinephrine-containing normal saline (1:200,000) until large flat areas are obtained. Powered dermatomes (Pagett or Zimmer) are used. The larger guards should be used to obtain good-quality grafts with appropriate width. The assistants should hold the head and the anesthetist control the ET tube while the harvesting is in process. Assistants must change the position of their hands during harvesting. Pressure must be exercised on the opposite part of the head to maintain the countertraction. Two assistants are necessary, maintaining pressure on the periphery of the skull to leave the entire area around the top of the scalp ready for harvest. After harvesting, epinephrine-soaked (1:10,000) Telfa dressings are immediately applied and left in place for 10 min. The scalp is then dressed in the standard fashion (either Biobrane or Acticoat dressings). When the entire face must be grafted, the scalp will not provide enough skin grafts. An alternative donor site is chosen (the back provide large amounts of good quality skin), and *all* skin grafts necessary to graft the entire face are taken from the same area to provide excellent color match. It is important to preserve the donor site that might be used for face grafting in order to provide the best quality of skin. A master plan is developed shortly after admission, and, if at all possible, the donor area to be used for face burns is spared. Donor sites are also infiltrated with large amounts of normal saline with epinephrine and powered dermatomes are used. The manual Padgett dermatome is the best instrument to obtain skin for cheeks and forehead, but it is cumbersome and difficult to use. Common thicknesses for face burns skin grafting are as follows:

Eyelids: 16/1000 inch
Children (all other areas): 14–18/1000 inch
Adults (all other areas): 18–21/1000 inch

The grafts are then carefully stitched into place with 4/0 and 5/0 plain catgut or Vycril rapide. Key stitches are placed at the corners to position the graft. Running sutures are then inserted on each side of the graft. Quilting stitches are not necessary. Bolsters are used on the eyelids, but the rest of the face is left exposed. Grafts should be stitched with slight tension to return grafts to their normal physical properties and avoid wrinkles. Darts are commonly used on the lateral aspect of the neck when the graft joins normal skin.

An alternative to skin autografts is the use of synthetic skin substitutes or dermal templates. Many groups have started to use Integra to close deep dermal and full-thickness face burns. Results differ among them, but common problems are still color match and graft texture. Even though their use is becoming more common practice in other anatomical locations, the routine use of synthetic skin substitutes in the management of face burns is still evolving and subject to intense research. At present, their use should be reserved for cases in which the entire face is to be grafted.

POSTOPERATIVE CARE

Grafts are normally exposed unless an elastomer mold can be applied with interim pressure garments. If the use of elastomers is feasible (depending on the capabilities of the rehabilitation services), a negative impression is made at the end of the excision and application of homografts (stage one). It allows the occupational and physical therapists to fabricate an elastomer that is applied under interim and permanent pressure garments.

In general, graft care includes the application of antimicrobial ointments on graft seams and petrolatum or antimicrobial creams on the graft surface to prevent desiccation. Grafts are inspected twice daily for seromas and hematomas. If these develop, they are drained through small incisions placed in the relaxed skin tension line. When hematomas are large, the patient is returned to the operating room so that surgeons can lift the graft, remove the hematoma, and stitch the graft back with the patient under general anesthesia.

Patients are kept from any oral intake for 4 days, and are fed via a nasogastric or nasojejunal tube. Patients should refrain from talking for 5 days, and 48 h ventilatory support should be considered in children and noncompliant adults. The head of the bed should be elevated 45 degrees and all manoeuvers that may increase head and neck pressure or systemic pressure should be avoided. A calm and comfortable environment should be maintained to decrease the patient's stress and facilitate the postoperative care. In case elastomers are not used during the immediate postoperative period, interim pressure garments should be used, followed by custom-made pressure garments; face masks and splints should be used as soon as the grafts are deemed to be stable.

BIBLIOGRAPHY

1. Engrav LH, Donelan MB. Face burns: acute care and reconstruction. In: Operative Techniques in Plastic and Reconstructive Surgery. Vol. 4. Philadelphia: W. B Saunders, May 1997.
2. Luce EA. Burn care and management. Clin Plast Surg 2000; 27:1.
3. Remensynder JP, Donelan MB. Reconstruction of the head and neck. In. Total Burn Care Herndon DN, Ed. London: W. B. Saunders, 2002.
4. Achauer BM. Burn Reconstruction. New York: Thieme, 1991.
5. Achauer BM. General reconstructive surgery. In: Plastic Surgery, Indications, Operations, and Outcomes. St. Louis: Mosby, 2000.

13

Burn Wound Care and Support of the Metabolic Response to Burn Injury and Surgical Supportive Therapy

Kevin D. Murphy, Jong O. Lee, and David N. Herndon
Shriners Hospital for Children and The University of the Texas Medical Branch, Galveston, Texas, U.S.A.

The hypermetabolic response to burn injury is more profound than in any other surgical condition. Changes occur in the metabolism of carbohydrate, lipids, structural and functional proteins, thermal homeostasis, and water and electrolyte handling. The body aims to deliver the optimal supply of energy and substrate through the circulation to the burn wound at the expense of other tissues [1]. When the burn wound is large (>40% TBSA) the effects can be profound, involving the whole body. The surgical response to trauma involves pharmacological manipulation of the internal hormonal milieu to attempt to achieve homeostasis while healing is achieved. Control of pain and anxiety, support of thermohomeostasis, and early burn wound closure are essential to ameliorate the hypermetabolic response to burn injury. Early closure of the burn wound is essential to control sepsis, which markedly augments the hypermetabolic response to trauma.

METABOLIC RESPONSE TO TRAUMA

Once a burn injury is sustained, the properties that the skin provides to help maintain body homeostasis are immediately lost. The loss of epithelium allows loss of water through the permeable burn eschar. Cytokine-mediated increased vascular permeability occurs in the burned area and in the surrounding zone of hyperemia, and in uninjured organs in patients who sustain large burns. This reduces intravascular volume and leads to signs of early shock. Venous return and cardiac output are reduced. Sympathetically mediated vasoconstriction of unburned areas such as the splanchnic and renal vascular beds attempts to maintain intravascular volume. The sympathetic system induces tachycardia and increased myocardial contractility, leading to increased cardiac work and increased oxygen consumption [2].

Catacholamines and cortisol are secreted from the adrenal medulla and cortex. Glucagon is secreted into the circulation by the pancreas. These so-called catabolic hormones are diabetogenic, having properties antagonistic to the actions of insulin. Under their influence glycogen is rapidly converted to glucose. This increases glucose flow rates markedly and quickly depletes limited carbohydrate stores in the liver. Fasting glucose levels become elevated. [3]. Catabolism of fats and protein also occurs, leading to breakdown of muscle protein and negative nitrogen balance at rates up to 30 grs/day for burns greater than 40 % total body surface area (TBSA) [4], with associated loss of potassium, zinc, and creatinine [5,6] (Fig. 1).

Constitutive serum protein levels (prealbumin, retinol-binding protein, transferrin) and circulating albumin levels are decreased, contributing to interstitial oedema. Type I (complement 3, alpha1-acid glycoprotein) and type II (haptoglobin, alpha1-antitrypsin) hepatic acute-phase proteins are increased. Cytokine-mediated T_1/T_2 cell ratios are reversed, with type II T-cell elevations leading to immune suppression and susceptibility to opportunistic infections such as herpes simplex virus and *Candida albicans*. Relative lack of substrate in the form of amino acids used to lay down collagen at the burn wound delays healing, further compounding the problem. In the longer term, constitutive protein exhaustion ensues, often followed by death.

If the patient survives, severe muscular weakness leads to problems with rehabilitation and subsequent scar contracture [7]. Muscular weakness increases the time to rehabilitation for patients with large burns. Animal studies, and occasional observations in starved humans, have indicated that loss of protein at these rapid rates ($\sim$20–25g/m^2/day) can be lethal within 3–4 weeks, when one-quarter to one-third of the body protein has been consumed. Prolonged periods of immobilization combined with greatly elevated cortisol levels lead to failure of bone deposition. Bone resorption may be mediated by cytokines. Serum osteocalcin, type I procollagen propeptide, parathormone, and 1,25 dihydroxycholecalciferol are all reduced [8], resulting in linear growth delays of up to 2 years [9], which are never fully regained.

During the first 5 days after severe burns, a cascade of events increases metabolic rates markedly. Oxygen consumption reaches a plateau at this time and re-

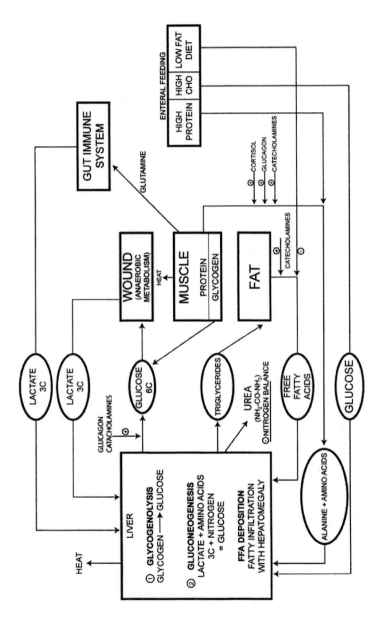

Figure 1 Metabolic pathways after severe burn injury.

mains elevated for approximately 9 months after the wound is healed. Carbon dioxide excretion rises in parallel with oxygen consumption. The initial postburn period is referred to as the ebb phase of the metabolic response and is followed by a flow phase. The flow phase of the response becomes significant on the fifth postburn day. In combination with raised levels of diabetogenic hormones, increasing glycogen degradation increases glucose flow rates markedly from 4mg/kg/min in the unburned subject to 10mg/kg/min with a burn of 50% TBSA [10]. Almost all of the flow is directed to the burn wound [11] as a result of increased cardiac output and vasodilatation in the burned area. Glucose is metabolized anaerobically at the burn wound by fibroblasts, inflammatory cells, and endothelial cells, producing large quantities of lactate. Lactate is metabolized in the liver by gluconeogenesis using amino acids (mainly alanine) derived from protein stores to replenish glucose levels [12] (Figure 1). Severe muscle catabolism persists for at least 6–9 months after burn injury [13,14]. This can be determined from cross leg nitrogen balance measurements. Actual metabolic rates depend on the total body surface area burned. Metabolic rates remain elevated but near normal for burns up to 25% TBSA. For burn of over 40% TBSA, metabolic rates are elevated to 1.4–2 times normal. Resting metabolic rates remain on average at 180% of resting metabolic rates during acute hospitalization, dropping to 150% when the patient's injuries are fully healed. Rates remain at 140% at 6 months postburn, 120% at 9 months, and 110% 1 year later [7] (Fig. 2).

THERMOHOMEOSTASIS

Loss of water from the burn surface by evaporation requires a significant amount of energy due to the large latent heat of vaporization of water, which is 4200

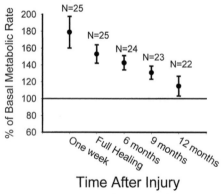

Error Bars Represent 95% Confidence Intervals

FIGURE 2   Resting energy expenditure. (From Ref. 62.)

kcal/L. Failure to increase body thermogenesis to counter these losses results in inevitable hypothermia. Core and surface temperatures in burned patients are elevated to 2°C above normal by a centrally mediated resetting of the hypothalamus. Energy to maintain body heat is provided by futile substrate cycling of carbohydrate and lipids at the expense of protein catabolism [15]. Stable isotope studies have identified simultaneous glycolysis and gluconeogenesis (using amino acids as substrate), and continuous cycling of triglycerides and fatty acids, which expend large amounts of energy in the form of heat. Carbohydrate and lipid cycling are 2.5 and 4.5 times normal, respectively, in patients with large burns.

NUTRITIONAL SUPPORT

Maintenance of body weight, lean body mass (muscle protein), electrolytes, and vitamin homeostasis are the primary objectives of nutritional support of the burned patient. Without proper nutritional support, hypermetabolic patients can lose up to 25% of their preadmission body weight in the first 3 weeks postburn. Weight loss of up to 30% of body mass was common in burn patients prior to the use of continuous feeding [16]. It is possible to maintain body weight, and/or lean body mass or achieve weight gain, using enteral and/or parenteral nutritional support. It has been demonstrated on many occasions that *body weight* can be maintained with milk- or soy-based formulations [17–20]. The amount of nutritional support required correlates well with resting energy expenditure (REE). REE can be measured directly at the bedside using portable calorimeters that analyze oxygen consumption and carbon dioxide excretion. Formulae have been derived from regression analysis of predicted caloric intake compared with measured weight loss in large patient series, or by direct measurement of metabolic rate using indirect calorimetry. These estimate the energy requirements of patients to maintain *body weight*. Body weight maintenance has been successfully demonstrated in large numbers of hospitalized patients using these formulae.

For an adult, the most commonly used formula calculates caloric needs in burn patients from body weight and TBSA burned. For children, the most appropriate formula differs with body surface area [21–23] (Table 1).

In patients with large burns this can equate to over 5000 kilocalories per patient per day for adults. Although these provide reliable guides, a better estimate of actual energy expenditure is made using a mobile calorimeter at the bedside. Double-labeled water techniques (which enable caloric balance to be studied over time, e.g., during hospital stay) have demonstrated that the actual energy expended is 1.2 times the REE for burns greater than 40% TBSA [25]. To maintain *lean muscle mass*, 1.2 times REE needs to be administered as food, although this does not maintain body weight [24]. Calories administered at 1.4 times REE maintain lean body mass and body weight [22]. Calories delivered at rates higher than this maintain lean body mass, but stimulate weight gain in patients only through

TABLE 1   Formulae to Estimate Caloric Requirements in Burn Injured Children and Adults

Galveston Infant	0-1 year	$2100 \text{ kcal/m}^2 + 1000 \text{ kcal/m}^2$ burned/day
Galveston Revised	1-11 years	$1800 \text{ kcal/m}^2 + 1300 \text{ kcal/m}^2$ burned/day
Galveston Adolescent	12 years	$1500 \text{ kcal/m}^2 + 1500 \text{ kcal/m}^2$ burned/day
Curreri Formula Adult	16-60 years	25 kcal/kg/day PLUS 40 kcal/%TBSA burned/day
Curreri Formula Seniors	> 60 years	25 kcal/kg/day PLUS 65 kcal/%TBSA burned/day

accretion of fat [24]. Optimal nutritional support in convalescent burn patients should be between 1.2 and 1.4 times measured REE [25]. Increasing the protein content of the diet from 1.15 to 3 g/kg/day does not stimulate muscle protein synthesis, and plasma urea, urea production, and urinary urea excretion are increased, rather than lean muscle mass [26]. Skin protein synthetic rates are increased, however, with enhanced wound and donor site healing [26]. Milk and the majority of available hospital diets are predominantly fat-based. A high-carbohydrate diet stimulates protein synthesis by increasing endogenous insulin. Enteral nutrition supplied predominantly as carbohydrate and protein (3% lipid, 82% carbohydrate, 15% protein) rather than as fat-based formula (44% lipid, 42% carbohydrate, 14% protein) improves the net balance of skeletal muscle protein in severely burned children [27]. Although body weight can be maintained with a fat-based diet, actual accretion of lean body mass is only achieved using high-carbohydrate, high-protein diets [28]. Muscle protein degradation is decreased with a high-carbohydrate protein diet due to increased endogenous insulin production. Burn patients may require exogenous insulin to control hyperglycemia. Tight euglycemic control with insulin improves wound healing and decreases infection and mortality [29,30].

The increased nutritional requirements in burn-induced hypermetabolism may be accomplished via enteral or parenteral routes. Nutritional support in severely burned patients is best accomplished by early enteral feeding where possible. Enteral feeding is less prone to complication and requires insertion of a feeding tube nasally. Nasogastric tubes are prone to limitation by gastric stasis, which is frequent in patients with burns, and nasoduodenal tubes are favored for this reason. Maximally tolerated enteral feeding may not deliver sufficient calories to the burned patient. However, attempts at parenteral hyperalimentation have been complicated by decreased liver function, reduced immune function, line sepsis, and increased mortality [31,32]. As a result, unless a true small bowel ileus also exists, the use of parenteral feeding has markedly decreased recently.

Enteral milk- or soy-based feeds have been shown to be sufficient to maintain body weight in the burned child, but high-carbohydrate diets have been shown to be superior. Early enteral feeding has been shown to reduce bacterial gut barrier translocation and attenuate the metabolic response significantly [33,34]. Enteral feeding intolerance and nasogastric aspirates in excess of hourly delivered nutrient correlate strongly with the presence of bacterial sepsis in the patient [35].

Under severe stress arginine and glutamine, which are nonessential amino acids, become essential dietary nutrients. Arginine enhances natural killer cell function, stimulates T lymphocytes, and stimulates synthesis of nitric oxide. Arginine appears to promote wound healing when given as a supplement. Glutamine is a primary fuel for enterocytes and appears to play an integral role in wound healing. Muscle glutamine formation is suppressed in severely hypercatabolic burned patients. There is increasing evidence that supplementation of arginine and glutamine is of benefit in critically ill patients [36]. A small quantity of fat is an essential component of nutritional support. A substantial proportion of calories delivered as fat improves glucose tolerance and decreases CO_2 production. However, the hormonal environment of the burn patient causes such a great degree of endogenous lipolysis that the extent to which excess lipid can be utilized in the burned patient is limited. Increased peripheral lipolysis results in fatty infiltration of the liver that can be exacerbated by overfeeding and the use of total parenteral nutrition. Released free fatty acids are oxidized for energy and re-esterified to triglycerides in the liver. They are either deposited in the liver or further packaged for transport to other tissues. Liver weight of burn children is increased up to twice that of age- and gender-matched controls [37]. Mochizuki et al. demonstrated an adverse effect on immune function in burned guinea pigs when diets contained more than 15% lipids [38]. Omega-6 fatty acids, derived from vegetable and animal oils, are metabolized to yield prostaglandin E1 (PGE1) and PGE2, which possess immunosuppressive properties. Omega-3 fatty acids from fish oil are metabolized to yield PGE3, which is immunologically inert. Postburn immunosuppression might be improved by replacing omega-6 with omega-3 fatty acids. Alexander et al. also showed that burned guinea pigs fed a diet high in fish oil had better cell-mediated immune responses [39].

ENVIRONMENTAL FACTORS

The high latent heat of vaporization of water normally causes large amounts of heat to be dissipated at the surface of the burn wound. This loss of heat is offset by an increased hypermetabolic response by the patient in the form of futile substrate cycling to generate heat. Modification of the patient's environment by heating allows environmental heat to provide energy for this obligatory water loss, thus reducing the metabolic demand on the patient. In large burns, loss of water can be appreciable, up to 2000 cc/m^2 burn/day [40,41]. In addition, the core and skin temperatures of burned patients are increased by 2° Centigrade under hypothalamic control. Thermal equilibrium can be achieved by elevating the external environmental temperature to 30–33°C (thermal neutrality). Given the ability to regulate environmental temperature, the burn-injured patient would select a temperature in the range 28°–38°C to achieve thermal neutrality and minimize metabolic demands on the body [42]. Conversely, attempts to decrease the patient's temperature with antipyretics merely exacerbate the hypermetabolic response. The metabolic requirements of the patient with burns greater than 40%TBSA is reduced from twice the REE to only 1.4 times REE with environmental heating alone (room temperature raised from 20 to 33°C).

Other agents contributing to hypermetabolism are pain and anxiety. Adequate analgesia is frequently not achieved for the burn-injured patient. Background pain results from the burn and is accentuated by surgical burn debridement at the recipient site and autograft harvesting. Procedural interventions that are painful for the patient include dressing changes, application of topical antimicrobial agents, and physiotherapy. Trauma and metabolic requirements can be effectively minimized by liberal usage of opioid analgesics such as morphine and fentanyl analogues, sedative agents, and anxiolytics [42a]. Psychological support of the burned patient is crucial in addition to pharmacotherapy.

PHYSICAL EXERCISE PROGRAM

Accretion of lean muscle mass requires, in addition to a high-carbohydrate diet, a resistance exercise program [43]. Formal supervision of this program by a physiotherapist or occupational therapist is required to direct attention to specific areas requiring greater attention, to prevent and minimize the effects of burn scar contracture and to ensure compliance. A supervised, coordinated 12 week inpatient program of resistance exercises has shown 50% greater accretion of lean muscle in patients who completed this program than in patients who followed standard exercise regimens as outpatients [44] (Fig. 3). Exercise programs in burned children undergoing rehabilitation appear to be safe, since children effectively dissipate the heat generated during exercise [45]. Children not only show significantly improved peak torque and stamina after undertaking an exercise program but also have notably improved pulmonary function [46].

COMPLICATIONS

Localized infection of the burn wound very frequently results in generalized septicemia. Sepsis can markedly increase the metabolic demands in the burned patient. Prevention of infection and sepsis are critical therapeutic manoeuvers to decrease the hypermetabolic response. Burn infection scores may be extremely useful to define infection, which is difficult to do clinically, in a hypermetabolic

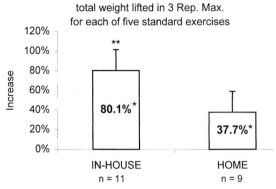

Muscle Strength
total weight lifted in 3 Rep. Max.
for each of five standard exercises
Increase
120%
100%
80%
60%
40%
20%
0%
**
80.1%*
37.7%*
IN-HOUSE
n = 11
HOME
n = 9
*Significant difference between IN-HOUSE and HOME exercise programs

Figure 3 Muscle strength after exercise. (From Ref. 44.)

burned patient. Scores defined by the Society of Critical Care Medicine or American Academy of Chest Physicians are useful (Fig. 4). Infection can increase the metabolic rate (as determined by stable isotope studies) in burn-injured patients by 40% relative to patients with like-sized burns that do not become septic. This large increase in metabolic rate persists throughout the patient's hospital stay and well into the rehabilitation period [13]. Local and systemic infection may be prevented by the early coverage of the burn wound by either split-thickness autograft or synthetic materials.

Clinical Definition of Burn Sepsis Scores

At least 3 of the following:
- T>38.5 or <36.5°C
- Progressive tachycardia
- Progressive tachypnea
- WBC > 12,000 or <4,000
- Refractory hypotension
- Thrombocytopenia
- Hyperglycemia
- Enteral Feeding Intolerance

AND
- Pathologic tissue source identified

Modified ACCP/SCCM Burn Sepsis Scores

At least 2 of the following:
- T>38.5 or <36.5°C
- HR>20% above NL for age
- RR>20% above NL for age / $PaCO_2$<32
- WBC > 12,000 or <4,000

AND
- Bacteremia or fungemia
- Pathologic tissue source identified–

Figure 4 Definitions of sepsis. (From Ref. 13.)

The other major therapeutic manoeuver shown to have a marked effect on metabolic rate is early excision and closure of the burn wound. Early burn wound excision and coverage with widely meshed autograft covered with cadaver skin, combined with cadaver skin used to cover all other non-grafted remaining areas, results in decreased operative blood loss [47], decreased length of stay, fewer septic complications, and decreased mortality in children and young burned adults compared to patients treated with serial debridement [13,48–50]. A significant reduction in catabolism and amelioration of the hypermetabolic response is also achieved [51].

Biobrane is a synthetic wound dressing that has been used successfully to cover superficial second-degree burns until spontaneous healing occurs. In burns greater than >40% TBSA, this has shown superior results to conventional dress-ings, expressed as a significant reduction in pain, time to healing, inpatient stay, and metabolic response to the burn [52]. Deep dermal burns (deep second-degree or deep partial-thickness) greater than 40% TBSA achieve superior healing when early coverage is achieved using cadaveric allograft compared to application of topical antimicrobial agents [53]. Hospital stay is reduced and significantly decreased pain levels and rates of infection serve to temper the hypermetabolic response markedly.

Early coverage of the debrided burn wound is the key to reduction of the hypermetabolic response exhibited by the burn-injured patient. Early debridement and coverage with either cadaveric skin or skin substitutes such as Integra or Dermagraft within 48 h of injury have shown results superior to delayed burn wound closure at 7 days [54,55]. Biological dressings and skin substitutes require subsequent autografting when the skin substitute has achieved sufficient biointe-gration with the wound bed. Metabolic response is diminished by 40%, resulting from improved rates of early closure [56].

In patients with large burns from whom insufficient donor skin is available for autografting, complete early closure of the burn wound by what is termed a sandwich technique has reduced intraoperative blood loss, infection rates, and hospital stay with resulting improved patient survival [48]. This involves early and complete debridement of the burn wound with application of widely meshed autograft covered with cadaver skin, and coverage of remaining areas with cadav-eric skin alone. Other studies have shown that other biosynthetic allograft materi-als such as Biobrane and Integra may be used to close the burn wound with equal efficacy. This is followed by delayed autografting later.

When phenylalanine clearance rate is used as a measure of loss of lean muscle mass protein, significant differences can be seen between groups treated by similar methods but for whom the timing of surgical intervention was different. Studies have compared three groups to assess metabolic rates as follows. The early group underwent surgery within 72 h of injury involving complete burn wound excision and complete coverage of the wound. The middle group had surgery deferred for 7–10 days postburn. The late group had did not undergo total excision and complete coverage until 10–21 days post burn. Rates of phenylal-anine loss were 0.03, 0.05, and 0.07 g/100 cc blood volume/min in the three respec-tive groups, representing a 66% and 130% increase in protein catabolism for the intermediate and late groups, respectively. Bacterial *log* counts for the groups were 3.0, 3.5, and 4.2, respectively, representing more than a tenfold increase in bacterial load in the late group compared with the early group. As a result, rates of wound sepsis in the respective groups were 20%, 35%, and 50% [51].

PHARMACOLOGICAL MANIPULATION OF SOFT TISSUE MASS

The physician's treatment of injury or surgical trauma should involve maintaining homeostasis of the patient's hormonal environment to prevent hypovolemia and promote stabilization of the cardiovascular systems, which is essential to survival. Corticotrophin-releasing hormone is secreted by the hypothalamus, promoting adrenocorticotrophic hormone (ACTH) release by the anterior pituitary. This acts on the adrenal cortex to increase greatly the levels of free cortisol, which is the active form of the hormone. Cortisol is essential to the stress response to maintain cardiovascular stability through glucocorticoid and mineralocorticoid activity. Catecholamines are secreted by the adrenal medulla, which immediately acts to maintain intravascular volume. Glucagon is secreted by the pancreas and enhances the effects of cortisol on carbohydrate metabolism. These hormones have cata-bolic actions. After trauma, activity of insulin and similar anabolic proteins, such as insulin-like growth factor (IGF), is reduced. These anabolic proteins increase anabolic activity by increasing transcription of deoxyribonucleic acids, intracellu-lar translation, and decreased efflux and increased uptake of amino acids into the cell. They also act to increase lipolysis as an alternative substrate to protein catabolism.

Attempts to reduce hypermetabolism beyond the clinical modalities previ-ously discussed have focused on the following:

1. 1. Anabolic proteins such as growth hormone, insulin, and insulinlike growth factor
2. 2. Anabolic steroids such as oxandrolone and testosterone
3. 3. Catecholamine antagonists such as propranolol and metropolol
4. 4. Glucocorticoid blockers (more recently)

Growth hormone and insulinlike growth factor

Growth hormone and insulinlike growth factor (IGF) levels are decreased follow-ing burn injury [70]. Growth hormone and IGF-1 promote protein synthesis by increasing the cellular uptake of amino acids, accelerating nucleic acid transcrip-tion, and enhancing cellular proliferation. Fatty acids are released from increased lipolysis of fat. There is a decrease in body fat with relative protein sparing [57,72]. The anabolic protein growth hormone (GH), administered as rhGH, and the anabolic steroids oxandrolone [58,58a] and testosterone [59] show promise in increasing lean body mass after burn injury. Catecholamine antagonists, such as propranolol and metoprolol, act to moderate the hypermetabolic effects of severe burn injury. In the acute setting, these anabolic properties can not only aid healing of the burn wound itself but also accelerate donor site healing. This allows for earlier recropping and ultimately earlier availability of autograft [60,61].

Growth hormone administered at a dosage of 0.2 mg/kg/day increases donor site healing by 25%. When hospital stay is adjusted to reflect percentage burn, hospital stay is reduced from 0.8 to 0.54 days/%TBSA burn, representing a decrease of 33% in length of hospital stay. For a burn of 60%, this allows patient discharge 2 weeks earlier than is possible for patients with burns of similar size treated with placebo. Scarring is similar to that experienced by untreated patients.

Burned children, once released from the hospital, administered rhGH at a dosage of 0.5mg/kg/day, by comparison with age-matched controls given placebo, achieved a greater weight, better linear growth, improved lean body mass, and increased mineralization of bone [62,62a] (Fig. 5).

Bone

Bone mass is decreased following severe burn injury (>40% TBSA) in adults and children. This is a result of reduced bone deposition and sustained hypercalciuria. High levels of endogenous corticosteroid released in response to major burn-induced stress, immobilization, bone marrow suppression, aluminium toxicity from antacids and albumin [63], and magnesium deficiency are postulated as

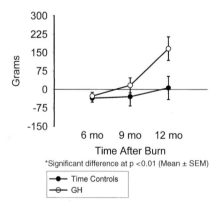

FIGURE 5   Changes in bone mineral content in major pediatric burns versus discharge from burn ICU. (From Ref. 62.)

being causative [64]. After severe burns, hypoparathyroidism also leads to additional loss of bone mass [65]. Long periods of immobilization lead to demineralization of bone, and bone marrow suppression results from sepsis and drug therapy. Magnesium depletion also occurs [66]. The consequences of bone loss are reduced peak bone mass, increased fracture risk, and loss of stature. Dual energy x-ray absorptiometry (DEXA) [67] shows that both bone mass and bone mineral density are delayed by 2 years in burned children compared to unburned age-matched controls [68,69]. Labeled tetracycline techniques show evidence of decreased bone formation, reduced surface area and osteoid area, and diminished reduced bone mineralization. Serum osteocalcin levels are also reduced.

TREATMENTS

GROWTH HORMONE & MEDIATORS

Burn injury greatly reduces endogenous levels of growth hormone and insulinlike growth factors such as IGF-1 [70]. When present in adequate quantities, protein synthesis is increased as a result of augmented cellular amino acid uptake, accelerated nucleic acid transcription and translation, and enhancement of cellular proliferation [71]. Body fat decreases with relative protein sparing [72]. Acute rhGH administration markedly reduces loss of essential and nonessential amino acids from muscle. Alanine efflux is attenuated, and efflux of glutamine and 3-methyl-histidine from muscle is abolished [73]. GH increases weight and height in burned children [74]. In a double-blind placebo-controlled trial of growth hormone administration at 0.05 mg/kg day for 1 year, children receiving the drug not only showed a significant increase in height and body weight over controls, but this gain was also continued in a divergent fashion over subsequent years after stopping the drug [75] (Fig. 6).

DEXA scanning demonstrated that this was attributable to significantly increased lean body (muscle) mass at 6, 9, and 12 months postburn [76]. GH has been administered to improve respiratory muscle strength in patients who have not responded to standard weaning from the respirator in the intensive care unit (ICU). GH allowed 81% of these patients to be weaned with a 76% survival rate. Mortality was reduced by almost 50% ($p < 0.05$) as predicted by APACHE II scores [77]. Bone mineral content is significantly increased at 9 and 12 months in patients treated with GH during rehabilitation. These increases were maintained in comparison with controls when measured at 3 years. Hypoparathyroidism-associated burn injury also improved with increased serum parathormone levels. Growth hormone ameliorates the production of acute-phase proteins, C-reactive protein, and serum amyloid-A, and increases levels of serum retinol-binding protein and albumin production by the liver [78,79]. GH decreases serum tumor necrosis factor -alpha and interleukin-1β, but not IL-1α, IL-6, or IL-10 compared with placebo. Free fatty acid levels are elevated.

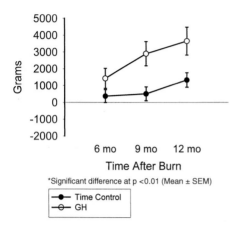

FIGURE 6   Changes in lean body mass in major pediatric burns versus discharge from burn ICU. (From Ref. 62.)

Growth hormone has a positive modulatory effect on immune function, improving production of the antiviral cytokine interferon gamma (IFN-γ), and suppressing populations of suppressor macrophages induced by burn injury [80]. Type I T-helper/type II T-helper cell ratios are increased: low ratios are associated increased susceptibility to infection [81,82]. Administration of GH aggravates existing hyperglycemia. In the acute setting administration of the peptide IGF-1, which is a mediator of GH effects, reduces catabolism while decreasing serum glucose. IGF-1 and IGF-binding protein 3 (IGF-BP3) levels are doubled in patients who receive growth hormone. Administered alone, IGF-1 improves protein metabolism but hypoglycemic episodes may be profound and frequent. These side effects are ameliorated remarkably by administration with its main binding protein, IGF-BP3. IGF-1 administration may be useful for the hyperglycemic catabolic patient, because it reduces blood glucose levels despite reduced levels of circulating insulin [83]. Hypermetabolism is decreased, and type I and II hepatic acute-phase proteins are reduced by simultaneous administration of IGF-1 and IGF-BP$_3$ [84,85]. Growth hormone ameliorates bone loss after burns and improves bone mineral density by comparison with untreated subjects [86]. Linear growth velocities are comparable to controls at 6 months postburn but significantly greater at 2 years in children treated acutely with growth hormone [87].

Failure of growth hormone to augment bone formation (mediated through IGF-1 and IGF-BP$_3$) may be due to increased circulating levels of the inhibitory peptide IGF-BP$_4$ [88]. This normalizes when the wound is healed. Loss of stature is prevented particularly in children not undergoing a growth spurt due to a physiological period of accelerated growth or puberty [89] (Table 1).

While early trials in burned adults showed improved survival [90], several large European trials have established increased mortality in *adults* treated acutely with GH [91,92]. This has not been seen with children [74], in whom hypoglycemic episodes are infrequent and protein kinetics improved [78]. Animal studies have shown increased renal scarring but the quality of burn scarring in randomized controlled trials is similar in patients receiving GH [93]. Recent studies have not found any adverse effects of GH on cosmetic or punctual outcomes [93a].

ANABOLIC STEROIDS

In male patients with burns, blood testosterone levels are decreased. Restoration of this androgenic hormone to normal levels improves protein synthesis twofold and reduces catabolism by half. Anabolic steroids may be used to improve protein kinetics after burn injury. Oxandrolone, an anabolic steroid, has been successfully used for this purpose. Because its androgenic potential is only 5% that of testosterone it can be used safely in female patients, in whom testosterone levels are normally low compared with males. Administered at an oral dosage of 0.1 mg/kg/day twice daily it significantly increases muscular protein synthesis [94,94a] (Fig. 7). Oxandrolone has also been shown to ameliorate the hepatic acute phase during rehabilitation [94b].

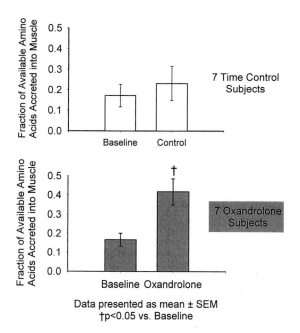

Data presented as mean ± SEM
†p<0.05 vs. Baseline

FIGURE 7   Protein synthetic efficiency. (From Ref. 94.)

INSULIN AND RELATED POLYPEPTIDES

Serum insulin levels are decreased by burn injury. Hyperglycemia and insulin resistance are associated with increased mortality in burn patients [95]. Insulin infusion in the intensive care setting markedly decreases mortality, particularly in patients with sepsis and multiorgan failure. The overall mortality, incidence of sepsis, transfusion requirements, and incidence of renal failure requiring dialysis are each decreased by 30–50% [96]. Continuous infusion of insulin in burn patients at a rate of 25–49 units/h achieves plasma insulin levels of 400–900 μ/ml. Continuous infusion acutely for 7 days stimulates protein synthesis without increasing hepatic triglyceride production [97,98]. Dextrose solution (50%) is infused continuously to maintain euglycemia at a rate of 20–50 ml/h. Donor site healing can be decreased from 6.5 $+/-$ 1 days to 4.7 $+/-$ 1.2 days (p < 0.05). This reduction in time for donor site healing decreases overall time to healing, reduces hypermetabolic response and reduces hospital stay by 2 weeks in patients with a 60% TBSA burn.

The natural hyperglycemia of acute burn injury may be sufficient to eliminate the need to infuse dextrose to maintain euglycemia when submaximal dosages of insulin are given [99]. Maintenance of tight euglycemic control in burn injury increases graft take by reducing infection, and decreases mortality [100]. For these applications, dichloroacetate and metformin may also have clinical utility in burn injury but further evaluation and trials are required [101]. IGF-1 reduces protein catabolism by reducing oxidation of amino acids and improving glucose uptake. Insulin secretion is reduced in response to a glucose challenge [102].

CATECHOLAMINE ANTAGONISTS

Catecholamines are the primary mediators of the hypermetabolic response to burn injury [103]. Serum catecholamine levels are increased 10-fold in response to severe burns and are the mediators of a hyperdynamic circulation [104]. Increases in REE [105] and rates of catabolism of skeletal muscle protein correlate directly with serum catecholamine levels. Stimulation of β-2 receptors increases lipolysis with consequent deposition of fatty acids in the liver [106,107]. This results in a doubling of liver size within 3 weeks of burn in patients sustaining a 60% TBSA burn [108]. Adrenergic blockade with propranolol results in a decrease in heart rate [109], reduced cardiac work [110,111], decreased lipolysis [112], diminished REE, and less thermogenesis [113] (Fig. 8). The cold-stress response is unaffected by adrenergic blockade [114].

Titration of propranolol to achieve a reduction of 20% in heart rate safely reduces cardiac work and diminishes the rate of adverse cardiac events. Less lipolysis peripherally results from β-2 blockade, and a decline in peripheral and splanchnic blood flow reduces palmitate delivery and uptake by the liver [106] in patients on a high-protein, high-carbohydrate diet [115]. Triacyl glycerol storage by the liver is decreased, resulting in less hepatomegaly and mesenteric

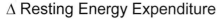

Δ Resting Energy Expenditure

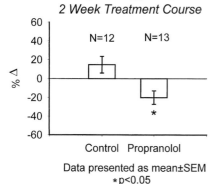

FIGURE 8 Change in resting energy expenditure in major burns with adrenergic blockade. (From Ref. 113.)

hypertrophy. Fat secretion and oxidation are not appreciably diminished. Treatment with propranolol reduced palmitate storage in the liver of severely burned pediatric patients from 1.53 ± 1.3 to 0.76 ± 0.58 mm/kg/min [116]. Patients accrete a greater lean body mass due to decreased skeletal muscle wasting. Increased recycling of amino acids *within* the cell can be demonstrated by isotope studies, which show enhanced amino acid reincorporation into intracellular proteins. These catecholamine-mediated effects are only demonstrated in catabolic subjects and propranolol does not result in these changes when administered in normal subjects [117]. Heavy muscular individuals are most prone to the effects of the hypermetabolic response [13]. Children less than 2 years old and elderly subjects show less catabolism than older children and younger adults. Significant protein catabolism does not usually occur in burns less than 40% TBSA unless the patient is septic; patients with burns larger than 40% invariably display marked muscle protein wasting.

SUMMARY

Severe burn injury exhibits a profound hypermetabolic response with disturbances in height, weight, linear growth, bone mineralization, and skeletal muscle wasting in children and adults. Peripheral lipolysis is increased with central deposition of fatty acids in the liver and mesentery. Muscle wasting and peripheral lipolysis lead to an emaciated pseudocushingoid appearance. Continuing catabolism may profoundly hamper rehabilitation. These metabolic changes are markedly increased by pain, sepsis, and delayed closure of the burn wound. Strategies aimed to reduce the metabolic affects of burn injury include early excision and closure of the burn wound leading to a reduction in the rate and extent of wound sepsis.

Wound infection is actively sought and treated aggressively. The hypermetabolic response is ameliorated by supportive measures, which include maintenance of thermal equilibrium by environmental heating to 30–32 °C. Early enteral feeding should be instituted on the day of burn with a high-protein, high-carbohydrate diet to reduce bacterial translocation across the compromised gut–blood barrier to reduce sepsis and to increase amino acid incorporation into muscle to prevent muscle wasting and aid rehabilitation [51,118]. A resistive exercise program in a supervised maximally compliant inpatient setting is essential to augment lean body mass, improve function, and minimize contracture. Pharmacological support with anabolic agents such as rhGH, insulin, or oxandrolone help enormously to improve donor site healing, eventual time to burn wound healing, and maintenance of muscle mass. These agents and propranolol mitigate the effects of the hypermetabolic response to burn injury. At present propranolol and oxandrolone are the most cost-effective with few side effects [119] (Tables 2–3 available). Research now underway aims to increase the effectiveness of present therapies and develop new treatment modalities to improve inpatient care and postoperative rehabilitation of patients with severe burns.

REFERENCES

1. Wilmore DW, Aulick LH. Metabolyic changes in burned patients. Surg Clin North Am 1978; 58:1173–1187.
2. Harrison TS, Seton JF, Feller I. Relationship of increased oxygen consumption to catecholamine excretion in thermal burns. Ann Surg 1967; 165:169–172.
3. Long CL, Spencer JL, Kinney JM, Geiger JW. Carbohydrate metabolism in man. Effective elective operations and major injury. J Appl Physiol. 1971; 31:110.
4. Soroff HS, Pearson E, Artz CP. An estimation of the nitrogen requirements for equilibrium in burn patients. Surg Gynecol Obstet 1961; 112:159.
5. Cuthbertson DP. The disturbance of metabolism produced by bony and non-bony injury with notes of certain abnormal conditions of bone. Biochem J 1930; J24: 144.
6. Kinney JM, Long CL, Gump FE, Duke JH. Tissue composition of weight loss in surgical patients, 1 Elective operation. Ann Surg 1968; 168:459.
7. Hart DW, Wolf SE, Mlcak R, Chinkes DL, Ramzy PR, Obeng MK, Ferrnado AA, Wolfe RR, Herndon DN. Persistence of muscle catabolism after severe burn. Surgery 2000; 128(2):312–319.
8. Klein Gl, Herndon DN, Goodman WG, Langman CB, Phillips WA, Dickson IR, Eastell R, Naylor KE, Maloney NA, Desai M. Histomorphometric and biochemical characterization of bone following acute severe burns in children. Bone 1995; 17(5): 455–60.
9. Rutan RL, Herndon DN. Growth delay in post-burn pediatric patients. Arch Surg 1990; 125(3):392–395.
10. Wilmore DW, Mason AD, Pruitt BA. Insulin response to glucose in hypermetabolic burn patients. Ann Surg 1976; 183:314.

11. Wilmore DW, Aulick LH, Mason AD, Pruitt BA. Influence of the burn wound on local and systemic response to injury. Ann Surg 1977; 186(4).

12. Jahoor F, Desai MH, Herndon DN, Wolfe RR. Dynamics of protein anabolic responses to burn injury. Metabolism 1998; 37(4):330–337.

13. Hart D, Wolf S, Chinkes D, Gore D, Mlcak R, Beauford RB, Obeng MK, Lal SO, Gold W, Wolfe RR, Herndon DN. Determinants of skeletal muscle catabolism. Ann Surg 2000; 232(4):455–465.

14. Hart DW, Wolf SE, Mlcak R, Chinkes DL, Ramzy PI, Obeng MK, Wolfe RR, Herndon DN. Persistence of muscle catabolism after severe burn. Ann Surg 2000; 128(2):312–319.

15. Wolfe RR, Herndon DN, Jahoor F, Miyoshi H, Wolfe M. Effect of severe burn injury on substrate cycling by glucose and fatty acids. N Engl J Med 1987; 317:403–408.

16. Newsome TW, Mason AD, Pruitt BA. Weight loss following thermal injury. Ann Surg 1973; 178:215–217.

17. Hildreth M, Herndon DN, Desai MH, Duke M. Caloric needs of adolescent patients with burns. J Burn Care Rehab 1989; 10(6):523–526.

18. Hildreth M, Herndon DN, Parks D, Desai MH, Rutan T. Evaluation of caloric requirement formula on burn children treated with early excision. J Trauma 1987; 27(2):188–189.

19. Hildreth M, Herndon DN, Desai MH, Duke M. Reassessing caloric requirements in pediatric burns. J Burn Care Rehab 1988; 9(6):616–618.

20. Hildreth M, Herndon DN, Desai MH, Broemling LD. Caloric requirement of patients with burns under one year of age. J Burn Care Rehab 1993; 14:108–112.

21. Hildreth M, Herndon DN, Desai MH, Duke M. Reassessing caloric requirements in pediatric burns. J Burn Care Rehab 1988; 9(6):616–618.

22. Gore DC, Rutan RL, Hildreth M, Desai MH, Herndon DN. Comparison of resting energy expenditure in caloric intake in children with severe burns. J Burn Care Rehab 1990; 11:400–404.

23. Curreri PW, Richmond D, Marvin J, Baxter CR. Dietary requirements of patients with major burns. J Am Dietet Assoc 1974; 65:4.

24. Hart DW, Wolf SE, Herndon DN, Chinkes DL, Lal SO, Obeng MK, Beauford RB, Mlcak RTRP. Energy expenditure and caloric balance after burn: increased feeding leads to fat rather than lean mass accretion. Ann Surg 2002; 235(1):152–61.

25. Goran MI, Peters EJ, Herndon DN, Wolfe RR. Total energy expenditure in burned children using the doubly labeled water technique. Am J Physiol 1990; 259(4 Pt 1):576–85.

26. Patterson BU, Nguyen T, Pierre E, Herndon DN, Wolfe RR. Urea and protein metabolism in burned children: the effect of dietary protein intake. Metabolism 1997; 46(5):573–578.

27. Hart DW, Wolf SE, Zhang XJ, Chinkes DL, Buffalo MC, Matin SI, DebRoy MA, Wolfe RR, Herndon DN. Efficacy of a high-carbohydrate diet in catabolic illness. Crit Care Med 2001; 29:1318–1324.

28. Hart DW, Wolf SE, Zhang X-J, Chinkes DL, Buffalo MC, Matin SI, DebRoy MA, Wolfe RR, Herndon DN. Efficacy of high-carbohydrate diet in catabolic illness. Crit Care Med 2001; 29(7):1318–1324.

29. Ferrando AA, Chinkes DL, Wolf SE, Matin S, Herndon DN, Wolfe RR. A submaximal dose of insulin promotes net skeletal muscle protein synthesis in patients with severe burns. Ann Surg 1999; 229:11–18.

30. Van Der Berghe G, Wouters P, Weekers F, Verwaest C, Bruyninckx F, Schetz M, Vlasselaers D, Ferdniande P, Lauwers P, Bouillon R. Intensive insulin therapy in critically ill patients. N Engl J Med 2001; 345:1359–1367.

31. Herndon DN, Stein MD, Rutan T, Abston S, Linares H. Failure of TPN supplementation to improve liver function immunity and mortality in thermally injured patients. J Trauma 1987; 27(2):195–204.

32. Herndon DN, Barrow RE, Stein M, Linares H, Rutan T, Rutan R, Abston S. Increased mortality with intravenous supplemental feeding in severely burned patients. J Burn Care Rehab 1989; 10(4):309–313.

33. Dominioini L, Trocki O, Fang CH, Mochizuki H, Ray MB, Ogle CK, Alexander JW. Enteral feeding in burn hypermetabolism: nutritional and metabolic effects at different levels of calorie and protein intake. JPEN J Parenter Enteral Nutr 1985; 9(3):269–279.

34. Mochizuki H, Trocki O, Dominioini L, Brackett KA, Joffe SN, Alexander JW. Mechanisms of prevention of post-burn hypermetabolism and catabolism by early enteral feeding. Ann Surg 1984; 200(3):297–310.

35. Wolf SE, Jeschke M, Rose K, Desai MH, Herndon DN. Enteral feeding intolerance an indicator of sepsis-associated mortality in burned patients. Arch Surg 1997; 132: 1310–1314.

36. Biolo G, Fleming RYD, Maggi SP, Nguyen TT, Herndon DN, Wolfe RR. Inhibition of muscle glutamine formation in hypercatabolic patients. Clin Sci 2000; 99: 189–194.

37. Barret JP, Jeschke MG, Herndon DN. Fatty infiltration of the liver in severely burned pediatric patients: autopsy findings and clinical implications. J Trauma. 2001; 51:736–739.

38. Mochizuki H, Trocki O, Dominioni L, Ray MB, Alexander JW. Optimal lipid content for enteral diets following thermal injury. JPEN J Parenter Enteral Nutr 1984; 8:638–646.

39. Alexander JW, MacMillan BG, Stinnett JD, Ogle CK, Bozian RC, Fischer JE, Oakes JB, Morris MJ, Krummel R. Beneficial effects of aggressive protein feeding in severely burned children. Ann Surg 1980; 192:505–517.

40. Zawacki BE, Spitzer KW, Mason AD, Johns LA. Does increased evaporative water loss cause hypermetabolism in burned patients?. Ann Surg 1970:171–236.

41. Barr PO, Birke G, Liljedahl SO, Plantin LO. Oxygen consumption and water loss during treatment of burns with warm dry air. Lancet 1968; 1:164.

42. Wilmore DW, Mason AD, Johnson DW, Pruitt BA. Effective ambient temperature on heat production and heat loss in burned patients. J Appl Physiol 1975; 38: 593–597.

43. Suman OE, Spies RJ, Celis MM, Mlcak RP, Herndon DN. Effect of a twelve week resistant exercise program on skeletal muscle strength in children with burn injuries. J Appl Physiol 2001; 91:1168–1175.

44. Cucuzzo N, Ferrando AA, Herndon DN. The effects of exercise programming versus traditional outpatient therapy and rehabilitation in severely burned patients. J Burn Care Rehab 2001; 22:214–220.

45. Mlcak RP, Desai MH, Robinson E, McCauley RL, Robson MC, Herndon DN. Temperature changes during exercise stress testing in children with burns. J Burn Care Rehab 1993; 14:427–430.

46. Suman OE, Mlcak RP, Herndon DN. Effective exercise training improves pulmonary function in severely burned patients. J Burn Care Rehab 23(4):288–293.

47. Desai MH, Herndon DN, Broemling LD, Barrow RE, Nichols RJ, Rutan RL. Early burn wound excision significantly reduces blood loss. Ann Surg 1990; 211(6): 753–762.

48. Herndon DN, Barrow RE, Rutan RL, Rutan TC, Desai MH, Abston S. A comparison of conservative versus early excision therapies in severely burned patients. Ann Surg 1989; 209(5):547–553.

48a. Murphy KD, Lee JO, Herndon DN: Current pharmacotherapy for the treatment of severe burns. Expert Opin Pharmacother. 2003 Mar; 4(3):369–384.

49. Gray DT, Pine RW, Harnar TJ, Marvin J, Engrav L. Early surgical excision versus conventional therapy in patients with 20 to 40% burns — a comparative study. Am J Surg 1982; 144(1):76–80.

50. Merrell SW, Saffle SR, Sullivan JJ, Larsen CM, Warden GD. Increased survival after major thermal injury — nine year review. Am J Surg 1987; 154:623.

51. Hart DW, Wolf SE, Chinkes DL, Beauford RB, Mlcak RP, Heggers JP, Wolfe RR, Herndon DN. Effects of early excision and aggressive enteral feeding on hypermetabolism, catabolism and sepsis after severe burn. J Trauma:(in press).

52. Barret JP, Dziewulski P, Ramzy PI, Wolf SE, Desai MH, Herndon DN. Biobrane versus 1% sulfadiazine in second degree pediatric burns. Plast Reconstr Surg 2000; 105(1):62–65.

53. Rose JK, Desai MH, Mlakar JM, Herndon DN. Allograft is superior to topical antimicrobial therapy in the treatment of partial-thickness scald burns in children. J Burn Care Rehab 1997; 18(4):338–341.

54. Wainwright D, Madden M, Luterman A, Hunt J, Monafo W, Heimbach D, Kagan R, Sittig K, Dimick A, Herndon DN. Clinical evaluation of an acellular autograft dermal matrix in full thickness burns. J Burn Care Rehab 1996; 17(2):124–136.

55. Purdue GF, Hunt JL, Still JM, Law EJ, Herndon DN, Goldfarb IW, Schiller WR, Hansborough JF, Hickerson WL, Himel HN, Keeley GP, Twomey J, Missavage AE, Solem LD, Davis M, Totoritis M, Gentzkow GD. A multi centered clinical trial of biosynthetic skin replacement Dermagraft TC compared with cryopreserved human cadaver skin for temporary coverage of excised burn wound. J Burn Care Rehab 1997; 18(1 Pt 1):52–57.

56. Heimbach D, Luterman A, Burke J, Cram A, Herndon DN, Hunt J, Jordan M, McManus W, Solem L, Warden G, Zawacki B. Artificial dermis for major burns: a multi-center randomized clinical trial. Ann Surg 1988; 208(3):313–320.

57. Moskowitz JA, Fain JN. Stimulation by growth hormone and dexamethasone of labeled cyclic adenosine 3′,5′-monophosphate accumulation by white fat cells. J Biol Chem 1970 10; 245(5):1101–7.

58. Sheffield-Moore M, Urban RJ, Wolf SE, Jiang J, Catlin DH, Herndon DN, Wolfe RR, Ferrando AA. Short term oxandrolone administration stimulates muscle protein synthesis in young men. J Clin Endocrinol Metab 1999; 84(8):2705–2711.

58a. Murphy KD, Thomas S, Mlcak RP, Chinkes DL, Klein GL, Herndon DN: Effects of long term oxandrolone administration in severely burned children. Surgery 2004 Aug; 136(2) pp.

59.   Ferrando AA, Sheffield-Moore M, Wolf SE, Herndon DN, Wolfe RR. Testosterone administraton in severe burns ameliorates muscle catabolism. Crit Care Med 2001; 29(10):1936–1942.

60.   Herndon DN, Hawkins HK, Nguyen TT, Pierre E, Cox R, Barrow RE. Characterization of growth hormone enhanced donor site healing in patients with large cutaneous burns. Ann Surg 1995; 221(6):649–659.

61.   Herndon DN, Barrow RE, Kunkel KR, Broemeling L, Rutan RL. Effects of recombinant human growth hormone on donor site healing in severely burned children. Ann Surg 1992; 12:424–431.

62.   Hart DW, Klein GL, Lee SB, Celis M, Mohan S, Chinkes DL, Wolf SE. Attenuation of post-traumatic muscle catabolism and osteopenia by long-term growth hormone therapy. Ann Surg 2001; 233:827–834.

63.   Klein GL, Herndon DN, Rutan TC, Barnett JR, Miller NL, Alfrey AC. Risk of aluminum accumulation in patients with burns and ways to reduce it. J Burn Care Rehab 1994; 15(4):354–8.

63a. Murphy KD, Wu X, Thomas S, Sanford DN. Long-term growth hormone treatment improves metabolic variables and incrementally improves hormone levels in severely burned children. Crit Care Med. Dec 2003; 31(12) Suppl pA20.

64.   Klein GL, Herndon DN, Rutan TC, Sherrard DJ, Coburn JW, Langman CB, Thomas ML, Haddad JG, Cooper CW, Miller NL, et al. Bone disease in burn patients. J Bone Miner Res 1993; 8:337–345.

65.   Klein GL, Langman CB, Herndon DN. Persistant hypoparathyroidism following magnesium repletion in burn-injured children. Pediatr Nephrol 2000; 14:301–304.

66.   Klein GL, Herndon DN. Magnesium deficit in major burns: role in hypoparathyroidism and end-organ parathyroid hormone resistance. Magnes Res 1998; 2(2): 103–109.

67.   Klein GL, Herndon GL. The role of bone densitometry in the diagnosis abd management of the severely burned patients with bone loss. J Clin Densitom 1999; 2(1): 11–15.

68.   Rutan RL, Herndon DN. Growth delay in post-burn pediatric patients. Arch Surg 1990; 125(3):392–395.

69.   Klein GL, Herndon DN, Langman CB, Rutan TC, Young WE, Pembleton G, Nusynowitz M, Barnett JL, Broemling LD, Sailer DE, McCauley RL. Long term reduction in bone mass after severe burn injury. J Pediatr 1995; 126:252–256.

70.   Jeffries MK, Vance ML. Growth hormone and cortisol secretion in patients with burn injury. J Burn Care Rehabl 1992; 13:391–395.

71.   Shotwell MA, Kilberg MS, Oxender DL. The regulation of neutral amino acid transport in mammalian cells. Biochim Biophys Acta 1983; 737:267–284.

72.   Van Vliet G, Bosson D, Craen M, Du Caju MV, Malvaux P, Vanderschueren-Lodeweyckx M. Comparative study of the litholytic potencies of pituitary derived and biosynthetic human growth hormone and hypopituitary children. J Clin Endocrinol Metab 1987; 65:876–879.

73. Mjaaland M, Unneberg K, Larsson J, et al. Growth hormone after abdominal surgery attenuated from glutamine, alanine, 3methylhistine, total parenteral nutrition. Ann Surg 1993; 217:413–422.

74. Ramirez RJ, Wolf SE, Barrow RE, Herndon DN. Growth hormone treatment in pediatric burns: a safe therapeutic approach. Ann Surg 1998; 228(4):439–448.

75. Jeffries MK, Vance ML. Growth hormone and cortisol secretion in patients with burn injury. J Burn Care Rehab 1992; 13:391–395.

76. Hart DW, Herndon DN, Klein GL, Lee SB, Celis M, Mohan S, Chinkes DL, Wolfe SE. Attenuation of post-traumatic muscle catabolism and osteopenia by long-term growth hormone therapy. Ann Surg 2001; 233:827–834.

77. Knox JB, Wilmore DW, Demling RH, Sarraf P, Santos AA. Use of growth hormone for postoperative respiratory failure. Am J Surg 1996; 171(6):576–80.

78. Jeschke MG, Barrow RE, Herndon DN. Recombinant human growth hormone treatment in pediatric burn patients and its role during the hepatic acute phase response. Crit Care Med 2000; 28(5):1578–1584.

79. Jarrar D, Wolf SE, Jeschke MG, Ramirez RJ, DebRoy M, Ogle CK, Papaconstantinou J, Herndon DN. Growth hormone attenuates the acute-phase response to thermal injury. Arch Surg 1997; 132(11):1171–1175.

80. Takagi K, Suzuki F, Barrow RE, Wolf SE, Kobayashi M, Herndon DN. Growth hormone improves the resistance of thermally injured mice infected with herpes simplex virus type 1. J Trauma 1998; 44(3):517–522.

81. Takagi K, Suzuki F, Barrow RE, Wolf SE, Kobayashi M, Herndon DN. Growth hormone improves immune function and survival in burned mice infected with herpes simplex virus type 1. J Surg Res 1997; 69(1):166–170.

82. Takagi, Suzuki F, Barrow RE, Wolf SE, Herndon DN. Recombinant human growth hormone modulates Th-1, T-2 cytokine response. Ann Surg 1998; 228(1):106–111.

83. Clements DR, Smith–Banks A, Underwood LE. Reversal of diet induced catabolism by infusion of recombinant insulin-like growth factor (IGF-1) in humans. J Clin Endocrinol Metab 1992; 75:234–238.

84. Jeschke MG, Barrow RE, Herndon DN. Insulin-like growth factor 1 plus insulin-like growth factor binding protein-3 attenuates the proinflammatory acute phase response in severely burned children. Ann Surg 2000; 231(2):246–252.

85. Spies M, Wolf SE, Barrow RE, Jeschke MG, Herndon DN. Modulation of types 1 and 11 acute phase reactants with insulin-like growth factor-1/binding protein-3 complex in severely burned children. Crit Care Med 2002; 30(1):83–88.

86. Klein GL, Wolf SE, Goodman WG, Phillips WA, Herndon DN. The management of acute bone loss and severe catabolism due to burn injury. Horm Res 1997; 48(Suppl 5):83.

87. Low JFA, Barrow RE, Mittendorfer B, Jeschke MG, Chinkes DL, Herndon DN. The effect of short-term growth hormone treatment on growth and energy expenditure in burned patients. Burns 2001; 27(5):447–452.

88. Klein GL, Wolf SE, Langman CB, Rosen CJ, Mohan S, Keenan BS, Matin S, Steffen C, Nicolai M, Sailer DE, Herndon DN. Effects of therapy with recombinant human growth hormone on insulin-like growth factor system components and serum levels of biochemical markers of bone formation in children after severe burn injury. J Clin Endocrinol Metab 1998; 83(1):21–4.

89. Low JF, Herndon DN, Barrow RE. Effect of growth hormone on growth delay in burned children: a 3-year follow-up study. Lancet 1999; 354(9192):1789.

90. Knox J, Demling R, Wilmore D, Sarif P, Santos A. Increased survival after a major thermal injury: the effect of growth hormone therapy in adults. J Trauma 1995; 39: 526–532.

91. Ruokonen E, Takala J. Dangers of growth hormone therapy in critically ill patients. Ann Med 2000; 32(5):317–22.

92. Takala J, Ruokonen E, Webster NR, Nielsen MS, Zandstra DF, Vundelinckx G, Hinds CJ. Increased mortality associated with growth hormone treatment in critically ill adults. N Engl J Med 1999; 341(11):785–92.

93. Barret JP, Dziewulski P, Wolf SE, Desai MH, Herndon DN. Effects of recombinant human growth hormone on burn scar development. Plast Reconstr Surg 1999; 104(3):726–729.

93a. Oliverra GV, Sanford AP, Murphy KD, Chinkes DL, Hawkins HK, Herndon DN: Growth hormone effects on hypertrophic scar formation: a randomized controlled trial of 62 burned children. Wound Repair Regen. 2004 July-Aug; 12(4):[in press].

93b. Thomas S, Wolf SE, Murphy KD, Chinkes DL, Herndon DN: The long-term effects of oxandidone on hepatic acute phase proteins in severely burned children. J. Trauma 2004 Jan; 56(1):37–44.

94. Hart DW, Wolf SE, Ramzy PI, Beauford RB, Ferrando AA, Wolfe RR, Herndon DN. Anabolic effects of oxandrolone following severe burn. Ann Surg 2001; 233: 556–564.

95. Gore DC, Chinkes DL, Heggers JP, Herndon DN, Wolf SE, Desai MH. Association of hyperglycemia with increased mortality after severe burn injury. J Trauma 2001; 51(3):540–544.

96. Van Der Berghe G, Wouters P, Weekers F, Verwaest C, Bruyninckx F, Schetz M, Vlasselaers D, Ferdniande P, Lauwers P, Bouillon R. Intensive insulin therapy in critically ill patients. N Engl J Med 2001; 345:1359–1367.

97. Aarsland A, Chinkes DL, Sakurai Y, Nguyen TT, Herndon DN, Wolfe RR. Insulin therapy in burn patients does not contribute to hepatic triglyceride production. J Clin Invest 1998; 101(10):2233–2239.

98. Sakurai Y, Aarsland A, Herndon DN, Chinkes DL, Pierre E, Nguyen TT, Patterson BW, Wolfe RR. Stimulation of muscle protein synthesis by long-term insulin infusion in severely burned patients. Ann Surg 1995; 222(3):283–297.

99. Ferrando AA, Chinkes DL, Wolf SE, Matin S, Herndon DN, Wolfe RR. A submaximal dose of insulin promotes skeletal muscle protein synthesis in patients with severe burns. Ann Surg 1999; 229(1):11–18.

100. Mowlavi A, Andrews K, Milner S, Herndon DN, Heggers JP. The effects of hyperglycemia on skin graft survival in the burn patient. Ann Plast Surg 2000; 45: 629–632.

101. Ferrando AA, Chinkes DL, Wolf SE, Matin S, Herndon DN, Wolfe RR. Acute dichloroacetate administration increases skeletal muscle free glutamine concentrations after burn injury. Ann Surg 1998; 228(2):249–256.

102. Cioffi WG, Gore DC, Rue LW, Carrougher G, Guler HP, MacManus WF, Pruitt BA. Insulin like growth factor-1 lowers protein oxidation in patients with thermal injury. Ann Surg 1994; 220:310–319.

103. Wilmore DW, Long JN, Mason AD, Skreen RW, Pruitt BA. Catecholamines: mediator of the hypermetabolic response to thermal injury. Ann Surg 1974; 180:653–669.

104. Asch MJ, Feldman RJ, Walker HL, Foley FD, Popp RL, Mason AD, Pruitt BA. Systemic and pulmonary hemodynamic changes accompanying thermal injury. Ann Surg 1973; 178:218–22.

105. Reese W, Pearson E, Art CP. The metabolic response to burns. J Clin Invest 1956; 35:62–77.

106. Herndon DN, Nguyen TT, Wolfe RR, Maggi S, Biolo G, Muller M, Barrow RE. Lipolysis in burned patients is stimulated by the beta 2 receptor for catecholamines. Arch Surg 1994; 129:1301–1305.

107. Wolfe RR, Herndon DN, Peters EJ, Jahoor F, Desai MH, Holland B. Regulation of lipolysis in severely burned patients. Ann Surg 1987; 206(2):214–221.

108. Barret JP, Jeschke MG, Herndon DN. Fatty infiltration of the liver in severely burned pediatric patients: autopsy findings and clinical implications. J Trauma 2001; 51(4):736–739.

109. Minifee PK, Barrow RE, Abson S, Desai MH, Herndon DN. Improved myocardial oxygen utilization following propranolol infusion in adolescents with post-burn hypermetabolism. J Pediatr Surg 1989; 24:806–810.

110. Herndon DN, Barrow RE, Rutan TC, Minifee P, Jahoor F, Wolfe RR. Effect of propranolol administration on human dynamic metabolic response of the burned pediatric patients. Ann Surg 1988; 208(4):484–492.

111. Baron PW, Barrow RE, Pierre EJ, Herndon DN. Prolonged use of propranolol effectively decreases cardiac work in burned children. J Burn Care Rehabl 1997; 18(3):223–227.

112. Gore DC, Honeycutt D, Jahoor F, Barrow RE, Wolfe RR, Herndon DN. Propranolol diminishes extremity blood flow in burn patients. Ann Surg 1991; 213(6):568–574.

113. Hendon DN, Hart DW, Wolf SE, Chinkes DL, Wolfe RR. Reversal of catabolism by beta-blockade after severe burns. N Engl J Med 2001; 345(17):1223–1229.

114. Honeycutt D, Barrow RE, Herndon DN. Cold stress response in patients with severe burns after beta-blockade. J Burn Care Rehabl 1992; 13:181–186.

115. Morio B, Irtun O, Hendon DN, Wolfe RR. Propranolol decreases splanchnic triacylglycerol storage in burned patients receiving a high carbohydrate diet. Ann Surg 2002; 236(2):218–225.

116. Aarsland A, Chinkes DL, Wolfe RR, Barrow RE, Nelson SO, Pierre E, Herndon DN. Beta-blockade lowers peripheral lipolysis in burn patients receiving growth hormone. Ann Surg 1996; 223(6):777–789.

117. Gore DC, Honeycutt D, Jahoor F, Barrow RE, Wolfe RR, Herndon DN. Propranolol diminishes extremity blood flow in burn patients. Ann Surg 1991; 213(6):568–574.

118. Sheridan RL, Hinson MI, Liang MH, Nackel AF, Schoenfeld DA, Ryan CM, Mulligan JL, Tompkins RG. Long-term outcomes of children surviving massive injury. JAMA 2000; 283:69–73.

119. Hart DW, Wolf SE, Chinkes DL, Wolfe RR. Anabolic strategies after severe burn. J Am Coll Surg:(in press).

14

A Practical Approach to Acute Burn Rehabilitation

Michael A. Serghiou and Scott A. Farmer
Shriners Burns Hospital, Galveston, Texas, U.S.A.

INTRODUCTION

A significant burn injury may lead to a devastating functional outcome if it is not methodically and systematically managed by an experienced burn team. Physical rehabilitation is an essential component of the burn team. Its goal is to assist the burn survivor throughout the recovery process in order to achieve the most positive functional outcome at the completion of therapy. Immediate attention to serious burn injuries in the acute phase is critical in saving the patient's life and may be a predictor of a good rehabilitative outcome in the long run. Today, there are no standard guidelines or protocols that dictate the way a therapist should design and deliver treatment. Therapists achieve the common rehabilitation goal of optimal functional recovery in different ways. Over the years therapists have developed their own treatment techniques, some of which have objectively demonstrated good outcomes and produced positive therapeutic results clinically. This chapter discusses current treatment techniques utilized in the acute phase of rehabilitation, which is defined as the time the patient has been admitted to the intensive care unit (ICU) until the completion of all grafting procedures and wound closure. Positioning, splinting, wound and scar management, exercise, and functional activities will be discussed in the preoperative, intraoperative, and postoperative setting, as indicated in the acute phase. Also, patient and family education as it relates to rehabilitation during this phase of recovery will be addressed.

Once the patient has been admitted to the burn center, the therapist conducts a comprehensive evaluation to assess the patient's needs for physical rehabilitation and design the most effective plan of care. The initial evaluation is critical and should be carefully documented by the therapist in the medical record. Initial observations made at that time, such as risk for pressure areas and special positioning needs, may affect the outcome of therapy later on in rehabilitation.

POSITIONING IN THE ACUTE PHASE

Correct positioning of the burned patient is vital early on after the injury and in some cases would almost guarantee positive functional outcomes at the completion of rehabilitation. Positioning should begin immediately upon admission to the burn center and should be continued until all the scars from the last operative procedure have matured (reconstructive phase of rehabilitation).

Preoperative Positioning

Positioning is initially designed to aid in edema reduction, promote wound healing, preserve function, and prevent contractures. It may be accomplished with the use of pillows, foam pads, cut out mattresses, overhead trapeze mechanisms, and splinting.

Head

Head elevation above the level of the heart decreases edema in the emergent phase of rehabilitation. In cases of large total body surface area burns (TBSAB) shock blocks may be utilized to achieve elevation of the entire bed (Fig. 1). With the use of these wooden (12 × 12 inch) blocks placed beneath the feet at the head of the regular bed, the entire bed comes to an incline of approximately 30 degrees. This aids in head edema reduction without having to position the patient's injured hips in the compromising flexion position. A wooden board padded with foam is placed at the foot of the bed (Fig. 1) to prevent the patient from sliding downward. The described positioning technique is impossible to achieve when the patient is positioned in a Clinitron bed.

Antitorticollis Head Strap

In preventing lateral neck flexion and cervical spine rotation, which may lead to the development of so-called burn torticollis, the therapist may design and fabri-

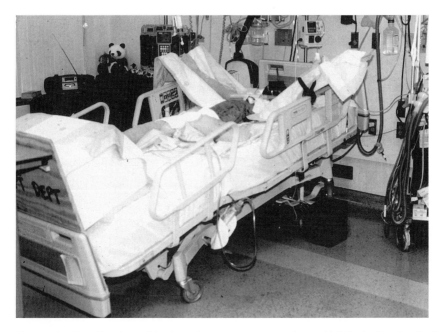

Figure 1 Total body positioning of an acute burn patient which includes detail of each individual body segment and addresses edema of the upper body.

cate a dynamic strap mechanism that achieves a head midline position (Fig. 2) while the patient is lying supine in bed. The dynamic strap includes a Velfoam headband attached to TheraBand elastic, which, in turn, is tied to the side of the bed and provides enough tension to bring the head/neck in the neutral position.

Ear Cups

The ear cartilage, if involved, may be easily damaged further by rubbing on the mattress or pillows if not protected. Ear cups may be fabricated to protect the ears and serve as anchors for tubes to be tied on, rather than wrapping around the head tightly and damaging the ears.

Neck

The neck should be positioned in neutral or in slight extension (10–15 degrees) with the use of towel rolls or foam pads behind the neck or on the scapular line. A foam mattress may be cut short and placed on top of the regular bed mattress, allowing the patient's neck to drop into extension, in so-called short mattress supine position. If the patient is in a Clinitron bed, weights may be placed on either side of the neck to allow it to slightly extend. A patient with injuries to the head and/or neck should not be allowed to use pillows. Special attention

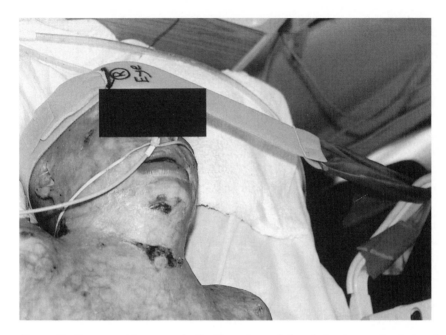

FIGURE 2   To prevent burn scar torticollis, a dynamic head sling is constructed and attached to the bed rail to bring the patient's head in to the midline.

should be given to the intubated patient when positioning the head and the neck accurately so that ventilation is not obstructed.

Shoulders

Both shoulders, if involved, should be positioned in the scaption position: the plane between shoulder flexion and shoulder abduction (Fig. 1). Positioning the shoulder in approximately 90 degrees of abduction with approximately 30 degrees of horizontal flexion alleviates stress on the brachial plexus. A nerve palsy may occur when the shoulder is positioned in plain abduction and the neck is rotated toward the contralateral side over a period of time. Bedside tables or metal troughs padded with foam may be utilized initially to achieve this position.

Elbow and Forearm

The elbow is positioned in extension with the forearm in neutral or in supination depending on the distribution of the injury. It is important not to lock the elbow into maximum extension when positioning it into a splint to prevent future elbow capsular tightness. Positioning of the elbow may be achieved through the use of anterior elbow conformers or metal bed conformers padded with foam.

Wrist and Hand

For the short term, the wrist and the hand may be placed in a functional burned hand position that may include wrist extension (0–30 degrees), metacarpophalangeal (MCP) joint flexion (70–90 degrees) placing the collateral ligaments of these joints into a stretched position to prevent future tightness, and the interphalangeal (IP) joint in full extension (0 degrees), placing the collateral ligaments and the volar plate into a stretched position to prevent future tightness and contracture. The thumb may be positioned into a combination of radial and palmar abduction, preventing future cupping of the hand created by volar skin contractures between the thenar and hypothenar eminence. The hand position described (Fig. 3) is a suggestive one with existing variations and may be accomplished using the burn hand splint.

Hips

The hips should be positioned in neutral rotation, approximately 10–15 degrees abduction and full extension (Fig. 1). When the hips are injured, elevation of the head of the hospital bed should be avoided to prevent flexion contractures. The hip position described may be accomplished through the use of wedges, pillows, or a hip spica splint.

Knees

The knees are positioned in extension, avoiding locking the joints in full extension, and thus preventing future capsular tightness. Positioning is commonly achieved with the use of hard thermoplastic posterior knee conformers.

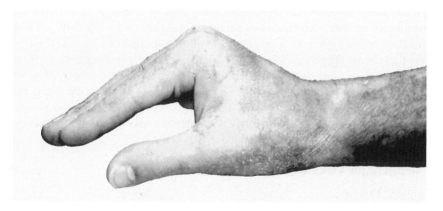

FIGURE 3 The burned hand functional position includes 0–30 degrees of wrist extension, 70–90 degrees of MCP joint flexion, 0 degrees IP joint, and a combination of CMC joint palmar and radial abduction.

Ankles

The ankles are positioned in the neutral position (0 degrees dorsiflexion) with the use of padded footboards (Fig. 1) or splints. Special attention should be given to the heel of the foot to prevent pressure ulcers.

Patients who have sustained a large burn injury require extensive custom positioning regimens, that are closely monitored and altered as dictated by the their medical status. The key to preventing skin breakdown and pressure ulcers is to reposition the patient frequently. This alleviates excessive and prolonged pressure on certain anatomical locations. A written comprehensive positioning and shifting regimen with photographs should be posted in the patient's room. The entire team along with the patient's family should be educated on how to implement this positioning program. When the patient is medically stable he or she should be spending a lot of time in the upright position ambulating or sitting in a chair with frequent shifting, in order to minimize the risk of pressure ulcers on already compromised body surface areas.

Intraoperative Positioning

In the operating room (OR) the patient must be carefully positioned to accommodate the physician's needs and to prevent complications from incorrect positioning such as iatrogenic pressure sores and nerve palsies. The problems associated with handling a patient with burn wounds are always a concern. Even transferring to and from an operating table can cause graft loss. Most frequently, patients may be positioned supine, prone, sidelying or, in the cases of special operative procedures, they may be suspended by traction. Skeletal traction may be utilized intraoperatively for delicate skin grafting procedures during which shearing may damage or destroy the new skin or skin substitute applied. This can be achieved by hoisting the patient's top four-corner traction frame up in the OR (Fig. 4). The traction's pulley system is disengaged and all four extremities are tied directly to the top frame. The therapist's role is to monitor closely the forces exerted on the extremities during suspension and to fabricate a special head sling (Fig. 4) to position the suspended head correctly in relation to the rest of the body. No matter how positioning in the operating room is approached, the team should make sure that the patient's entire body is positioned correctly and not focus only on the positioning of the operative site.

Postoperative Positioning

Skeletal Traction

After a skin grafting operation the patient may be placed on bed rest according to the unit's immobilization protocol. Postoperative positioning is very similar to preoperative positioning, with the emphasis on protecting the newly applied

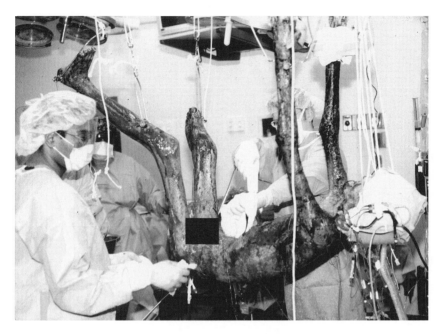

FIGURE 4 Skeletal traction can be used as an intraoperative suspension system for successive skin grafting procedures and must account for head suspension.

skin while preventing contractures and preserving function. Therapists are often called upon to design skeletal traction systems that minimize the need for direct handling of patients with large burn injuries (Fig. 5). The successful construction of a traction frame begins with an understanding of biomechanics and the ability to control the forces acting upon the skeletal system. Cardinal plane motion is desired as much as possible when designing a pulley system. Force vectors perpendicular to the bone are most effective at producing a desired position. Some deviation is required when force vectors are desired in a common direction. When deviation occurs it is best to determine the motion of greatest concern and provide a vector most advantageous for that joint. Key points of control are maintained due to the strong cortical bone that holds the traction pins. This issue of control makes skeletal traction such a valuable management tool. A list of benefits that this system provides includes the following:

> Elevates extremities off the supporting surface
> Provides an alternative means of handling
> Maintains functional positions
> Provides a slight distraction force to the joint capsules
> Can be used as an intraoperative suspension system

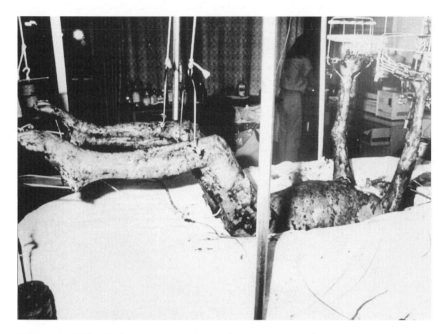

FIGURE 5 This skeletal traction design incorporates a Clinitron airbed into the support frame and requires less direct handling of the patient.

Elevation of the Extremities off of the Supporting Surface

One of the most crucial aspects of burn care is saving the skin grafts in large burns. As the size of a burn increases, the need to preserve donor tissue and limit repeated grafting procedures becomes more important. In this system, the extremities can be elevated and free from contact pressures. While in this position the hands can be addressed several different ways. Some of the more common hand management traction techniques include the banjo, hay rake, and halo. These all provide an appropriate hand position and assist with application of wound dressing.

Traction as an Alternative Means of Patient Handling

The stability and control provided by cortical bone allow the patient to be manipulated using the traction pins. A caregiver can lift directly on the bows that connect to the pins or pull down on the pulley system to lift the patient for any assessed need. This will limit much of the pressure associated with other handling techniques that require pressure to be applied directly to the superficial tissues. This can be a visually disturbing process: to see a patient being lifted by pins that are protruding from the extremities. However, the skeletal system is much less innervated than the superficial tissue and it can actually be less painful and safer than direct handling of the patient.

Maintenance of Functional Positions

Elevation of the extremities primarily occurs in the sagittal plane. The pulley design that controls the skeletal system is positioned so that the patient will have 90 degrees of flexion at the glenohumeral joint (Fig. 5). This places the arms in a functional plane for long periods of time to allow modeling of the periscapular scar tissue. Since the functional position for the legs is closer to extension, the resting position is maintained at 45 degrees and metatarsal pins pull the ankle into a neutral position (Fig. 5). Once the positions have been determined, weights are applied via the pulley system to maintain the position. The positions are alternated in opposing directions on a 2 h schedule. The resistance that maintains the extremities can also be used to supply resistance to the traction pins for an active exercise program. Traction may be a good alternative to conventional positioning after delicate grafting techniques such as Integra or cultured epidermal autografts (CEAs).

ORTHOTICS AND SPLINTING

Splints and other orthotics are widely accepted means for correctly positioning the burned patient. They are utilized to prevent or correct contractures and deformities, preserve function, maintain or increase range of motion (ROM), depress hypertrophic scars, promote wound healing, protect skin grafts or flaps, and decrease edema. The burn rehabilitation therapist must be well aware of the anatomy and kinesiology of the body surface to be splinted to avoid further injury such as joint dislocation. Splints should be constructed along the continuum of care as needed to be most effective and produce, the most desirable outcome. Orthotics and splints should be constructed of appropriate materials; be functional, cosmetically appealing, easy to apply, and remove; should not cause pain; and they need to be monitored frequently and altered as indicated.

Preoperative Splinting

In the emergent phase (0–72 h from the injury) positioning of the patient may be accomplished through splinting to reduce edema and preserve function. During this time splinting for the head, face, neck, and shoulders may not be indicated if correct positioning is achieved through the use of pillows, foam troughs, and cut-out foam mattresses.

Burn Hand Splint

One of the most frequently utilized splints in the early stages of burn rehabilitation and later is the burn hand splint (Fig. 6). Positioning of the hand within the splint may include wrist extension (0–30 degrees), MCP joint flexion (70–90 degrees), and IP joint maximum extension (0). The thumb is positioned in a combination of palmar and radial abduction. Initially this splint may be worn at all times, especially if the edema is very significant to prevent further damage to hand structures from movement attempts by the patient. As edema subsides, the splint may only be worn at night only so that the patient can perform activities of daily living (ADLs) independently during the day.

Elbow Conformer

An anterior elbow conformer (Fig. 1) may be fabricated to prevent elbow flexion contractures. It is made out of thermoplastic materials on top of dressings and must be frequently monitored and altered to accommodate the various dressings

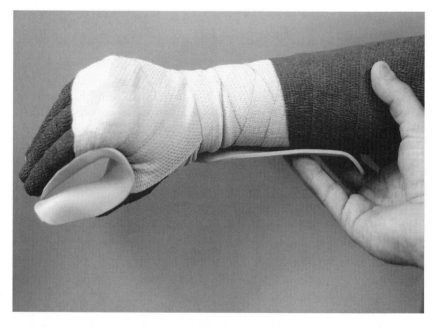

FIGURE 6 The burn hand splint positions the hand appropriately and aids in preventing hand stiffness by positioning the collateral ligaments at the MCP joints and the collateral ligaments and the volar plate at the IP joints in maximal stretch. The combination of palmar and radial abduction at the thumb helps to prevent cupping of the palm.

thicknesses and presence of edema. The splint should clear the wrist joint distally and the axillary region proximally by 1–2 in. In most cases the elbow splint is combined with the hand splint in an overlapping fashion. It is important to designate which splint is worn on top by marking the thermoplastic material.

Posterior Knee Conformer

To prevent flexion contractures at the knee, the therapist may construct a hard thermoplastic posterior knee splint. The splint should clear the Achilles tendon and heel distally and the buttocks and perineal area proximally by 1–2 in. to avoid proximal and distal pressure when the splint shifts.

Foot Drop Splint

Most commonly during this stage of recovery a posterior foot drop splint is fabricated out of thermoplastic materials (Fig. 7a) or a prefabricated (Fig. 7b) splint is utilized to prevent plantar flexion while protection the heel from breakdown. The splint positions the ankle in neutral and suspends the heel, thus preventing pressure acting upon it. The therapist should adjust the foot and knee splint in order to be applied together in cases in which both splints are required at the same time and designate which splint is worn on top by marking the thermoplastic material.

Intraoperative Splinting

Splinting in the OR, when needed, is beneficial because the anesthetized patient will not actively resist splinting that may damage freshly applied skin grafts. Care should be given to minimize the OR dressing in order for constructed splints to fit correctly and functionally.

Neck Conformer

The patient may be fitted with an anterior hard neck splint over bulky dressings (Fig. 8). The splint is not removed until the first postoperative dressing change is performed.

Airplane Splint

After undergoing axillary releases and skin grafting, the patient may be required to wear an airplane splint. These splints may be custom-made or prefabricated and they are applied in the OR at the completion of the surgical procedure to immobilize and protect new skin grafts. The benefits of the prefabricated airplane splint, which unfortunately comes in only one adult size, is that it minimizes OR splinting time and allows for different abduction ranges. This is achieved by unlocking the goniometric mechanism and changing the abduction setting manually, thus eliminating future time-consuming splint adjustments by the therapist. Other splints most commonly fabricated in the OR include the hand splint, elbow,

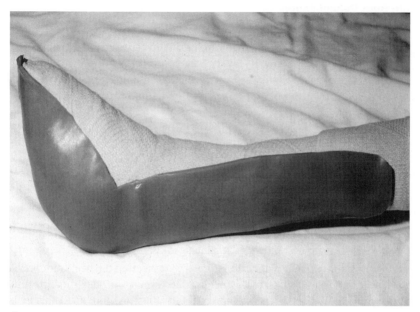

A

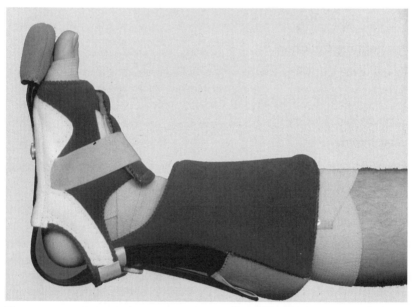

B

FIGURE 7 (a) A posterior custom-made foot drop splint or (b) a prefabricated posterior foot drop splint helps to maintain the foot in the neutral position and suspend the heel thus protecting it from unwanted pressure and skin breakdown.

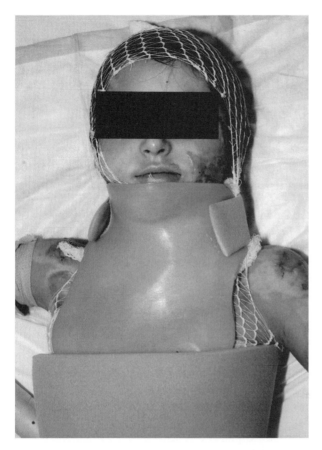

FIGURE 8 Postoperatively, the neck is positioned appropriately with the use of an anterior hard neck splint.

and knee conformers. The key to successful OR splinting is to minimize the postoperative dressing without compromising the grafted sites. When intraoperative splinting is scheduled in advance, the therapist makes the necessary preparations prior to entering the OR, this minimizing the splint fabrication time and not prolonging the anesthesia time.

Unna's Boot

To protect a fresh graft best until the first dressing change, the grafted site may be immobilized and protected at the same time with an Unna's boot intraoperatively. This resembles a soft cast that eliminates the need for hard thermoplastic application for immobilization.

OR Casting

After a contracture release and skin grafting, immobilization may be achieved through the application of a fiberglass or plaster cast. The hard cast helps to maintain the position achieved by the surgeon in the OR. In the case of hands or feet that have been operated on, it may help to prevent pinning of digits or joints.

Postoperative Splinting

The patient's operated-on sites are immobilized for approximately 4 days according to the unit's protocols. Once the grafts take and wounds close, the focus of splinting is on counteracting the contractile forces of by the newly formed scar. The therapist must choose appropriate thermoplastic materials prior to the construction of splints. Materials with memory allow for multiple adjustments of splints and are best suited for serial splinting. At this time dynamic splints are introduced to provide traction and aid in reversing scar contractures, maintain and/or increase ROM, and allow for functional use of the splinted joints. In the case of peripheral nerve injuries to the upper extremity, dynamic splints may help the hand perform ADLs until muscle innervation and functional strength return.

It is imperative that the therapist be knowledgeable about the anatomy of the body part to be splinted before constructing a splint in order to prevent further injury to the already compromised joints. The basic mechanical principles of splinting need to be consider prior to splinting. As the physical status of the patient continues to change, and depending on the stage of scar maturation, all splints must be closely and frequently monitored for fit and be adjusted or modified as indicated.

Splint application schedules should also be assessed on a regular basis and modified to allow the patient to function independently as much as possible.

In cases of severe circumferential injuries, splints need to provide stretching to the agonist and antagonist muscles and stretch the scar in all directions.

Ear Obturators

Active scars may contract around the ear canal, causing it to begin to close circumferentially. Ear obturators (Fig. 9a) are fabricated out of hard thermoplastics to maintain and increase the ear canal opening. Fast results in opening the ear canal with these serially adjusted splints have been observed.

External Ear Splint

Severe burns to the face and head may cause a contracture in the back of the ear, which may begin to contract toward the scalp. A splint resembling an oyster shell is formed behind the ear to prevent it from attaching to the scalp. The splint is made of thermoplastic materials directly fitted to the patient (Fig. 9b) or by

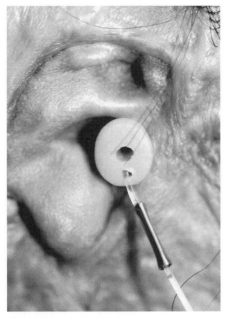

A

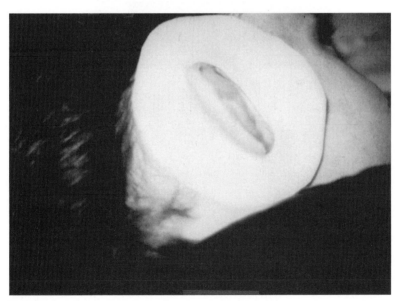

B

FIGURE 9 (a) Ear obturators prevent closure of the ear canal. (b) A low thermoplastic splint resembling an oyster shell may be formed behind the ear to prevent it from contracting to the scalp.

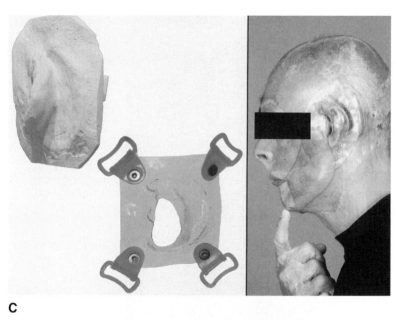

C

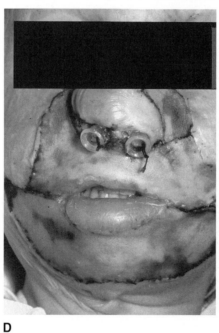

D

Figure 9 (Cont.) (c) A negative mold of the patient's ear is taken, from which a positive mold is constructed. Then a high thermoplastic transparent posterior splint is fabricated. (d) Nasal obturators can reverse burn scar stenosis of the nostrils.

utilizing the negative/positive mold technique to create a positive mold of the surface described above. A conformer made of high thermoplastic material is then created from the positive mold (Fig. 9c).

Nasal Obturators

Similarly to the ear obturators, these splints reverse the stenosis of the nostrils created by contracting scar around the nose. These splints produce fast positive results if they are worn continually when the scars are active (Fig. 9d).

Mouth Splints

Oral microstomia may develop as a result of perioral scar development. Several oral microstomia splints can be utilized to stretch the mouth horizontally, vertically, or circumferentially. The devices may be static or dynamic (Fig. 10). They need to be worn around the clock, except during meals and exercise, in order to produce the most positive results. A dynamic horizontal splint may be worn during the day to prevent drooling and a static splint at night when the patient is resting in the supine position. The tension at the oral commissures is adjusted to prevent skin breakdown or pressure sores during prolonged application of these devices.

Neck Splints

In addition to the traditional anterior hard neck conformer, other types of neck splints may be used. Open-phase neck designs include lateral, anterior, or posterior neck splints, which are specifically constructed to position the neck appropriately postoperatively while protecting fragile autografts or skin substitutes (Fig. 11).

Figure 8 Axillary Pads

As scar begins to form, contractures may be caused in the axilla anteriorly, posteriorly, or on both surfaces. These contractures may negatively affect the ROM of both shoulders and lead to functional limitations. In addition to the airplane splint, figure 8 axillary pads may be fabricated to keep the axillary skin surface stretched and prevent webbing of the skin on the anterior or posterior surfaces. These pads are made of foam are attached to a strapping mechanism that promotes good postural control by bringing the scapulae into correct retraction and adduction.

Deformities of the Hand

During the acute post operative phase wounds continue to heal and overabundance of collagen laid at the wound site for healing leads to the formation of contracting hypertrophic scars. As a result of these scars, different deformities may begin to

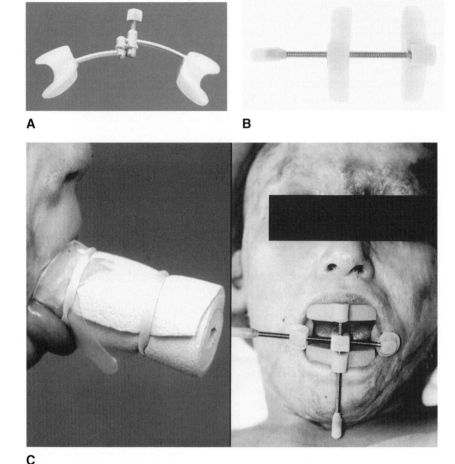

FIGURE 10 Mouth splints are used to prevent or correct oral microstomia; (a) static horizontal mouth opening splint, (b) static vertical mouth-opening splint, (c) circumferential microstomia device.

develop in the hand that, if left untreated, may lead to devastating functional limitations.

Claw Hand Deformity

As burn wounds on the dorsum of the hand begin to close they may cause MCP joint hyperextension and IP joint flexion, leading to what is known as a claw

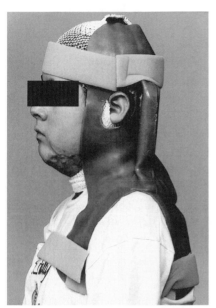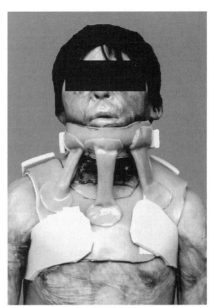

A   **B**

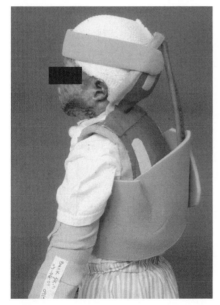

C

FIGURE 11   Open phase neck splints are constructed to position the neck appropriately after skin grafting and prevent shearing of the newly applied skin or skin substitute; (a) lateral neck splint, (b) anterior neck splint, (c) posterior neck splint.

hand deformity. The hand becomes flat in its palmar surface and the definition of the palmar arches is lost. A burn hand splint or a dorsal block splint adjusted in a serial fashion should be utilized to correct this deformity. In extreme cases in which the deformity has significantly progressed, serial casting may be prescribed. The cast resembles a dorsal block splint that allows the digits to flex freely. If a cast fails, surgical pinning may take place to reverse this contracture. A dynamic composite hand flexion splint may be considered after serial casting or pinning to bring the hand progressively into flexion (Fig. 12). The dynamic and static splints should be used in combination on a 24 h basis until this deformity is reversed. When the patient has lost fingernails, a unique method of attaching hooks to the digits may be used. A contour hook and Coban are used to attach the hook to the distal surface of the digit (Fig. 13). The attachment of rubber bands to the hooks distally and to a D-ring proximally on a volar wrist splint provide for composite closure of the hand.

Boutonniere Deformity

Damage to the extensor hood mechanism of a digit may cause a disruption of the central slip, leading to the development of boutonniere deformity during which

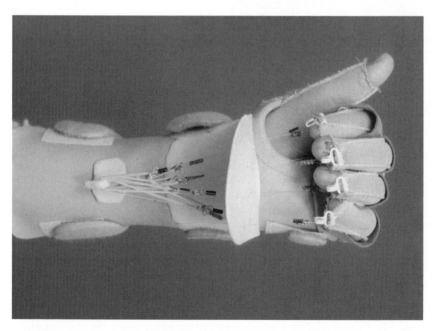

FIGURE 12   A dynamic composite hand flexion splint provides adequate traction to stretch and remodel scar adhesions.

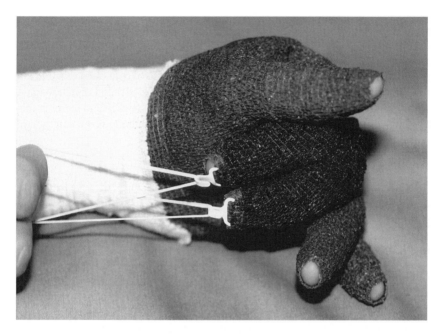

FIGURE 13 A contour hook and Coban mechanism is constructed to provide the digits without nails with hooks for dynamic flexion.

the proximal IP (PIP) joint contracts into flexion and the distal IP (DIP) joint hyperextends. If the contracture is mild, a digital gutter splint may be fabricated and serially adjusted to bring the digit into a functional position until the involved structure heals and scars mature. The digit should be immobilized in the splint while the rest of the hand is allowed to function normally. A gutter splint may also be utilized in the presence of a tendon exposure in any digit until re-epithelialization occurs.

Swan Neck Deformity

Severe injury to the digits may result into an imbalance of forces acting on the phalanges, causing a collapse of a digit. This so-called swan neck deformity presents as hyperextension at the PIP joint and flexion at the DIP joint. The affected digit needs to be protected in a custom-made and serially adjusted Figure 8 finger splint or using prefabricated Murphy rings. These splints allow for the functional use of the digit and maintain the PIP joint into a position of function while being corrected. These splints must be worn for as long as the scars are active and the affected structures are healing.

Cupping of the Palm

Active scar in the palm of the hand may begin to pull the thenar and hypothenar eminence together, causing a cupping of the palm deformity. The deformity, in some cases, may be severe enough to cause the thumb to hyperextend or subluxed at the MCP joint. A resting pan splint with the thumb in a radial abduction and the palm stretched open or a thumb spica splint is fabricated to correct this deformity. A thumb spica serial cast may be fabricated initially if the contracture is severe prior to splinting.

Mallet Finger

Volar finger burns or damage to the extensor tendon at the DIP joint level may result into a flexion contracture at the DIP joint known as mallet finger. A Stax splint may be used to position the DIP joint in neutral while the tendon is healing, or a volar gutter splint may be fabricated to serially reverse the DIP flexion contracture.

Dynamic Hand Extension Splint

Volar hand contractures respond positively to dynamic traction that provides a gentle and prolong stretch to remodel scar tissue. Peripheral nerve injuries involving the radial nerve will significantly affect function: the hand is able to close but not open correctly. In cases of volar hand contractures or radial nerve injury, a dynamic hand extension splint may be indicated. Based on the principles of achieving proximal stability to allow for distal mobility, the dorsal static component of this splint may be extended over the middle of the proximal phalanges to create the base for a dynamic PIP extension outrigger when the volar contractures involve the PIP joints.

Digital Dynamic Springs

Flexion or extension contractures to the digits may, in addition to the static gutter splints, be managed with dynamic flexion or extension spring splints. These digital splints allow for the continuation of normal functional activities of the rest of the hand.

Other Body Areas

Hip Spica

Large body surface area burns involving the whole body may significantly affect the patient's ability to ambulate correctly. Hip flexion contractures may occur during this time due to improper positioning while supine in bed over a period of time. An anterior hip spica splint (Fig. 14) is fabricated and worn at all times while the patient is in bed. The splint may be serially adjusted to achieve the hip neutral position and allow the patient to resume normal ambulation.

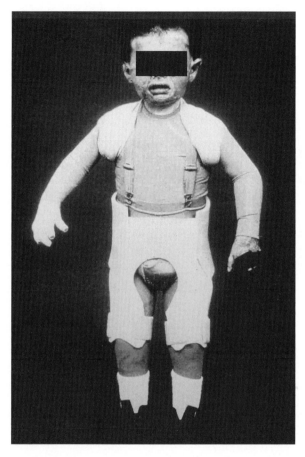

FIGURE 14 Hip flexion contractures may be corrected with the use of an anterior hip spica splint.

Knee Conformers

Knee flexion contractures may be corrected with the use of custom thermoplastic posterior knee splints or a soft circumferential prefabricated conformer. These splints are mostly worn when the patient is in bed or resting. They should be removed for ambulation to prevent further injury.

Foot Splints

Positioning appropriately in bed in the acute phase of recovery will help to prevent dorsiflexion, plantar flexion, inversion and eversion of the foot, and prepare the patient to resume normal ambulation when appropriate. Circumferential burns to the feet require splinting of the anterior or posterior surfaces (Fig. 15). Foot plates

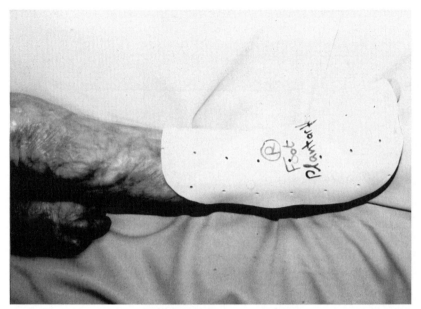

A

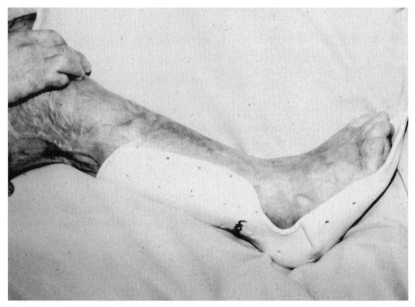

B

FIGURE 15   Circumferential burns to the feet require splinting of both the (a) anterior and (b) posterior surfaces to prevent both dorsiflexion and plantar flexion contractures.

340

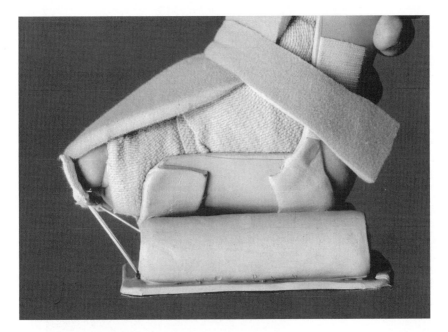

FIGURE 16 The dynamic metatarsophalangeal flexion boot may be fabricated to allow for ambulation and stretching of the toes in flexion at the same time.

are worn at night to prevent toe hyperextension. Special shoes may also be needed to prevent toe hyperextension. When the dorsum of the foot is released and toe hyperextension is corrected post operatively, a unique dynamic toe flexion custom splint can be fabricated. This splint is applied in the operating room and allows for immediate postoperative ambulation and simultaneous dynamic toe flexion through a tunnel attached to a posterior foot splint (Fig. 16).

SERIAL CASTING

In some cases, scar tissue does not adequately respond to the therapeutic measures designed to prevent joint contracture. Serial casting is an effective method of treating joints with progressive loss of motion. This technique involves the use of plaster or fiberglass casting material to apply a static low-load stress along the length of restrictive scar tissue. Traditional casting procedures are designed to immobilize a segment over an extended period of time. Casting procedures that address scar tissue must be applied several times over an extended period to allow incremental improvement. Complete healing of the target tissue is not

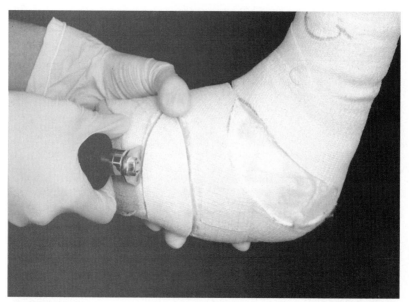

A

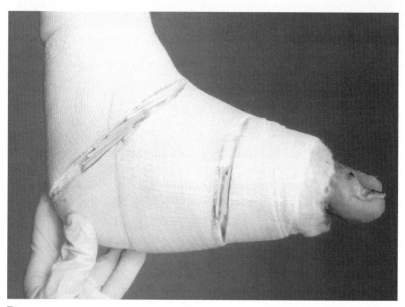

B

FIGURE 17 The force and duration of a serial cast can be increased with a spacer system. (a) Wedge-shaped slits are cut into the medial and lateral surfaces of the cast to obtain a greater degree of eversion. (b) Small wooden spacers maintain the improved position.

a requirement if proper wound dressing and relief techniques are followed. A typical protocol will last 2–3 weeks, with a staggered application schedule that begins
daily and extends to every 3 days to allow for skin assessment and active exercise.

Almost every joint in the extremities is capable of being casted. However,
the larger joints tend to respond more favorably to casting due to longer leverage
arms. Regardless of the joint being treated, it is extremely important to provide
sufficient padding to protect bony landmarks and the edges of the cast. As the
cast is applied, the joint is positioned so that 5–10 degrees of motion are gained
and held until the material hardens. Since healing tissues are more fragile than
intact tissue, extra protection should line the surfaces that are cut for the removal
process. If skin integrity is well established, a wedge design can be used to
prolong the use of a single cast. Wedge-shaped sections are cut into the medial
and lateral surfaces of the cast to allow for repositioning (Fig. 17). The new
position is maintained by placing small rigid spacers on the restricted side, which
applies additional stress to the restrictive tissue. Once the new position is attained,
the wedges are recast without replacing the entire cast.

The disadvantage of this routine is that active motion and strength are
compromised while the cast is in use. Serial casting procedures are used in the
context of a larger program. As soon as a cast is removed, the patient should
participate in active mobility exercises that strengthen the newly gained range of
motion. Scar management is critical for the rest period between casting procedures
to condition the tissue and prevent excessive dryness or maceration. Balancing
periods of stressed immobility and active functional motion is the key to a successful serial casting routine. If applied in appropriate parameters, the contracted joint
should respond positively in both available motion and muscular strength.

EXERCISE AND PERFORMANCE OF ACTIVITIES OF DAILY LIVING

Physical activity is typically avoided following a grafting procedure to ensure
viability of the skin graft. If strength is an issue, isometric exercise, which does
not produce joint motion, can be attempted earlier in the postoperative phase.
Patient compliance is required to prevent shear forces due to excessive motion.
In cases of small partial-thickness burns, activity may begin following initial
wound management, which may include application of bio-occlusive dressings.
Once the grafts or skin substitutes are sufficiently incorporated, which may take
about 3 days, active movement should be encouraged. Activity can begin in
several forms. Passive, active, or active assistive exercises are all appropriate
techniques to begin an activity program. Resistive motion is a higher-level skill
that can improve performance and tolerance for functional mobility; however, it
should only be used after the burn team is satisfied with the graft's viability.
Resistance can be introduced manually by the therapist in a static fashion with

the use of weights or dynamically with elastic bands. Another alternative to static weights is the skeletal traction exercise program described earlier.

The intensity of an exercise program is always based on the patient's tolerance as dictated by the physiological condition and current state of skin replacement material. A rehabilitation therapist is often confronted with the dilemma of when to proceed with an active exercise program. In the early stages there can be an inverse relationship with the amount of active, movement and the successful adherence of skin grafts. The question that must be posed is: What is more important, improving the deconditioned state of this individual, or preventing loss of wound coverage? The answer to this question will provide the team with the appropriate direction. In some cases, both goals can be met with moderate results if the program consists only of isometric muscle contractions performed at joint angles that represent a full arc of motion.

Many considerations go into the planning of an exercise program that includes active exercise, range of motion, and performance of daily living skills. There is a direct relationship between the type of exercise performed and the ability to perform daily living skills successfully. Active exercise can strengthen the muscles that combat restrictive scar tissue. This form of exercise can lead to improved range of motion that allows participation in skilled activity. Once the physiological requirements needed to complete a task are achieved, practice and repetition are needed to reinforce the patient so that the skill can be performed over time.

AMBULATION AND MOBILITY TRAINING

Ambulation and all other out-of-bed activities should not begin until viability of the skin replacement procedure is established. Ambulation is typically initiated by one of two means. Orientation to the vertical position is introduced either by gradual tilting on a table, or standing at the bedside. Depending on the duration of bed rest, a patient may be at risk for orthostatic hypotension. In noncomplicated cases a normal time for beginning mobility training is 3–7 days. In some instances of cadaver skin grafting patients may begin mobilizing as early as postoperative day 1.

Regardless of when the patient is allowed to participate in mobility training, it is very important to maintain appropriate handling techniques. Acute burn wounds and grafts need to be dressed with an appropriate interface to minimize adherence of the wounds to the dressings, which should allow for gas exchange and avoid adhering to the surrounding tissue. Once the proper dressings are applied, elastic wraps can be placed on the extremities and torso to assist with regulating blood pressure. Some have advocated for double-wrapping the lower extremities to assist further with the gravity-dependent position.

Ambulation training should be preceded by training for mobility in bed. Functional mobility evaluations should include all gross motor movement in both the horizontal and vertical planes. Each individual will present with unique barriers to mobility. The rehabilitation therapist should be responsible for analyzing the strengths and weakness of each situation to determine the most efficient means of accomplishing mobility. This type of training will relate closely to strength training, since both are required to combat the negative effects of bed rest.

Bed mobility is mainly concerned with a patient's ability to transfer into and out of the sleeping surface. This activity may become increasingly difficult due to the softer and more conforming surfaces common in acute hospital facilities. A patient may need to be transferred to a firm surface, such as a mat-table, to decrease the difficulty of accomplishing the task. If this is not an option, progress would be somewhat slower than expected. Airbeds, such as the Clinitron, are so difficult to transfer from that mobility training may need to be postponed until a more suitable surface is available.

The ability to transfer is evaluated and assessed based on the amount of assistance required to complete the task. The range of assistance varies from total dependence to complete independence. Other patients may be independent with the use of assistive devices such as an overhead bar or raised side rails. Advancing an individual who requires assistance typically involves greater amounts of functional exercise and development of more efficient movement strategies. These techniques are typically safe to perform in the absence of compounding factors. One area of concern is the management of peripheral equipment, such as intravenous lines, physiological monitoring devices, catheters, and nasogastric tubes. As the patient is asked to move, it is very important to inspect closely all the equipment that could get dislodged.

Once the transfer is complete, ambulation is the next taste to be mastered. If the patient is standing, ambulation is initiated with the appropriate amount of assistance. Assistive devices are all considered, from axillary crutches to walking canes. Tolerance for duration and intensity are closely monitored by the rehabilitation department and progression is determined by the patient's overall ability to tolerate increasing amounts of exercise.

SCAR MANANGEMENT

The unrelenting progressive nature of scar formation following a burn injury has the potential for drastically altering an individual's biomechanics. Collagen fibers are aggressively formed to assist with wound closure in the early stages of wound healing. One of the major goals of rehabilitation therapists is to limit the impact of scar formation on mobility. Scar management must be addressed during all phases of the patient's treatment by the acute burn service. The techniques involved will change as the healing process progresses. Early in the preoperative stage, soft tissue length is preserved with the use of splints and positioning, which are important in maintaining a resting functional length. Those techniques have been described earlier. There is considerable overlap with the discussion of scar management, since patients will need to continue with aggressive splinting and positioning programs throughout their entire recovery process.

Basics

Whatever the technique applied, some basic rules apply to scar management. Perhaps the most important rule is that the resting position tends to become the position of contracture. The burn care team should always strive to bring an individual out of a resting position to prevent scars from limiting the natural arc of motion a joint produces. The rule that therapists should never ignore is that scarring is a metabolic process that is quite aggressive and does not fatigue. If careful attention is not provided on a 24 h basis, a scar can quickly form a contracture that limits range of motion and has a negative impact on function (Fig. 18a). As burn wounds are inspected, it is a good idea to remember that small and vulnerable body areas are more seriously affected by scar formation. Hand and foot burns are good examples of how devastating scars at the digits can be (Fig. 18b). Large flat areas tend to have the potential to form long bands that affect multiple segments such as the neck, chest, and hip. It is also important to realize that a scar forms three-dimensionally and has the ability to bind with the deeper tissues. The process is not always the same in every case and some individuals will scar with greater intensity than others. A therapist should evaluate a scar knowing that size and thickness are closely correlated with degree of disability. Some scars left untreated can grow so large and thick that a joint's function can be completely disrupted. The scars will typically contract until an opposing force is encountered; once encountered, the balance of that force can redirect a scar. Fortunately for the burn team, scars tend to respond to the external forces applied. A therapist must provide an external force that exceeds the internal contracture force of the scar. This concept must be strictly adhered to once an increase resting length is established, or the progressive nature of scar tissue will reclaim the gains achieved.

A basic scar management program should include pressure therapy, scar massage, passive stretching, the use of various treatment modalities, and education for the patient or caregiver. The initial stages of the program will usually be addressed by a rehabilitation therapist. However, as the healing tissues become more durable, more responsibility is placed on the patient or caregiver to manage the scars. The parameters suggested for each individual program would vary depending on the aggressiveness and overall surface area of the scar tissue. A general recommendation will be based on realistic expectations of time involvement balanced against other conflicting events common to a typical daily schedule. Once a patient is mostly covered and has few open areas remaining, it should be emphasized that scar management is a crucial tool in the recovery or preserva-

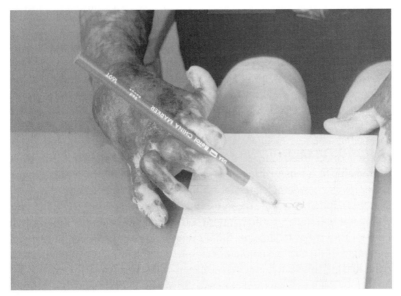

A

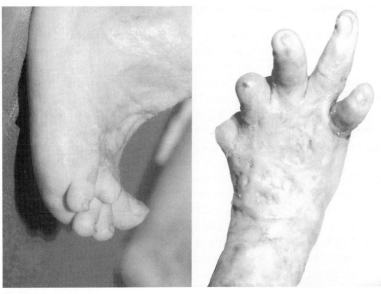

B

Figure 18 Burn scar contractures can have a negative impact on function as range of motion becomes compromised. (a) Note how difficult midline activity appears to be for a patient with limited motion in both upper extremities. (b) Hand burns resulting in partial amputation and loss of functional mobility in the remaining fingers, and dorsal foot burns can lead to extension contractures of the toes.

347

tion of functional mobility. The key components of the program should be performed a minimum of twice daily and can even provide greater benefit if increased to three or four times daily. A treatment session should continue for a minimum of 20 min to achieve the desired response. Treatment sessions that fall short of the 20 min goal may not have the carry over effect that allows for the plastic changes necessary to sustain improvements in functional mobility. They may also result in a need to increase the intensity of a treatment, which can cause excessive tissue trauma. Longer treatment sessions that continue up to an hour in duration are also acceptable, if intensity remains low enough to prevent local tissue trauma. Pressure therapy is considered separately from this discussion of treatment duration. Pressure is applied on a more rigorous schedule, which will include whenever the patient is not bathing or participating in other scar management procedures. The intensity of all these treatments should remain low to allow the scar tissue to accommodate to the stress supplied during treatment. It has been well established in the rehabilitation literature that collagen-based scar tissue responds most favorably to low-load, long-duration stress.

Pressure Therapy

The role of pressure therapy evolves along with the healing process. In the emergent preoperative phase, pressure is applied with elastic bandages to control the amount of edema associated with the inflammatory phase of wound healing. Several techniques can be used to wrap the extremities, including the spiral, figure eight, and modified figure eight. The modified figure eight is simply a combination of the spiral and figure eight wraps that crosses anteriorly and is spiral-warped posteriorly. This technique has been noted to provide a more evenly distributed pressure that prevents excessive force at any one point on the extremity. During the early stage of recovery, immobility may predispose the acute patient to orthostatic hypotension. Some therapists advocate double-wrapping the lower extremities to modulate the response of the vascular system to the upright position. The torso can be addressed with a spiral wrap that incorporates the axillae or pelvis as needed. Any wrap should begin at the distal end and progress proximally. Overlap of the wrap should remain at 50% of the entire length of the segment being covered. The hand should be wrapped so that the thumb is allowed to pass through a precut slit in the bandage. The fingers are not included in this wrap to prevent restrict on of individual movement. The fingers can be wrapped with a self-adhesive taping technique that also progresses from distal to proximal. The fingertips are excluded to allow for tactile stimulation and easier grasping. Narrow strips should also be applied between each finger to maintain the depth and slope of the web spaces (Fig. 19).

The use of elastic wraps and self-adhesive tape will continue until healing of the tissues allows for progression to the next phase of pressure therapy. Elastic

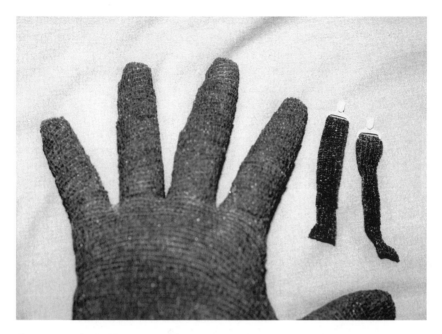

FIGURE 19 Self-adhesive taping can control edema and scar formation in the hand once wound closure is achieved. Note the soft inserts between the fingers to maintain the web spaces.

wraps are applied circumferentially so that the shear force is minimized during the application process, but they do not provide the most uniform pressure. Tubular elastic bandages provide a more uniform pressure, but they must be pulled on as a unit. This application process may increase shear forces and may be delayed until wound closure is complete. Some small open areas are acceptable, but when the tubular bandage is removed dried exudate can be problematic if the wound bed is pulled off by the bandage. Elastic bandages are more easily removed in the presence of adherent wounds because of the circumferential application and removal process. The application of tubular bandages can be assisted with cylindrical guides placed over the extremity. However, the guide must be larger than the extremity, which, in some cases, may cause excessive stretch of the material (Fig. 20).

As the healing process progresses, the inflammatory phase gives rise to the proliferative phase. This phase usually takes place in the postoperative stage of the acute burn care management as wound healing is taking place and few open areas remain. The time from initial injury may be from 2 weeks to 2 months, since wound healing phases tend to overlap, especially in large traumatic injuries.

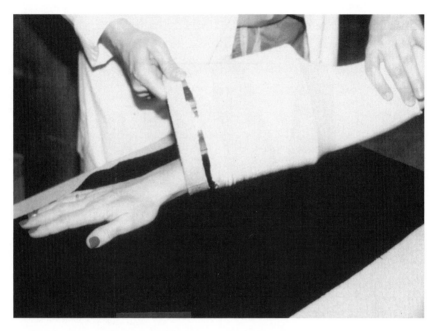

FIGURE 20   To lessen shear forces during application, tubular bandages can be applied using a cylindrical guide.

The goal of pressure therapy in the proliferative phase transitions from edema control to scar suppression. The pressure applied in this phase is intended to exceed capillary pressure to deprive the scars of nutrients and fluid. During this phase the circumferences of the body regions are almost stable and a more appropriate pressure therapy can include interim garments. Interim garments are prefabricated pressure garments applied like regular garments. These also include face masks, gloves, and stockings. These garments are also available in individual body segments. The advantages of these garments are durability and even pressure distribution.

Pressure garments may not be able to apply therapeutic pressure over irregular body surfaces. Various insert materials are utilized underneath the pressure garments to aid in depressing hypertrophic scars. Inserts utilized in combination with pressure garments may be custom-made or preformed. Customized inserts are liquids or putties that require a catalyst to create semi-rigid or rigid material molded as it hardens to fit specific contoured or concave body surfaces. Soft insert materials such as strapping material, foam, and silicone gels may be utilized initially in scar management, to treat the fragile and sensitive hypertrophic scar.

The final stage of wound healing includes remodeling of the scar tissue. Open areas are mostly healed at this stage, but a few may remain. These areas should be covered with a drying solution such as Mercurochrome if infection is not suspected. In this stage the goal of nutrient and fluid restriction remains; however, the additional goal of reorienting collagen fibers begins to be addressed. Now that extremity girth is mostly stable, customized pressure garments can be applied. These garments are measured for each individual and can be fabricated for any body region (Fig. 21). These garments are applied over stable scars. The application process can be made easier with the use of zippers or hook and loop closures. These garments encourage the orientation of collagen fibers by creating a customized template over the scars to prevent excessive proliferation and growth.

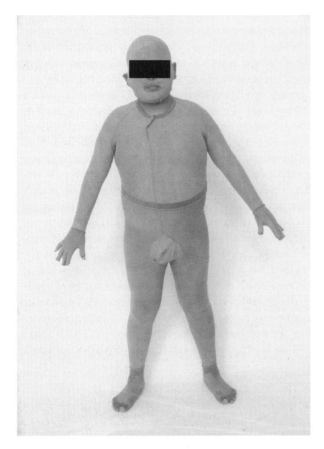

FIGURE 21 Customized pressure garments are measured to fit each unique individual and can be obtained for any body surface region.

Regardless of when pressure therapy is applied, the problems remain the same. The tissues must be inspected daily for breakdown, maceration, or blistering. If problems arise, pressure should be diverted from the local regions if possible. If inserts are used, they can be discontinued for short periods of time to encourage healing. Excessive pressure can also become an issue and each patient should be educated to detect the signs and symptoms of ischemia.

Scar Massage

Burn wounds that limit the natural lubrication of tissues produce scars that become excessively dry. Lack of lubrication also adversely affects the pliability of viable tissues and hampers mobility. Individuals who experience these circumstances benefit from scar massage. This form of massage typically begins with water- or oil-based lubricating lotion. This process facilitates an increase in pliability, which assists tissue mobility. The techniques involved in scar massage evolve along with the stages of wound healing. Early in the inflammatory phase, lubrication is typically not an issue due to the use of topical antibiotic medications. Massage techniques may be used more for relaxation and pain modulation because direct manipulation of a fresh burn wound is contraindicated. Following a grafting procedure, as the proliferative stage is causing growth of the scar, aggressive massage may accentuate the growth by causing local vasodilatation. In this stage, gentle techniques that assist with lubrication and pain control are advised. Massage is always discouraged directly to open areas because the lotion can contaminate the wound bed. Scar management is most advantageous in the remodeling phase of wound healing. During this stage, deep and cross friction massage techniques target adhesions that can form between scar tissue and the surrounding tissues. Longitudinal techniques assist in the realignment of collagen when performed in conjunction with passive stretching techniques. Vibrating massage units are commonly used in the later phases of recovery to assist with scar massage and often come with a thermal head. The attachments for these units can be changed depending on the area being treated: flat broad heads for large areas, moderate size heads for small regional areas, and blunt pointed heads for recessed areas. This technique is appropriate to use in conjunction with the actual stretch and is effective in regaining the end range of a restricted motion. This is also a technique easily taught for home use to provide the caregiver with a more effective home program.

Passive Stretching

The concept of passive stretching is defined as an external force that provides a resting tension across scar tissue. Initially, this tension force is supplied by splints and positioning techniques. Once a patient has been evaluated for joint integrity and all tissues have been cleared for activity, a patient is typically ready for passive stretching. This may take place in the postoperative phase of recovery while proliferation or remodeling is occurring in the scar tissue. The parameters of low-load long-duration stretch should be applied at all times when passively manipulating scar tissue. A restriction that has been assessed will need to be evaluated in each available plane of joint motion (Fig. 22). Scar tissue can affect a joint asymmetrically and they should be addressed in each cardinal plane. A risk involved in passive stretch is exceeding the elastic limit of the scar. If this occurs, depending on the amount of force applied, a nonsurgical release of the tissue can occur. This situation should be inspected by a physician to assess the immediate wound needs. Often it only requires local wound treatment and a large increase in joint range of motion is observed. In some cases, a nonsurgical release will require a skin graft to cover the defect. This type of release can be prevented if close attention is given to the passive stretch. The extremity should be moved passively until blanching of the scar is observed. Excessive blanching in an area of restriction is a warning sign that the elastic limit has been reached.

Treatment Delivery Methods

The use of various treatment delivery methods in burn care can be somewhat limited due to the changes that occur during the formation of scar tissue. Most of the literature includes subjects with intact skin. The parameters for healing burn injuries need to be modified from typical protocols because there are changes in resistance to current, temperature regulation, thickness, resilience, and pliability. These techniques are applied to the burn scars prior to stretching in an attempt to prepare the tissue for the procedure. The goal is to apply a moderate amount of energy that will facilitate collagen realignment within the scar tissue.

Delivery systems that apply heat may include moist hot packs, paraffin baths, and ultrasound. Heat can be applied once the proliferative phase of wound healing has slowed down. Applying heat early in the proliferative phase may increase blood flow to the developing scar and accelerate scar formation. In the remodeling phase, heat allows for relaxation of resistive contractile tissue and prepares the scar for stretching procedures. Close inspection is important, because heat can also cause more wounds if the intensity is too high. Moist heat packs can be applied for 12–20 min with six layers of towel for protection. Paraffin wax baths are used for the hands and feet prior to activity for up to 10 min. Ultrasound has been much less investigated in burn wounds than other modalities and should only be used following a complete review of the current literature.

AMPUTATION

Full-thickness burn injuries can lead to amputation of nonviable tissue. Cell death is typically caused either by a direct flame injury or anoxia resulting from in-

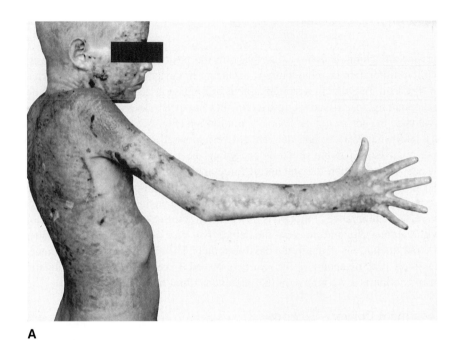

A

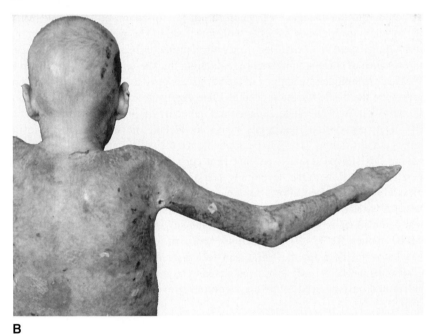

B

Figure 22 Restricted joints should be managed in multiple planes. (a) Shoulder flexion. (b) Shoulder abduction.

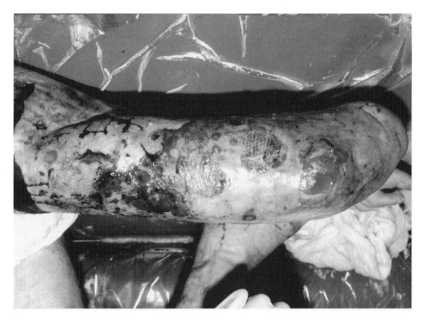

FIGURE 23   Burn injuries that lead to amputation will typically produce fragile residual limbs.

creased compartmental pressures. The role of a rehabilitation therapist on the acute burn service following amputation should be to:

Control the initial edema and shrink the residual limb
Maintain proximal joint mobility
Initiate weight bearing and tolerance
Facilitate use of the definitive prosthesis

This list of responsibilities is performed under different circumstances than traditional traumatic amputation protocols because the residual limb will have an associated burn injury that complicates progression (Fig. 23). One of the major obstacles to using prosthetics in acute burn care settings is the fragility of the residual limb. Prosthetic sockets provide a large amount of local pressure and use suspension mechanisms that are mostly occlusive. Depending on the amount of time required to prepare an individual properly for definitive prosthetic training, some of the acute care duties may have to be addressed in the outpatient setting.

Edema Control

Amputations may occur during any stage in the acute setting. It is common for physicians to evaluate an extremity over time to provide an opportunity for resuscitative measures to spare the compromised extremity. As a result, the residual limb may present in various phases of the inflammatory process. The final goal of applying a prosthetic device requires some stability of the residual limb. Edema will need to be managed prior to the application of a temporary prosthesis due to the fixed volume of the socket. Pressure therapy is the technique usually used to manage the edema in an amputated extremity. Elastic bandages are applied in what has traditionally been described as a stump wrap. This is an effective means of controlling edema; however, this wrap must also accompany a positioning protocol that elevates the residual limb to assist with postural drainage. In some cases, retrograde massage may also assist with edema control if the surrounding tissues have headed enough to withstand the treatment. The benefits of elastic bandages over interim garments have been described earlier in this chapter and the same benefits are found in this situation. As the residual limb progresses through the healing process, open areas and the distal suture line respond most favorably to the stump wrap with elastic bandages. Once the tissues are closed and wound healing is mostly complete, an interim garment known as a stump shrinker can be applied. Throughout the entire time it takes for an individual to be fitted for a definitive prosthesis, the residual limb should be monitored for fluctuations in girth. Daily fluctuations may be observed as great as 2 cm. These small changes can be accounted for with the number of socks used to cover the residual limb.

Maintenance of Proximal Joint Stability

Prosthetic devices have a terminal device that serves as a substitute for absent body parts. The different types of terminal devices available are too numerous to include in this discussion. However, it is extremely important that all remaining joints proximal to the terminal device have as much motion as possible. This helps to provide a greater functional range for the terminal device. One of the greatest hindrances to appropriate prosthetic function is joint contracture. Limited range of motion prevents the arc of motion available to the terminal device. The reason joint contracture is such an issue following amputation is because the shortened extremity lacks the leverage to maintain a resting length and the extremity typically contracts into a flexed position. Splints are used to maintain proximal joints in extension. The protocol is exactly the same as described earlier except that the construction is slightly modified to account for a shorter distal segment. These splints may require a more efficient application technique because there is less control of the distal segment and it may be possible for the joint to flex despite the splint.

Active motion of proximal joints must also be addressed. Contracture prevention and active mobility form a delicate balance that must be evaluated daily.

Suggestions for activity and splinting do not differ from those already presented in this chapter.

Weight Bearing and Tolerance

The suspension systems used by prosthetic devices along with the rigid sockets that accept the residual limb can be harsh to healing burn wounds. The end-bearing load is much less for upper extremity prosthetics than for the lower extremity; however, all residual limbs will require conditioning before the successful application of a prosthesis. The conditioning process begins with an evaluation of sensation. If an individual does not have the ability to self-monitor the pressure caused by a prosthesis, then a poor outcome is anticipated. Sensory integration techniques will assist patients with amputations to begin learning a new body image. The residual limb should be presented with a multitude of stimuli including light touch, vibration, temperature, and various textures. This will assist with desensitization of the extremity and address proprioception if performed at various joint angles. After functional tolerance has been established, it is important to reintroduce weight bearing to the extremity. This is also true for the upper extremity, when the weight of the prosthesis serves as the weight-bearing force. A protocol to address tolerance for pressure should begin by placing low loads on the extremity for short periods of time. For the lower extremity, a foam block or air cast can be placed on the residual limb and gradual pressure can be introduced by means of a tilt table (Fig. 24). A patient can provide upper extremity weight bearing by sitting at a table while leaning forward on a padded surface, using the residual limb for support. As with all burn care techniques, close inspection and gradual progression are the key to a successful program. The preprosthetic weight-bearing activities should continue until stability of the tissues is observed. When the residual limb is stable enough to accept a temporary socket, a wearing schedule is determined. A beginning schedule should not exceed 30 min and allow for ample opportunity to inspect the extremity. The wearing schedule can progress up to 1 h within the first couple of days and up to 3 h within the first week. Progression should not be allowed if excessive breakdown occurs. Some small areas of redness and a limited amount of blistering are acceptable.

Use of the Definitive Prosthesis

The final goal of rehabilitation for the patient with an amputation is learning how to use a prosthesis. Practicing functional tasks is the most efficient way to facilitate learning. The protocol should coincide with the wearing schedule and participation in functional activities is encouraged. The upper extremity program concentrates more on daily living skills (Fig. 25) and the lower extremity program focuses more on balance and mobility issues (Fig. 26). A program should mimic

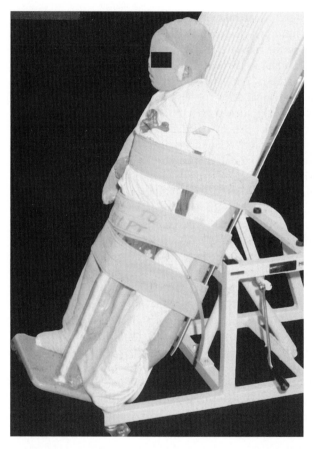

FIGURE 24 Modifications for those who are prepared to stand prior to complete coverage of a fragile residual limb may include an air cast or foam support to substitute for a lower extremity prosthesis.

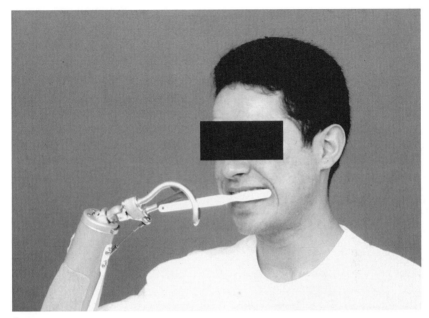

A

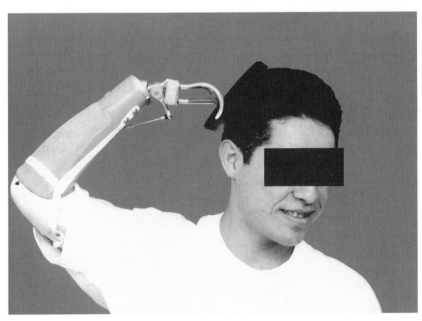

B

FIGURE 25 Practicing daily activities with an upper extremity prosthesis may include (a) brushing teeth, (b) combing hair and (continued)

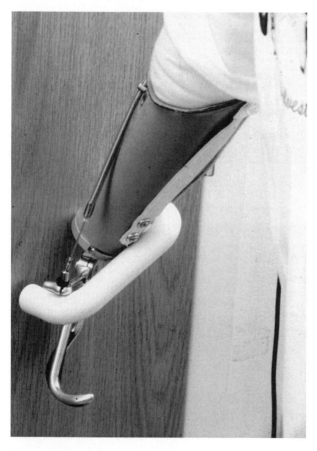

FɪGᴜʀᴇ 25 (**Cont.**)   (c) opening doors.

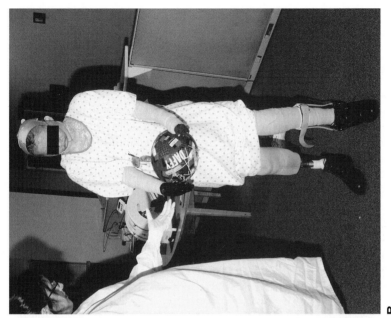

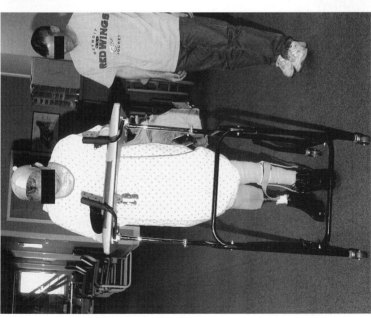

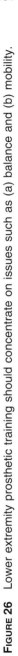

FIGURE 26 Lower extremity prosthetic training should concentrate on issues such as (a) balance and (b) mobility.

as closely as possible the patient's own living conditions and degree of support so that an appropriate transition can be made from the acute burn service.

SUMMARY

Burn rehabilitation is challenging and requires an experienced and innovative burn team to produce positive functional outcomes. Therapists work closely with physicians along the continuum of care to ensure the delivery of high-quality care for the burn survivor. Even though there are no uniform standards for burn physical rehabilitation, the primary goal of therapy is functional independence during performance of ADLs. It is extremely important for rehabilitation to begin as soon as possible after a significant burn injury and focus on the positioning and splinting of the patient to maintain function. As the patient's status stabilizes, therapy shifts focus to exercise, mobility, and performance of ADLs. Later in the acute phase of rehabilitation, scar management is introduced to minimize scar hypertrophy, correct contractures, and optimize function. The practical approach to burn rehabilitation presented in this chapter serves as a guide for therapists and may be adapted to fit the needs of any burn survivor.

BIBLIOGRAPHY

1. Serghiou MA, Evans EB, Ott S, Calhoun JH, Morgan D, Hannon LComprehensive rehabilitation of the burned patient. In Herndon D, Ed Total Burn Care. 2nd ed.. London: W.B. Saunders, 2002:563–592.
2. Malick MH, Carr JA. Manual on Management of the Burn Patient. Pittsburgh, PA: Harmarville Rehabilitation Center Educational Resource Division, 1982.
3. Richard RL, Staley MJ. Burn Care and Rehabilitation: Principles and Practice. Philadelphia: F.A. Davis, 1994.
4. Walters C, Splinting the Burn Patient. Laurel: RAMSCO, 1987.
5. Wilton JC. Hand Splinting: Principles of Design and Fabrication. London: W.B. Saunders, 1997.
6. Fess EE, Philips CA. Hand Splinting: Principles and Methods. 2nd ed. Part II. St. Louis: C. V. Mosby, 1987.
7. Miles WK, Grigsby L. Remodeling of scar tissue in the burned hand. In Hunter J , Schneider L , Callahan A, Eds Rehabilitation of the Hand: Surgery and Therapy. 3rd ed.. St. Louis: CV Mosby, 1990:841–857.
8. Grigsby-deLinde L, Miles WK. Remodeling of scar tissue in the burned hand. In Hunter J , Mackin E , Callahan A, Eds Rehabilitation of the Hand: Surgery and Therapy. 4th ed.. St. Louis: CV Mosby, 1995:1267–1303.
9. Salisbury RE, Utley-Reeves S, Wright P. Acute care and rehabilitation of the burned hand. In Hunter J , Schneider L , Mackins E , Callahan A, Eds Rehabilitation of the Hand: Surgery and Therapy. 3rd ed.. St Louis: CV Mosby, 1990:831–840.
10. Fisher SV, Helm PA. Comprehensive Rehabilitation of Burns. Baltimore: Williams & Wilkins, 1984.

11. Donnelan MB. Reconstruction of the burned hand and upper extremity. In: Plastic SurgeryMcCarthy MB, Ed. Philadelphia: WB Saunders, 1990:452–482.
12. Kisner C, Colby LA. Therapeutic Exercise: Foundations and Techniques. 2nd ed.. Philadelphia: F.A. Davis, 1990.
13. Michlovitz S. Thermal Agents in Rehabilitation. 2nd ed.. Philadelphia: F.A. Davis, 1990.
14. Shurr DG, Cook TM. Prosthetics & Orthotics. Connecticut: Appleton & Lange, 1990.

15

Psychosocial Support

Walter J. Meyer III and Patricia Blakeney
Shriners Burns, Hospital Galveston, Texas, U.S.A.

INTRODUCTION

The initial response of most individuals upon seeing a survivor of major burn injury is one of shock, followed by sympathy, and wondering how patients can live after their burns heal. Because even small burns can cause considerable disfigurement, the reactions of people who are naïve to burn sequelae are, after shock, to be curious and, being sympathetic, to feel reluctant to query the burn survivor. If caught staring, they feel awkward and at a loss for words. They look away, avoid eye contact, and pretend that they never noticed; or they ask questions of a nonburned person who is in the company of the burn survivor, as if the survivor can neither hear nor answer questions.

Burn survivors must cope on almost a daily basis not only with their own adjustment to the dramatic changes in their own bodies but also with the responses of other people to their burn scars. They are made visibly different from most other people around them, and each gaze from another person is a reminder of their differences. Trips to the supermarket, to the shopping mall, wherever they are likely to encounter strangers become emotionally charged interpersonal challenges. Any behavior that is likely to attract attention from other people requires the courage to tolerate and cope with the reactions they expect from others [1]. A young man (17 years old) who had been quite attractive to girls prior to his severe burns hinted at this process in describing his experiences. He had been out of the hospital for about a year when he said to us, ''I forget I was burned, and I start to flirt with girls ⋯ then I see the way they look at me and I remember.'' He went on to describe his despair at noticing the expressions of mixed horror and sympathy on the faces of the young women.

Although there is general agreement among outcomes studies that most survivors of burns, even the most massive injuries, adjust well over time, the struggle to achieve a good quality of life is sometimes very, very hard and very long. Some burn survivors do not ever achieve the quality of life to which they aspire. We hope in this chapter to describe that process, clarify what we know from research and what we have experienced clinically, and report interventions that appear to facilitate the process and enhance the long-term well being of burn survivors.

Psychological healing occurs across time commensurate with physical healing in a pattern that is relatively predictable and consistent [2–11]. Awareness of this pattern allows caregivers to anticipate the emergence of psychosocial issues and to prepare a patient for coping with those issues. Predicting problematic issues for patients enables them to view their concerns in a context of normal reactions rather than as symptoms of psychological impairment [2,12]. For convenience in describing this pattern, we have arbitrarily designated a preinjury phase and five phases of recovery: admission, critical care, in-hospital recuperation, reintegration, and rehabilitation (Fig. 1.)

PREBURN FACTORS

The cause of the burn is often a major factor in an individual patient's recovery and is sometimes predictive of problems the patient may exhibit later. Pertinent questions are: Did the person who was injured cause the injury? Was the injury accidentally received? Or was it intentional? Was it self-inflicted? Or did it occur consequent to an act of abuse by another person?

Psychiatric conditions

Pre-existing psychiatric disorders are relatively common in the histories of older burned patients, and frequently appear to have contributed significantly to the injury itself [13–18]. Certain psychiatric conditions characterized by impulsive behavior predispose one to be accidentally burned. Attention deficit disorder (ADD) usually with hyperactivity (ADHD) is a predisposing condition. Thomas et al. have identified that in a small series of children diagnosed with attention deficit disorder prior to being treated for burn injury at Shriners Burns Hospital in Galveston, the majority were on drug holiday at the time they were injured [12]. ADHD, when untreated, is characterized by not paying attention closely enough to avoid accidents involving fire. Many of these children are so impulsive

PRE-BURN--->IDEALLY ADAPTED
INDIVIDUAL

DOMAINS	ACUTE PHASE (3-6 mos post-burn) →	EARLY ADAPTATION (6 mos-2 yrs post-burn) →	INCORPORATION (1-5 years post-burn) →	IDEAL ADAPTATION (2+ years post-burn)
EMOTIONAL ISSUES	1.Pain 2.Fear 3.Anxiety 4.Sadness	1.Emotional lability-rapid shifts 2.Fear, 3.Sadness 4.Anger 5. Pride in accomplishment 6. Hope	1.Sadness 2.Anger 3.Pride 4.Spiritual renewal	1.Acceptance 2. Hope 3.Anger 4.Optimism
SELF-CONCEPT	Of pre-burn self with pre-burn body	1. Of pre-burn self with "temporary disfigurement" 2. Forgets that others see disfigurement 3. Rapid shifts 4. Seeking solution to regaining preburn features	1. As burned and scarred "hero" or victim 2. Scars prominent in self-concept as sources of shame and pride	As person who was burned and has important assets and roles
IMPORTANT EXTERNAL INFLUENCES	1. Parents 2. Other family 3. Hospital staff 4. Peers	1. Parents 2. Other family 3. Peers 4. Professional helpers	1. Peers 2. Parents 3. Other family 4. Other adults	1. Peers 2. Parents 3. Other family 4. Other adults

Figure adapted from figure presented Outcomes conference sponsored by

ABA/Shriners Burns Hospitals (55)

FIGURE 1   Psychosocial adaptation to burn injury. (From Ref. 55.)

that they do dangerous things with fire, never intending that the fire should hurt anyone including themselves.

Impulsive behaviors with risk taking are also characteristic of persons with bipolar disorder. For example, one young man with previously diagnosed bipolar disorder used a match to examine the inside of a large oil drum. When the match burned down to his fingers, he dropped it in the oil drum, creating an explosion in which he was badly burned.

Serious burn injuries from purposeful self-immolation are more rare, and are usually preceded by a psychiatric illness [19,20]. Individuals who deliberately set themselves on fire are typically suffering from major depression with psychotic features, including suicidal ideation [21,22]. In such a case, the patient's fears lead to feelings of hopelessness, isolation, panic, and despair. The families of such patients are often characterized by hyperreligiosity, rigidity, and denial or minimization of problems.

Substance abuse is associated with flame injury because of intoxication or poor judgment, leading to setting a fire [18]. One study found alcohol use disorder in 11% of hospitalized burn patients with almost all of those injuries considered to be preventable [23]. Patients intoxicated at the time of burn injury also suffer a higher rate of complications in their treatment [24]. We have seen, for example, several individuals who lit candles, became intoxicated, fell into a stupor, leaving the candles burning. The candles eventually set the room on fire, and the individual either failed to wake up or was so debilitated that his or her escape was prolonged.

Those abusing flammable inhalants are at particular risk for burn injury [25–27]. A not uncommon event, particularly among boys in the age range of 10 years and older, is to sniff gasoline in a setting in which the gasoline fumes can be ignited by such things as an electrical charge or a pilot light. A story we have heard too frequently is that the boy sniffed gasoline and, while intoxicated, decided to have a cigarette. Of course, he lit the cigarette and the fumes ignited. This type of injury can be identified by the severity of the inhalation injury associated with the burn. The most suspicious situation is when the inhalation injury occurs in an outside fire. The other drug-related burns that we have seen are attempted murder by burning after a drug deal has gone sour.

Burn patients with a history of any premorbid psychiatric disorders are more likely to have preventable injuries [23], require longer hospitalization [28], and have problems with adjustment early in their recovery [29,30]. The risk of psychiatric complications following burn injury is greater in patients with a previous history of affective, alcohol, or substance use disorders [30]. It is therefore important to screen for any pre-existing mental illness in burn patients.

Abuse by burning

Burning is a particularly horrible way of abusing another person, yet the evidence is clear that it occurs more often than we would like to believe. Deliberate injury

to children by burning has been identified and discussed in the professional literature for about 20 years [31]. Similar aggressive acts toward adults began to be
recognized as a concern more recently [32]; and abuse of adults by burning has
rarely been documented in empirical studies. Three articles have been found that
report abuse to adults by burning [31,33,34]. Two studies describe burn injuries
of adults due to violent assault [33,34]. Associated risk factors in these reports
were substance abuse and domestic violence. Although Purdue and Hunt [34]
report that there was no identifiable burn pattern, Krob [33] describes a pattern
of scald injury to the anterior trunk and upper extremity. Men and women seem
equally at risk for burning by assault.

Bowden [31] describes a population of older adults made vulnerable by
physical or mental impairment who were burned by abuse or neglect. All but 3
of their 26 subjects were burned while living in health care facilities or institutions.
Although this single article identifies abuse of the elderly by burning as a problem,
it is likely that such abuse occurs with greater frequency than presently documented, and that it occurs within family settings as well as the institutional settings
that dominate this Michigan sample. Elder abuse has been identified as a public
concern in the United States only in the last 15 years. Relatively little, however,
has been written about the subject in spite of the estimated 2.5 million persons
who suffer annually [35]. When such abuse does occur within a family, it is often
perpetrated by an adult child or spouse of the victim. The abusers are often
intoxicated and have a history of being abused as children [32]. Some abusers
of the elderly have no prior history of mental illness, but have become exhausted
by the demands of their lives, including caring for an aged parent as well as a
spouse and children of their own [36,37]. Passive neglect may also result in injury
to an elderly or vulnerable person, particularly if that person is disoriented or is
reluctant to ask for attention and physical care [35]. Risk factors of abuse for adults
are similar to those for children: physical dependence [31,36,37], psychological
dependence [35,37], accessibility as a target for abuse through institutional living
or living with a caregiver [31,35], caregiver(s) with a history of substance abuse
[38].

It seems highly probable that burning as a form of violence against adults
occurs with much greater frequency than reflected in the literature, but has long
been unrecognized. Unless adult patients are asked about abuse, they are unlikely
to volunteer the information [33]. As burn care professionals become increasingly
sensitive to the problem of abuse to adults, the reported incidence will probably
increase dramatically and replicate the pattern observed with child abuse: the
more we ask, the more we will discover [36].

Estimates posit that as many as 30% of children treated for burn injury
have incurred their burn injuries through abuse or neglect. This amounts to about
200,000 children each year abused by burning [39]. To screen and identify these
individuals better, a checklist of risk factors can be useful. Risk factors for abuse

occur across several domains, and so a useful checklist includes information about the injury characteristics, circumstances of injury, family factors, and family history. The Shriners Hospital has recently reviewed the usefulness of such a checklist [40]. The follow up of about 100 children who had been referred for investigation by Children's Protective Services (CPS) was conducted, with specific interest in identifying which interventions were made and documenting evidence of recurrence of abuse. We found in this study that without intervention the abuse often persists; the best estimate of recurring abuse and neglect is 50%. Others have reported that 30% of the children suffering recurrent abuse and neglect are eventually mortally injured [41]. Therefore, children are reinjured repeatedly over years until they die from abuse-related injuries.

Retrospective review of the clinical and research literature has identified a number of possible risk factors to be used prospectively to access risk for abuse and neglect [42–45]. The most obvious in the risk factor group relates to the appearance of the wound: forced immersion demarcation, injuries incongruent with the story, unusual areas of burn, whole areas of burn involving entire palms, genitals, or other areas. Also included are items related to the history of the injury, inconsistency of the burn story with the developmental age of the child, interrupted or lack of bonding between the child and caregiver, other nonburn injuries or sexual abuse in the same patient, poor family support with problems including domestic violence, unusually high number of "accidents", isolated family, caregiver history of being abused, inexperienced, no work history, among others. As few as two identified risk factors have been necessary to indicate whether abuse or neglect is more likely than not [46]. The risk factors for abuse and neglect are often obscure and difficult for health care professionals to appreciate.

Care-giving health professionals are trained to be positive and supportive with families rather than to be suspicious. Health care workers want to give the family the benefit of the doubt. Yet health care professionals are responsible for whether the abused individual will be injured again, or even die from the next abusive incident. The approach at our hospital is to refer to protective services for investigation and possible intervention any child who has two or more risk factors noted [38]. Protective services for children and adults exist as governmental agencies in every US state as they do in many countries. Interventions by these agencies can provide support to the family while also protecting the vulnerable member(s). The best of these agencies provide psychotherapy for parent(s), physical modifications to the home, psychotherapy for the abused individual, home visits by caseworkers, placement of the individual with relatives or in a temporary foster home, and parenting classes. These interventions can give the family support and provide psychosocial and safety monitoring after the patient is discharged [38].

TIMING OF PSYCHOLOGICAL INTERVENTION

Initial treatment: ensuring survival acutely during critical care

Patient support

Immediately following a serious burn injury, the patient is usually so focused on their acute pain and fear (of death, of the hospital, etc.) that they do not think about the long-term questions of scars and lost capacity. They are first just trying to survive, although they often express a wish to die because of the severity of the pain and the stress of the intensive care setting. These suicidal expressions are usually not of great importance and can be eliminated by effectively and rapidly treating the pain and suffering.

The most distressing acute psychiatric problem for the staff is patient delirium. The major causes to assess for rapidly are sepsis, hypoglycemia, hyperglycemia, fever, and electrolyte imbalance [47,48]. Pain control, sleep deprivation, and medications including benzodiazapines, narcotics, and anabolic steroids should also be considered as possible offenders, but only after sepsis is treated and metabolic abnormalities are corrected. The verbalizations and visions of the delirious patient are often bizarre, and the staff may have difficulty dealing with their content. As such, they do not represent an emergency. However this psychotic behavior can lead to behaviors that are dangerous to the patient and threatening to their caregivers, such as trying to get out of bed, hitting staff, pulling off dressings, and so on. When these occur, regardless of cause, psychotropic medication may be required if correcting the sepsis or metabolic abnormality does not effect the necessary change. Talking therapy per se is not very useful during this time; however, reassurance and orientation of the patient are very important. Familiar voices are often reassuring and calming.

During delirium, ensure that the patient's pain is adequately treated. Once the pain is managed well, if the patient is still delirious, the alleviation of anxiety should be assisted with a benzodiazapine or phenothiazine [49,50]. For the adult, haloperidol has been used more than any other medication. It is usually effective in dosages of 5 mg repeated as needed. Some major burn centers for young children also use haloperidol liberally [51]. The side effects of haloperidol are significant [52,53] and, in teenagers, are not uncommon in our experience. In cases where haloperidol is to be avoided, higher dosages of lorazapam are used instead. The most frequent side effect of phenothiazines that occur in this clinical setting is a dystonic reaction associated with a stuperous state and/or oculogyric crisis [52,53]. The most dangerous side effect is hyperthermia. This should be treated aggressively with rapid cooling and dantrolene [54].

Sometimes the patients are not delirious but are vocalizing their acute stress disorder symptoms such as illusions, vivid flashbacks, or nightmares. The patients may be literally too afraid to remain in the bed or room. This extreme anxiety should be treated aggressively. The diagnosis of acute stress disorder should be considered. Its identification and treatment are described below.

Family support

An extremely important part of the acute psychological support of the burn victim is the psychological evaluation and support of their immediate family. The family is distressed about the severity of the life-threatening event but also are focused on the losses. Often the loss of the patient's life is not their only fear. They are also focused on the changes in appearance of their loved one. In many instances the family is also distracted by the loss of other loved ones in the fire or loss of property. They may be facing the loss of a wage earner, or the awareness that the costs of medical care may push the family into financial failure. While they are attending to the patient, they are also missing work and may be threatened by the possibility of losing their own jobs. Even at hospitals where the medical care is free of charge to the families, the attendant costs of lost wages, travel expenses, and special arrangements to care for the patient postdischarge can be extremely high and cause family distress. As one mother of a burned child told us, "They quit delivering my mail in the usual way and began bringing it to me in big bags ⋯ almost all bills related to the accident."

Getting well: after the wound is closed

Once the wound is closed, a new series of challenges arises. This protracted phase includes a succession of stages that span several years.

The acute period begins with the patient usually still in the hospital. In this stage immediately postburn, the patient may express a variety of psychiatric or psychological problems [13,56–63]. The most prominent symptom during this period is anxiety, initially related to procedures that hurt, such as dressing change and exercise. During the first year postburn, the child is emotionally labile. He or she experiences rapid shifts in body image, thinking of himself or herself often as his or her preburn self and then being reminded, by a physical limitation or by a response from another person, that that self is different. These cognitive shifts are accompanied by rapid emotional shifts from happiness to anger to depression to happiness. The patient's adjustment occurs within the context of a family that is also changed by the injury. Feelings of guilt or anger related to the traumatic incident can drive family members apart.

The patient begins to realize that he or she is going to live and that his or her body is different. Such simple tasks as bathing the skin or participating in rehabilitation are painful.

Some patients experience depression that requires active cognitive behavioral-based psychotherapy as well as medication. Serotonin reuptake inhibitors are typically chosen because of their safety. However, their metabolism by the cytochrome p450 system raises some question when the patient is still having to receive other medications, such as certain antibiotics or hydrogen pump inhibitors for gastric distress. We usually use a once-a-day antidepressant such as fluoxetine rather than those that require more than daily dosing in order to keep the patient's medication regimen as simple as possible,

After passing through the early adaptation period of recovery, the individual begins to focus more on ordinary tasks of life and less on recovery from burns. The survivor has re-entered society and has begun to incorporate the burn scars into his or her self-image. Re-entry to school or work and society is a major issue.

Behavioral problems during the last two phases of recovery are observed at a mild to moderate rate, reflecting fairly good adjustment in the majority of survivors. Most studies of adults burned as adults document similar outcomes for survivors, with 20–30% of any sample expected to have moderate to severe psychological disturbance [64–74]. After about 2 years, results of standardized tests indicate that the majority of burned children make satisfactory adjustments with no more behavioral problems than age- and gender-matched cohorts of the published, nonclinical reference groups on which the tests were standardized. Also, only 20–30% of the pediatric burn survivors have clinically significant behavior problems [75–88]. Even fewer of those have such severe symptoms that they meet criteria for a psychiatric diagnosis [89].

About the same percentage, (20–30%) of each sample of pediatric burn survivors is additionally handicapped by social difficulties, as indicated by their poor scores on measures of competence, especially social competence [85,89]. There is some overlap, with the same children appearing to have poor competence and behavioral problems, so that 40–50% of any sample can be expected to have significantly high problem scores and/or significantly low competence scores. Of the small numbers of patients who qualify for psychiatric disorder diagnoses, the most frequently given diagnoses are anxiety disorders. During these late stages of recovery, the individual is no longer anxious about painful treatments, of course. Rather the anxieties typically center around social demands, manifesting in separation anxiety and social phobias [89,90].

In addition to posttraumatic stress disorder, other psychiatric illnesses also appear later in the process. Some researchers have found depression to be very prominent [57,91,92]. Others, as well as our own studies, have noted an increase in aggressive, angry behavior rather than depression [93–95]. The duration of these illnesses is not clear. In children, this is of special concern because of the tremendous influence such emotional states can have on the learning that must take place during the maturation process. The implications are not clear, but are suspected to be negative.

Social Reintegration

Families and patients are often ambivalent about leaving the safe environment of the hospital. Patients, including very young children, fear social rejection or ridicule because of their changed abilities or appearance [96–98]. Family members will probably express a desire to protect their patient from rejection or ridicule. Patients may doubt their abilities to resume their former activities. As the time of discharge approaches, anxieties intensify, and patients can be expected to evidence some regressive behaviors that, in turn, can reinforce the family's doubts.

Psychotherapeutic activities of this phase involve education of the patient and family about the difficulties that can be anticipated at discharge. The therapist may assist in problem-solving to develop a repertoire of alternative behaviors to address those problems. The psychotherapist can characterize the concerns as normal and usual, and proceed with a verbal rehearsal of problem solving: just in case without condescending or judging. Issues such as recurrence of symptoms of posttraumatic stress, including sleep disturbance and irritability, or fear of resuming sexual activities should be discussed during the days prior to discharge. This preparatory rehearsal enhances the probability that the patient/family will be less reluctant to ask for help if problems do occur. If problems do not occur, the staff has the opportunity to congratulate the patient/family on their strengths or skills in coping [2].

The re-entry of the burn survivor into society is extremely important to the recovery of a normal life. In addition to preparing a patient and family for discharge, the burn team may also prepare the community to which a patient will return. The community may include extended family, neighbors, church groups, social clubs, a patient's workplace or, in the case of a school-aged pediatric patient, the school. Although there are no empirical data to demonstrate that re-entry programs do, in fact, facilitate reintegration, anecdotal reports and clinical experience suggest that survivors have benefited from such efforts [98,99].

Preparing the school administrators, teachers, and school mates for a child's return can be very helpful to the burn survivor [98,100–103]. In order to do this five issues need to be addressed: preparation should be done as soon as possible; planning must include the family and patient; programs need to be individualized; return should be done as quickly as possible after discharge from the hospital, even if it is only part time; the burn team should be available as consultants to the school [99]. The interaction with the school can be done effectively with either a video picturing the child and his or her treatment or by a direct visit to the school by members of the burn team. Sometimes both are used. These interactions assist the child's peers in more comfortably welcoming the child with his or her new appearance that may involve masks and/or other covering garments. The programs seem to reduce the intense questioning and curiosity that are occasioned when the child returns to school, and, it is hoped, increase the acceptance of the child back into society. Research is needed in this area to refine further the techniques for facilitating reintegration.

The situation with adult survivors is often more complicated. Although there is no evidence that adult burn survivors are in less need of assistance reintegrating into their social worlds, published information about organized re-entry programs for adults is scarce [100,104,105]. Re-entry programs for adults and children involve the same fundamental elements and address the same issues [98]. They educate the community in a developmentally sensitive fashion. They address both the intellectual and emotional aspects of burn injury, provide generic information about burn injuries and burn treatment, and emphasize a survivor's abilities as well as clarify the ways in which a survivor may need assistance.

With adult burn injuries, a number of factors complicate the process for the patient. Many times the injury occurred at work, so there is an associated phobia concerning the work place and posttraumatic stress disorder, (PTSD) is triggered when return is attempted. At other times there is an associated disability issue that augurs significant financial implications to the employer and thereby prevents the patient's return. If return to work is delayed more than 6 months, it often does not happen.

A major effort in the United States to enhance the employability of survivors is being led by the National Institute for Disability and Rehabilitation Research (NIDRR) [106], the principal source of federal funds for burn rehabilitation research. NIDRR's so-called new paradigm for conceptualizing and conducting rehabilitation research places environmental factors on an equal footing with characteristics of the person. This is based on the understanding that an individual may be able to function very effectively in some situations while his or her so-called impairments (e.g., disfigurement, restricted range of motion) only limit him or her in certain situations. Environmental factors are defined broadly to include interpersonal factors (e.g., social support) and socioeconomic structure (e.g. insurance coverage, training opportunities). NIDRR has identified five substantive research areas related to the goals of their long-range plan [106]; employment, community integration, technology for access and function, health and function, and associated disabilities. Among the goals of the research NIDRR will fund are applied programs to enhance access to the physical and social environment by removing barriers to full integration in the community and the workplace. We hope that NIDRR's efforts will result in increased research into interventions that succeed in facilitating the process of reintegration.

Anxiety disorders

Most patients in intensive care settings are anxious. It is the nature of these settings to be loud, very active, and have many intrusions into the patient's world, if for nothing more than to measure vital signs. However, for many reasons the burn patient usually continues to exhibit significant anxiety after leaving the intensive care setting. Patients must adapt to a new view of themselves. They must adapt to what are often painful or at least uncomfortable exercises and/or dressing changes. They are anxious about how they will be accepted by their families as well as the public at large. They often meet the following criteria for generalized anxiety disorder [107]: excessive anxiety and worry for more days than not for at least 6 months; difficulty controlling the worry; anxiety and worry associated with three of more of the following six symptoms—restlessness or feeling keyed up or on edge, being easily fatigued, difficulty concentrating or mind going blank, irritability, muscle tension, sleep disturbance; broad-based worry.

Although most burn care professionals are aware of such pervasive anxieties and may routinely prescribe medications to alleviate anxiety, most do not assess for anxiety in a structured way. In 2000 Robert [108] published a survey of burn units and how they approached anxiety. Eighty-nine percent reported that they did not formally measure anxiety in their patients: they use direct observation and/or dialogue with the patient. Based on our research in preparing to conduct that survey, we chose to use the fear thermometer [109] to assess anxiety.

The treatment for this anxiety can take two forms: psychological and pharmacological. The psychological or social techniques involve imagery and relaxation, whereas medications include minor tranquilizers such as benzodiazapines and antidepressants such as serotonin reuptake inhibitors and tricyclic antidepressants. Both approaches are useful, Benzodiazapin give more immediate relief to the patient whose anxiety is acute. For short-term treatment we use lorazapam; for more chronic treatment we use diazepam, particularly if muscle relaxation is also indicated in the treatment program. If anxiety persists and often takes the form of PTSD, specific phobias, or social phobia then the antidepressants are very useful.

Patients several years post burn, often have phobias. Social phobia is the most common and has eight characteristics [107]: a marked and persistent fear of social or performance situations, social situations provoke anxiety, patient recognizes that his or her fear is excessive, avoidance of social situations, this avoidance interferes with life; duration is at least 6 months; not due to direct physiological effects of substances or general medical condition; fear is not related to the medical condition. Some patients have the same symptoms but related only to specific experiences, such as heights, fire, closed spaces, animals, or insects. These conditions usually require more than just medication, but can demonstrably benefit from psychotherapy such as cognitive–behavior therapy including desensitization.

Sleep Disturbance

Sleep problems are a common complaint of the burn survivor. They first occur on the intensive care unit as part of the frequent and significant interruptions secondary to the care procedures [110–112]. Sometimes this leads to intensive care unit (ICU) psychosis [113]. Sleep polysomnographic studies done at the Cincinnati Shiners Burn Hospital with pediatric burn survivors indicate an adequate length of time in sleep but a reduction in slow-wave sleep and rapid eye movement (REM) [114]. Several groups have reported a relationship between sleep quality and healing [111,115], emphasizing the importance of treating the sleep disorder. One study examined the effect of sleep on energy expenditure in the child recovering from burn injury and found no specific effect of sleep per se [116]. These sleep disorders are sometimes relieved by changing the number of patient interruptions, or the use of short-term sleep inducing medications such as chlorohydrate or benzodiazapines. At other times they are just one of the symptoms of acute stress disorder, which must be directly treated (see below).

Follow up studies in burn survivors indicate the persistence of sleep disorder for months after hospitalization [117–119]. Possible causes of this persistent sleep problem are continued poorly controlled pain related to positioning at night, poorly controlled itching, undiagnosed depression, and Post Traumatic Stress Disorder (PTSD). The treatment of pain with acetaminophin, ibuprofen, or opiates, and the treatment of itch with antihistamines should be addressed first. The specific effects of these medications on polysonography are minor. Some patients also benefit from medications that help with muscle relaxation, such as diazepam, which is known to decrease slow wave sleep.

Acute Stress Disorder and Posttraumatic Stress Disorder

An extremely common complication of the course of recovery from a severe burn injury is the presence of acute stress disorder (ASD). This disorder has several criteria [120]:

> Exposure to a traumatic event in which both of the following were present: the person experienced, witnessed, or was confronted with an event that involved actual or threatened death or serious injury; the person's response involved intense fear, helplessness, or horror.
> The person has developed three or more of the following dissociative symptoms: a subjective sense of numbing, detachment, or absence of emotional responsiveness; a reduction in awareness of surroundings; derealization; depersonalization; dissociative amnesia.
> The event is persistently re-experienced in one of the following ways: recurrent images, thoughts, dreams, illusions, flashbacks, or a sense of reliving the event.
> There is marked avoidance of stimuli that arouse recollections of the trauma.
> There are marked symptoms of anxiety to increased arousal.
> There is clinically significant distress or disruption of life.

The disturbance lasts 2 day within 4 weeks after the event.

The condition is not due to direct physiological effect of a substance.

In our patient population of children, the incidence of ASD ranged from 9 to 13%. More aggressive treatment of pain, generalized anxiety, and itch resulted in a reduction in incidence.

The same criteria apply to posttraumatic stress disorder except that they persists beyond 4 weeks after the event.

Adults who survive trauma frequently also experience emotional sequelae. The best estimate of lifetime prevalence of PTSD in adults is 25% [121], making it one of the most common psychiatric disorders in the United States. Adults with ASD and PTSD were identified after the Viet Nam War. Numerous trials revealed that two classes of drug were useful in treatment: tricyclic antidepressants and serotonin reuptake inhibitors. Clinicians who have documented the use of imipramine with adults who have PTSD symptoms postburn report promising findings, with efficacy rates ranging from 67 to 100% [122]. The dosages associated with response were often lower than those needed for treatment of depression. Fluoxetine's effectiveness in treating patients with PTSD has been examined in at least three open clinical trials. Nagy and colleagues Charney [123] found that fluoxetine significantly reduced all three major symptom categories in veterans with PTSD. Shay [124] concluded that 61% of the veterans responded positively to fluoxetine. In a double-blind placebo–control study, Van der Kolk [125] included civilians with PTSD who had recently experienced a traumatic event. Van der Kolk concluded that fluoxetine was effective and speculated that it would prove to be more effective than previously utilized pharmacotherapies.

Recently Robert has conducted a series of studies in pediatric burn survivors and found a similar response [126]. The acute distress disorder symptoms were resistant to benzodiazapine therapy. The specific medication used was imipramine and it outperformed chlorohydrate, which had previously been used in our hospital for anyone with a sleep disorder [127]. These initial findings suggested that low dosages of imipramine assisted children with ASD symptoms by improving sleep patterns and decreasing the frequency of nightmares. In the past year SSRI's have been used in children with PTSD from a variety of causes. They may not respond as frequently to SSRIs as the adults did [128–130]. The specific SSRIs tested were fluoxitine and sertraline.

LONG-TERM INTERVENTIONS

As described earlier in this chapter, most survivors of burn injury do not experience psychiatric illnesses, and, when they do, they are in the form of anxiety disorders related to social situations. Burn survivors themselves describe their most difficult moments as involving the responses of other people to their appearance. As we obtain more empirical data about pediatric and adult burn survivors, the evidence grows that the most significant limitation on the long-term quality of life for the burn survivor is not in functional impairment of the body [131] but at the interface of the disfigured burn survivor (even if the disfigurement is not easily apparent) and other, nonburned people. The survivor's inhibitions in taking initiative in interpersonal situations is reinforced by rejecting or demeaning attitudes of others. This creates huge barriers to the success of many burn survivors. Thus, the recent work of our team, as well as that of Fauerbach, Lawrence, and their group at Johns Hopkins, has been in studying stigmatization, body image dissatisfaction, and interventions to assist survivors in coping with these social obstacles.

Social Learning Theory

The framework of social learning theory suggests that both diminished social competence and increased behavioral problems (especially the anxiety disorders such as separation anxiety) might be related to coping techniques that burned individuals have utilized in an attempt to deal with their disfigurement. Both behavioral problems and social competence could be improved if the survivors could learn new, and more appropriate, skills in interacting with others. Social learning theory, more specifically social cognitive theory, emphasizes that the individual forms a vision of self and reality through reciprocal interaction (i.e., the impact of the individual upon his or her environment and vice versa) and feedback (the reaction of the environment to the individual) [132]. A person's behavior will determine the aspects of their environment to which they are exposed and to which they attend; and their behavior is, in turn, modified by that environment. Based on learned preferences and competencies, humans select whom they interact with and the activities they participate in from a vast range of possibilities. Human behavior also influences their environment, such as when an aggressive person creates a hostile environment. Thus, the individual's behavior determines which of many potential environmental influences come into play.

Humans evoke diverse reactions from their social environment as a result of their physical characteristics, such as age, size, race, gender, and physical attractiveness. Through interactions with the social environment, the individual forms cognitions: beliefs, values, and expectations used to guide his or her behavior. Cognitions can change over time as a function of maturation and experience (i.e., attention span, memory, ability to form symbols, reasoning skills). The individual's interpretations or perceptions of the reactions of the social environment feed into his or her concepts of self and expectations of the future.

In order to understand how this theory applies to burned individuals, it is helpful to imagine a hypothetical burned child who leaves the hospital in bandages and splints. He returns to school, in spite of his parents' anxieties, feeling timid, and unsure of himself because he knows his body looks and functions differently than it did in the past and differently from others'. In the school cafeteria, he notices that some of the older children stare at him, but look away when he looks at them. He interprets that behavior as indicating that he looks like a freak. When he walks by those children, one of the boys says "Hey, Freddy Krueger," referring to an evil, burned character from a horror film. This is, for the child, further evidence that he looks like a freak or monster. The child begins to incorporate this feedback into his image of himself as he modifies his self-concept to adapt to his burn injuries. With recurrent similar experiences, the burned child is likely to misinterpret any looks from others as being related to his appearance, without considering other possible explanations (such as his own perceptible misery). Because he cannot change his appearance and does not know how to behave to decrease their discomfort, he may well decide that he should not approach people whom he expects to be uncomfortable. He may decide to stay away from other people to the extent possible; he may decide to avoid any situation in which he is likely to call attention to himself; or, he may decide to attack others before they can hurt him. Depending on many factors including what he has learned from watching others, the child will develop strategies to maintain to the degree possible his own comfort. The strategies developed may facilitate successful interactions with others, but they are just as likely to work against his successful adjustment. The more strategies the child develops and the more helpful feedback he receives, the more likely he is to identify strategies that are effective in specific situations involving social interactions.

Although our vignette is written around a typical experience of a child, the same process applies to the adult survivor struggling to become comfortable with a new, dramatically changed body.

Maturational Transition

During the process of maturing from an embryonic self-image to a well-established one, numerous factors have an impact on survivors, both demanding and limiting adaptive change. They must, over time, solve a number of problems. They must define themselves intellectually, emotionally, socially, and sexually; three out of four of these tasks depend heavily upon social skills and techniques for coping well in social situations. Family values provide the anchor for the individual to try on different values, roles, and strategies, but peers are of great influence in the individual's self-definition and self-evaluation. The well-adjusted adult is expected to have a positive self-concept, to continue solid relationships with friends, and to withstand negative peer group influence [133]. Sexual experimentation, control over impulses, and interest in developing emotional intimacy are characteristics of the well-adjusted person [134].

The discussion of social learning and social cognitive theory above shows that there are many reasons to believe that survivors of severe burn injuries, even those who appear well adjusted as children, will be impeded in their abilities to develop into well-adjusted adults. And there are many reasons to expect them to experience a diminished quality of life, suffer psychological pain, and present with symptoms of psychological ill health. Years of rehabilitation and reconstructive surgeries follow the acute injury, and are not only painful physically but also separate the burn survivor from his or her peers. Pressure garments, masks, and splints worn to combat burn scar contractures also call visual attention to the individuals who wear them, further singling them out as different from others. Even after years of work in rehabilitation, disfigurement is the norm for individuals with burn scars. The years of special treatment for the severely burned person create major disruptions for his or her family of and create situations that would be expected to interfere with the survivor's normal psychological development and social integration.

Yet the majority do not develop significant psychopathology. They adapt; but there are indications that they have particular struggles. Only five studies examine the adjustment of adults burned as children. Bowden [135] indicated that adults burned as children had more self-esteem problems than adults burned as adults. Love [136] found in a group of 42 adult survivors of pediatric burns lower adjustment correlated with visible disfigurement and less peer support rather than with severity of burn. Blakeney [83] included survivors as old as 32 (mean age = 19.6) and found most of them to be progressing appropriately for age, with positive adjustment largely dependent on family support. Cain and Cahners [137] reported positive outcomes for a group of 150 young adults (ages 21–38) who had been burned as children. They report positive outcomes to be related to emotional and social support. Sheridan [138] also report generally positive outcomes for young adults who had survived massive burn injuries (total body surface area [TBSA] greater than or equal to 70%), noting that care by a multidisciplinary burn team and family support were important influences in the success of that group.

The family support system emerges as the consistently recognized contributing factor in determining quality of psychosocial adaptation [76,79,83, 139–144] but peer support is also reported as critical [136,137].

Personality characteristics of the child are likely additional predictors of outcome. One study by Moore [145] indicates two personality factors—extroversion and social risk taking—to be highly related to psychosocial adjustment of a sample of burned adolescents. Although the factor of family support accounted for most of the variance, when these two personality characteristics were factored in, more than 80% of the variance in the teens' adjustment outcomes was accounted for. Both extroversion and social risk taking imply skills in social interactions.

One strategy that many burned children seem to employ to adapt to their injuries is to rationalize, denying the importance of those things that they cannot change and turning their attention and energy to areas where they can succeed. In two separate studies, we have found the self-esteem of burned children to be high and not different from the nonburned comparison group [146–148]. Where the burned children did differ from the non-burned children was in the values they placed on the aspects of self they were describing. In comparison to the nonburned adolescents, the burned group rated personal appearance, athletic competence, and social acceptance as less important than scholastic competence, job competence, and romantic appeal.

The findings of diminished social competence among our patients suggest that another strategy they may use in their adaptation to disfigurement is to try not to attract attention: to withdraw and to try to blend in with the background and not excel or otherwise draw attention to oneself. This would explain why symptoms of disturbed behavior in burned children are more likely to be noted by parents (who observe their children in private) than by other observers [87].

Faber and Egeland [149] made the important distinction between competent behavior and emotional health, describing strategies and adaptive behaviors that would earn positive scores on behavioral rating scales (i.e., no significant, observable behavioral problems) but would not be emotionally healthy on measures of internalizing symptoms. This is likely to be the case for burn survivors. A comparison of standardized test scores (representative of the public facade) of burned children with the scores on the Rorschach Ink Blots (representative of the private, internal feelings) indicated the children to be significantly more depressed internally than was apparent externally [150]. It seems likely that persons with severe burns manage their behaviors in such a way that their public observable ''selves'' appear to be healthy while internally they suffer. This would, of course, require social distance from others, including peers and potential role models, and thus impede the availability of social and peer support.

If these deductions are valid, many burned survivors are failing to develop a range of skills, techniques, and strategies to assist them with successfully negotiating the social environment. These adaptive behaviors are critical for the transition to successful adult living.

In summary, successful accomplishment of maturational tasks is heavily dependent upon social skills and techniques for coping well in social situations. Peers are influential in the individuals' self-definitions and self-evaluations. People face a marked disadvantage unless they have developed strategies to elicit peer support, to take social risks, and to overcome social shyness. Burned individuals have the additional burden of scars that differentiate them from their peers and that may attract negative attention. If their strategies for maintaining self-esteem are to withdraw and to tell themselves that social acceptance is unimportant, they cannot satisfactorily develop the capacity for intimate relationships with friends and family. They will be vulnerable to negative peer group influences, lowered self-esteem, and symptoms of psychological distress.

It seems likely that this is an important part of the underlying process for the significant portion of the burned population that exhibits behavioral problems and/or social incompetence. Although from one vantage point it seems remarkable that so many burned persons recover so well, it appears that we have an important opportunity to improve the psychosocial outcomes even more by teaching the skills and strategies that will facilitate their greater success in interpersonal social situations.

Humans have the ability to learn vicariously: to learn not only from direct experience but also from the observation of others. Observational learning allows one to develop an idea of how a new behavior is formed without actually performing the behavior oneself [132]. This information can be used as a guide for future action. Vicarious learning is important in that it enables humans to form patterns of behavior quickly, avoiding time-consuming trial and error. Observational learning is more likely to be effective if the observer can identify with the person they are observing. Through feedback, a person is able to control or adjust their efforts and goals to make them more feasible and realistic. In addition, receiving feedback on performance accomplishments will improve a person's belief in their own ability for that behavior. A third important factor that influences learning via its impact on motivation is the anticipated time to goal attainment. Proximal goals are more effective than distal goals in enlisting motivation. Therefore, we propose an intervention that facilitates observational learning of skills utilized by other persons with disfigurements to interact comfortably in a variety of social situations, provides the subjects with practice and feedback in a supportive atmosphere, and keeps the focus on proximal and attainable goals.

Two studies of older adolescents and young adults reported that 40–50% of the individuals presented as well-adjusted while 50–60% presented with some degree of psychological distress; 25% presented with symptoms severe enough to warrant clinical attention [83–85]. Most of both populations had not undergone separation from their families at the time of study.

Sheridan [138] used the SF-36 to assess the quality of life in a group of 60 adults, average age 24 ± 8, who were pediatric burn survivors treated at the Boston Shriners hospital. These subjects were similar to normal population in all areas except that they had significant physical disability.

More recently we were funded by NIDDR of the Department of Education to study in a cross-sectional manner more than 90 subjects with 30% or greater burns between the ages of 18 and 28 [151]. Their mean IQ was normal with a normal standard deviation. Their current educational status was reflective of the referral population. Most are dating and had had sexual experience; 23% have a current significant other and 10% had children. In terms of employment, 73% are employed and half of the remainder are in school. Compared to reference groups published by Achenbach in 1997 in the YASR Manual [152], the male burn survivors reported significant increases only in the somatic complaints subscale; the female survivors reported significant increases in withdrawn, somatic complaints, thought problems, aggressive behavior, and delinquent behavior subscales [151]. The subjects were further assessed using the Suicide Probability Scale [153], a 36-item, paper and pencil self-report. Burn survivors were compared to three normative samples: normal adults, psychiatric inpatients, and suicide attempters. Elevated suicide probability was not associated with age, years postburn, or percentage TBSA. Although the burn survivor group was found to be significantly more distressed than the normal comparison group, this group is less distressed than both the psychiatric inpatient and suicide attempter groups [154]. Despite being many years postburn, adult survivors of major pediatric burn injury appear to be at greater risk than their nonburned cohorts and to have need for long-term access to mental health services. When the pediatric burn survivors were asked about their personal concerns, 75% mentioned physical, social, or health issues [151]. Overall, most young adult survivors of serious childhood burn injury are functional in work and school and have experience with adult relationships. The women seem to be having more psychosocial problems than the men.

Developmental psychology struggles to define and refine the term resilience in reference to individuals who survive and succeed in some way in spite of mitigating circumstances [155]. Faber and Egeland [149] described strategies and adaptive behaviors that would earn positive scores on behavioral rating scales for individuals who might not be emotionally healthy on measures of internalizing symptoms. Only an in-depth study, which elicits information of both sorts, can help us to understand this phenomenon.

Our society places great emphasis on an individual's ability to meet his or her own self-care needs, such as dressing, feeding, hygiene, and mobility. Persons who experience burns often become dependent, for a time, in these self-care areas. We investigated the self-care skills of the young adults who were pediatric burn survivors. Twenty-six self-care skills were assessed by a physical therapist, and none was found to be related to age at burn; a few of the self-care skills had fair correlations ($r = 0.25–0.38$) with TBSA [156]. The results suggest that a vast majority of children experiencing moderate to severe burns will be able to address their own self-care needs as young adults. These are in agreement with the SF-36 findings of Sheridian [138] and ourselves [157]. In contrast Rosenberg [158] found that young adults who were pediatric burn survivor rated their quality of life at least one standard duration below a reference population in almost all area using the Quality of life Questionnaire by Evans and Cope [159]. In summary, however, the pediatric burn survivors are able to function well in society in spite of their burn scars and other residual physical problems.

Outcome of Intervention

Very few studies have examined the outcome following psychological or social intervention for burn survivors. However, these very limited studies do suggest some potential for success. Studies of chronically ill pediatric camp populations have shown that the camp experience is beneficial in increasing the self-esteem of children. Studies specific to the effectiveness of pediatric burn camps have been limited. CBCL scores, obtained from 55 pediatric burn survivors several months before a 2 week camp, were significantly lower 1 year after the camp experience [160]. The camp utilized age-similar groups to work on real life issues. The decrease was significant for total problems (p = 0.02) and aggressive behavior (p = 0.05). Further analysis revealed that the total group change occurred in boys 12 and 18 years old. Their total problems decreased and externalizing behaviors improved significantly. A matched group of pediatric burn survivors who did not attend camp did not have significant improvement in the CBCL scores over a 1 year period. This study indicates that a focused short intervention can have a measurable impact on a group of burn survivors 1 year later. More recently Rimmer [161] and Gaskell [162] have reported improvement of self-esteem and psychological well-being, respectively, after a burn camp experience. These studies of the effect of burn camp and that of Partridge [163] support the idea that a relative brief intervention focused on life skills can influence adaptive behaviors in adolescents and young adults and therefore support use of such an intervention.

SUMMARY

Psychological support is extremely important for the burn patient and the team of professionals who work with these severely injured population. Although comprehensive psychosocial services are provided at only a few burn centers, psychiatric and psychological staff have a central role in patient care and as members of the multidisciplinary burn team. Many of the problems experienced by patients and families require a combination of psychology and psychiatry. These problems include coping with grief, disfigurement, and functional losses. In addition, these staff are helpful in dealing with problems of adherence, obstacles to decision making, and maladaptive coping. In some hospitals they are in charge of assessing pain and identifying and treating delirium, acute stress disorder, depression, and other psychiatric disorders. The psychological professionals should, on a regular basis, be an integral part of patient rounds with the full multidisciplinary team to assist in treatment and discharge planning. They are helpful in making sure that the planned outpatient setting meets all the patient's needs. One of the major role of such psychosocial personnel is to work with families to understand the illness and the impact of the injury on the person's psychological recovery. In some patients their work is never done. It continues for years postburn as the individual struggles to become integrated back into society and to accept themselves as they now appear with burn scars.

REFERENCES

1. Knudson-Cooper MAdjustment to visible stigma: the case of the severely burned. Soc Sci Med 1981; 15:31–44.
2. Blakeney P, Robert R, Meyer W. Psychological and social recovery of children who have been disfigured by physical trauma: elements of treatment indicated by empirical data. Int. Rev Psychiatry 1998; 10:196–200.
3. Mendelsohn I. Liaison psychiatry and the burn center. Psychosomatics 1983; 24: 235–243.
4. Tucker P. Psychosocial problems among adult burn victims. Burns 1987; 13:7–14.
5. Knudson-Cooper M. Emotional care of the hospitalized burned child. J Burn Care Rehab 1982; 3:109–116.
6. Watkins P, Cook E, Mary R, Ehleben C. Psychological stages in adaptation following burn injury: a method for facilitating psychological recovery of burn victims. J. Burn Care Rehab 1988; 9:376–384.
7. Meyer W, Blakeney P, Robert R, Murphy L. Longitudinal view of psychosocial recovery of pediatric burn survivors and their parents. Proceedings of the 14th International Congress of the International Association for Child and Adolescent Psychiatry and Allied Professions, Abstract #2480–5112, Stockholm, Sweden, Aug. 15, 1998.
8. Shenkman B, Stechmiller J. Patient and family perception of projected functioning after discharge from a burn unit. Heart Lung 1987; 16:490–496.
9. Luther S, Price J. Burns and their psychological effects on children. J Sch Health 1981; 51:419–422.
10. Blakeney P, Moore P, Meyer W, Murphy L, Herndon D. Early identification of long-term problems in the behavioral adjustment of pediatric burn survivors and their parents. Proc Am Burn Assoc: Abstract 27 1995.
11. Meyer W, Murphy L, Robert R, Blakeney P. Changes in adaptive behavior among pediatric burn survivors over time. Proc. Am Burn Assoc: Abstract 84 1998.
12. Thomas C, Ayoub M, Villarreal C, Rosenberg L, Robert R, Meyer W. Attention deficit hyperactivity disorder and pediatric burn injury. Burns, 2004; 30:221–223.
13. Chang F, Herzog B. Burn mortality: a follow-up study of physical and psychological disability. Ann Surg 197; 183:34–37.
14. Vanderplate C. An adaptive coping model of intervention with the severely burn-injured. Int J Psychiatr Med 1984; 14:331–341.
15. Patterson D, Everett J, Bombardier C, Questad K, Lee V, Marvin J. Psychological effects of severe burn injuries. Psychol Bull 1993; 113:362–378.
16. Ward H, Moss R, Darko D. Prevalence of post-burn depression following burn injury. J Burn Care Rehab 1987; 8:294–298.
17. Blakeney P, Meyer W. Psychological aspects of burn care. Trauma Quaterly 1994; 11:166–179.

18. Barillo D, Goode R. Substance abuse in victims of fire. J Burn Care Rehab 1996; 17:71–76.
19. Garcia-Sanchez V, Palao R, Legarre F. Self-inflicted burns. Burns 1994; 20(6): 537–38.
20. Erzurum V, Varcellotti J. Self-inflicted burn injuries. J Burn Care Rehab 1999; 20: 22–24.
21. Stoddard FJ, Pahlavan K, Cahners SS. Suicide attempted by self-immolation during adolescence; I Literature review, case reports, and personality precursors. J Adolesc Psychiat 1985; 12:251–265.
22. Stoddard FJ, Cahners SS. Suicide attempted by self-immolation during adolescence; II Psychiatric treatment and outcome. J Adolesc Psychiatry 1985; 12:266–80.
23. Powers PS, Cruse CW, Boyd F. Psychiatric status, prevention, and outcome in patients with burns: a prospective study. J Burn Care Rehab 2000; 21:85–8.
24. Grobmyer SR, Maniscalco SP, Purdue GF, Hunt JL. Alcohol, drug intoxication, or both at the time of burn injury as a predictor of complications and mortality in hospitalized patients with burns. J Burn Care Rehab 1996; 17:532–9.
25. Ho WS, To EWH, Chan ESY, King WWK. Burn injuries during paint thinner sniffing. Burns 1998; 24:757–59.
26. Sheridan RL. Burns with inhalation injury and petrol aspiration in adolescents seeking euphoria through hydrocarbon inhalation. Burns 1996; 22(7):566–67.
27. Oh SJ, Lee SE, Burm JS, Chung CH, Lee JW, Chang YC, Kim DC. Explosive burns during abusive inhalation of butane gas. Burns 1999; 25:341–44.
28. Van Der Does AJW, Hinderink EMC, Vloemans AFPM, Spinhoven P. Burn injuries, psychiatric disorders and length of hospitalization. J Psychosom Res 1997; 43:431–435.
29. Fauerbach JA, Lawrence J, Haythornthwaite J, McGuire M, Munster A. Preinjury psychiatric illness and postinjury adjustment in adult burn survivors. Acad Psychosom Med 1996; 37:547–55.
30. Fauerbach JA, Lawrence J, Haythornthwaite J, Richter D, McGuire M, Schmidt C, Munster A. Preburn psychiatric history affects posttrauma morbidity. Psychosomatics 1997; 38:374–385.
31. Bowden M, Grant S, Vogel B, Prasad J. The elderly, disabled and handicapped adult burned through abuse and neglect. Burns 1988; 14:447–450.
32. Rathbone-McCuan E. Elderly victims of family violence and neglect. Soc Casework 1980; 61:296–304.
33. Krob M, Johnson A, Jordan M. Burned and battered adults. J Burn Care Rehab 1986; 7:529–531.
34. Purdue G, Hunt J. Adult assault as a mechanism of burn injury. Arch Surg 1990; 125:268–269.
35. Sukosky DG. Elder abuse: a preliminary profile of abusers and the abused. Fam Violence Sexual Assault Bull 1992; 8:23–26.
36. Pedrick-Cornell C, Gelles RJ. Elder abuse: the status of current knowledge. Fam Rel 1982; 31:457–465.
37. Fulmer T. Elder mistreatment: progress in community detection and intervention. Fam Commun Health 199; 14:24–26.

38. Robert R, Blakeney P, Herndon D. Abuse, neglect and fire setting: when burn injury involves reporting to a safety officer. Second Edition In Herndon DN, Ed Total Burn Care. London: W. B. Saunders Company, Harcourt Publishers Limited, 2002:774–782.

39. Hight D, Bakalar H, Lloyd J. Inflicted burns in children: recognition and treatment. JAMA 197; 242:517–520.

40. Teague R, Meyer W, Bishop S, Robert R. Assessing abuse and neglect in burn injury. ISBI Abstract, Seattle, WA, August, 2002.

41. Weimer C, Goldfarb I, Slater H. Multidisciplinary approach to working with burn victims of child abuse. J Burn Care Rehab 1988; 9:79–82.

42. Doctor M. Abuse through burns. In Carrougher G, Ed Burn Care and Therapy. St. Louis. MO: CV Mosby, 1998:359–380.

43. Giardino A, Christian C, Giardino E. A Practical Guide to the Evaluation of Child Physical Abuse and Neglect, Thousand Oaks. CA: Sage Publications, 1997:74–96.

44. Rivara F. Developmental and behavioral issues in childhood injury prevention. Dev Behav Pediatr 1995; 16:362–370.

45. Bakalar H, Moore J, Hight D. Psychosocial dynamics of pediatric burn abuse. Health Soc Work 1981:27–32.

46. Hammond J, Perez-Stable A, Ward C. Predictive value of historical and physical characteristics for the diagnosis of child abuse. South Med J 1991; 84:166–168.

47. Andreasen N, Nayes P, Hartford C. Factors influencing adjustment of burn patients during hospitalization. Psychosom Med 1972; 34:517–525.

48. Steiner H, Clark W. Psychiatric complications of burned adults: a classification. J. Trauma 1977; 17:134–143.

49. Moore DP. Rapid treatment of delirium in critically ill patients. Am J Psychiatry 1977; 134:1431–1432.

50. Teicher MH, Glod CA. Neuroleptic drugs: indications and guidelines for their rational use in children and adolescents. J Child Adolesc Psychopharmacol 1990; 1:33–56.

51. Brown R, Henke A, Greenhalgh D, Warden G. The use of haloperidol in the agitated, critically ill pediatric patient with burns. J Burn Care Rehab 1996; 17:34–38.

52. Huang V, Figge H, Demling R. Haloperidol in burn patients. J Burn Care Rehab 1987; 8:269–273.

53. Still J, Friedman B, Law E, Deppe S, Epperly N, Orlet H. Neuroleptic malignant syndrome in a burn patient. Burns 1998; 24:573–575.

54. May DC, Morris SW, Stewart RM. Neuroleptic malignant syndrome: response to dantrolene sodium. J Clin Psychiatry 1991; 48:739–745.

55. Meyer W. Psychosocial Factors of the Child and Famiy. Agency for HealthCare Research and Quality and ABA. Leesburg. VA: Research Development/Consensus Conference, November 7–8, 2001.

56. Bergman A, Fritz G. Psychiatric and social work collaboration in a pediatric chronic illness hospital. Soc Work Health Care 1982; 7:45–55.

57. Kavanagh C. Psychological intervention with the severely burned child: report of an experimental comparison of two approaches and their effects on psychological sequelae. J Am Acad Child Psychol 1983; 22:145–156.

58. Meyer W, Blakeney P. Psychiatric disorders associated with burn injury In Total Burn Care D. N. Herndon, Ed. London: W. B. Saunders, 1995:544–549.

59. Pavlovsky P. Occurrence and development of psychopathologic phenomena in burned persons and their relation to severity of burns, age and premorbid personality. Acta Chir Plast 1972; 14:112–119.

60. Stoddard FJ, Norman DK, Murphy M, Beardslee WR. Psychiatric outcome of burned children and adolescents. J Am Acad Child Adolesc Psychiatry 1989; 28: 589–595.

61. Tarnowski K, Rasnake L, Drabman R. Behavioral assessment and treatment of pediatric burn injuries: a review. Behav Ther 1987; 18:417–441.

62. Thompson R. Where we stand: twenty years of research on pediatric hospitalization and health care. Child Health Care 1986; 14:200–210.

63. Zetterstrom R. Responses of children to hospitalization. Acta Paediatr Scand 1984; 73(3):289–295.

64. Andreasen N, Norris A, Hartford C. Incidence of long-term psychiatric complications in severely burned adults. Ann Surg 1971; 174:785–783.

65. Andreasen N, Norris A. Long-term adjustment and adaptation mechanisms in severely burned adults. J Nerv Ment Dis 1972; 154:352–362.

66. Bernstein NR. Psychosocial results of burns: the damaged self-image. Clin Plastic Surg 1982; 9:337–346.

67. Bernstein N. Marital and sexual adjustment of severely burned patients. Med Aspects Human Sexuality 1985; 19:91–101.

68. Blumenfield M, Reddish P. Identification of psychologic impairment in patients with mild-moderate thermal injury: Small burn, big problem. Gen Hosp Psychiatry 1987; 9:142–146.

69. Kjaer G. Psychiatric aspects of thermal burns. Northwest Med, 1969; 68:537–41.

70. Mlott S, Libra F, Miller W. Psychological assessment of the burn patient. J Clin Psychiatry 1977; 33:425–430.

71. Simons R, Green L, Malin R, Suskind D, Frank H. The burn victim: his psychosocial profile and post-injury career. Burns 1979; 5:97–100.

72. Malt U. Long-term psychosocial follow-up studies of burned adults: review of the literature. Burns 1980; 6:190–197.

73. Roca R, Spence R, Munster A. Posttraumatic adaptation and distress among adult burn survivors. Am J Psychiatry 199; 149:1234–1238.

74. Williams E, Griffiths T. Psychological consequences of burn injury. Burns 1991; 17:478–480.

75. Meyer W, Robert R, Murphy L, Blakeney P. Evaluating the psychosocial adjustment of 2- and 3-year-old pediatric burn survivors. J Burn Care Rehab 2000; 21:179–184.

76. Davidson T, Bowden M, Feller I. Social support and post-burn adjustment. Arch Phys Med Rehab 1981; 62:274–277.

77. Seligman R, MacMillan B, Carrol S. The burned child: a neglected area of psychiatry. Am J Psychiatry 1971; 128:84–89.

78. Knudson-Cooper M. The antecedents and consequences of children's burn injuries. Adv Dev Behav Pediatr 1984; 5:33–74.

79. Byrne C, Love B, Browne B, Roberts J, Steiner D. The social competence of children following burn injury: a study of resilience. J Burn Care Rehab 1986; 7:247–252.

80. Brown B, Roberts J, Browne G, Byrne C, Love B, Steiner D. Gender differences in variables associated with psychosocial adjustment to a burn injury. Res Nursing Health 1988; 11:23–30.

81. Knudson-Cooper M, Thomas C. Psychosocial care of the severely burned child. In Carvajal H , Parks D, Eds Burns in Children: Pediatric Burn Management. Chicago. IL: Year Book Medical Publishers, 1988:345–362.

82. Tarnowski K, Rasnake L, Linscheid T, Mulick J. Behavioral adjustment of pediatric burn victims. J Pediatr Psychiatry 1989; 14:607–615.

83. Blakeney P, Herndon DN, Desai MH, Beard S, Wales-Seale P. Long-term psychosocial adjustment following burn injury. J Burn Care Rehab 1988; 9:661–665.

84. Blakeney P, Meyer W, Moore P. Psychosocial sequelae of pediatric burns involving 80% or greater total body surface area. J Burn Care Rehab 1993; 14:684–689.

85. Blakeney P, Meyer W, Moore P, Broemeling L, Hunt R, Robson M, Herndon D. Social competence and behavioral problems of pediatric survivors of burns. J Burn Care Rehab 1993; 14:65–72.

86. Meyer W, LeDoux J, Blakeney P, Herndon D. Diminished adaptive behaviors among pediatric burn survivors. J Burn Care Rehab 1995; 9:511–518.

87. Meyer W, Blakeney P, Moore P, Murphy L, Robson M, Herndon D. Inconsistencies in psychological assessment of children post major burn. J Burn Care Rehab 1995; 9:559–568.

88. Meyer W, Doctor M, Robert R, Murphy L, McShan S, Blakeney P. Psychosocial outcome of 327 pediatric burn survivors. Proceedings, American Burn Association 1997.

89. Blakeney P, Thomas C, Berniger F, Holzer C, Meyer W. Long term psychiatric disorders in adolescent burn survivors. European Burns Association, Lyon, France, Abstract 41, 2001.

90. Stoddard FJ, Norman DK, Murphy M. A diagnosis outcome study of children and adolescents with severe burns. J Trauma 1989; 29:471–477.

91. Campbell J, LaClave L. Clinical depression in pediatric burn patients. Burns 1987; 13:213–217.

92. Miller W, Gardner N, Mlott S. Psychosocial support in the treatment of severely burned patients. J Trauma 1976; 16:722–725.

93. Martin H. Parents' and children's reactions to burns and scalds in children. Br J Med Psychol 1970; 43:183–191.

94. Sutherland S. Burned adolescents' descriptions of their coping strategies. Heart Lung 1988; 17:150–156.

95. Blakeney P, Moore P, Meyer W, Broemeling L, Robson M, Herndon D. Are burned adolescents more depressed than non-burned adolescents?. Proceedings, Amer Burn Association 1992.

96. Langlois JH, Downs AC. Peer relations as a function of physical attractiveness: the eye of the beholder or behavioral reality?. Child Dev 1979; 50:409–418.

97. Barden RC. The effects of cranio-facial deformity, chronic illness, and physical handicaps on patient and familial adjustment: research and clinical perspectives. In Lahey BB , Kazdin AE, Eds Advances in Clinical Child Psychology. Vol. 13. New York: Plenum, 1990:343–375.

98. Blakeney P. School reintegration. In K. Tarnowski, Ed Behavioral Aspects of Pediatric Burns, Plenum Press. 1994:217–241.

99. Blakeney P, Moore P, Meyer W, Bishop B, Murphy L, Robson M, Herndon D. Efficacy of school of reentry programs. J Burn Care Rehab 1995; 16:469–472.

100. Dobner D, Mitani M. Community reentry program. J Burn Care Rehab 1988; 9: 420–421.

101. Stein J. Comments from Maricopa Medical Center, Phoenix. J Burn Care Rehab 1988; 9:418–419.

102. Cahners S. A strong hospital–school liaison: a necessity for good rehabilitation planning for disfigured children. Scand J Plast Reconstr Surg 1979; 13:167–168.

103. Doctor ME. Returning to school after a severe burn. In J. A. Boswick, Ed The art and science of burn care, Aspen Press. 1987:323–328.

104. Walls Rosenstein DL. A school reentry program for burned children. Part I: Development and implementation of a school reentry program. J Burn Care Rehab 1987; 8:319–322.

105. Blumenfield M, Schoeps M. Reintegrating the healed burned adult into society: Psychological problems and solutions. Clin Plast Surg 1992; 19:599–605.

106. National Institute on Disability and Rehabilitation Research. Long Range Plan and the New Paradigm. NIDRR, 1999.

107. Liebowitz M, Barlow D, Ballenger J, Davidson J, Foa E, Fyer A, Koopman C, Kozak M, Spiegel D. DSM-I. V. anxiety disorders: Final overview. In Widiger T , Frances A , Pincus H , Ross R , First M , Davis W , Kline M(), Eds DSM-IV Sourcebook, American Psychiatric Association. 1998; 4:1047–1076.

108. Robert R, Blakeney P, Villarreal C, Meyer WJ. Anxiety: Current practices in assessment and treatment. Burns 2000; 26(6):549–552.

109. Silverman W, Kurtines W. Anxiety and Phobic Disorders: A Pragmatic Approach. NY: Plenum Press, 1996.

110. Shilo L, Dagan Y, Smorjik, et al Y. Patients in the intensive care unit suffer from lack of sleep associated with the loss of normal melatonin secretion pattern. Am J Med Sci 1999; 317:278–281.

111. Krachman SL, D'Alono GE, Criner GJ. Sleep in the intensive care unit. Chest 1995; 107:1713–1720.

112. Culpeper RK, Bairnsfather L. A description of night sleep patterns in the critical care unit. Heart Lung 1988; 17:35–42.

113. Easton C, MacKenzie F. Sensory–perceptual alternations: delirium in the intensive care unit. Heart Lung 1988; 17:237.

114. Gottschlich MM, Jendins ME, Mayes T, Khoury J, Kramer M, Warden GD, Kagan RJ. A prospective clinical study of the polysomnographic stages of sleep after burn injury. J Burn Care Rehab 1994; 15:486–492.

115. Rose M, Sanford A, Thomas C, Opp MR. Factors altering the sleep of burned children. Sleep 2001; 24:45–51.

116. Gottschlich MM, Jenkins M, Mayes T, Khoury J, Kagan R, Wardin GD. Lack of effect of sleep on energy expenditure and physiologic measures in critically ill burn patients. J Am Diet Assoc 1997; 97:131–139.

117. Lawrence JW, Fauerbach J, Eudell E, Ware L, Munster A. Sleep disturbance after burn injury: a frequent yet understudied complication. J Burn Care Rehab 1998; 19:480–486.

118. Kravitz M, McCoy B, Tompkins D, Daly W, Mulligan J, Robert McCauley J, Robson M, Herndon D. Sleep disorders in children after burn injury. JBurn Care Rehab 1993; 14:83–90.
119. Boeve SA, Aaron LA, Martin-Herz SP, Peterson A, Cain V, Heimbach DM, Patterson DR. Sleep disturbance after burn injury. J Burn Care Rehab 2002; 23:32–38.
120. Marshall R, Spitzer R, Liebowitz M. Review and critique of the new DSM-IV diagnosis of acute stress disorder. Am J Psychiatry 1999; 156(11):1677–1685.
121. Robins L, Helzer J, Croughan J, Ratcliff K. National Institute of Mental Health interview schedule. Arch Gen Psychiatry 1981; 38:381–389.
122. Frank J, Kosten T, Giller E, Dan E. A randomized clinical trial of phenelzine and imipramine for PTSD. Am J Psychiatry 1988; 145:759–769.
123. Nagy L, Morgan C, Southwick S, Charney D. Open prospective trial of fluoxetine for posttraumatic stress disorder. J Clin Psychopharmacol 1993; 13:107–113.
124. Shay J. Fluoxetine reduces explosiveness and elevates mood on Vietnam combat vets with PTSD. J Traumatic Stress 1992; 5:97–110.
125. Van der Kolk B, Dryfuss D, Michaels M, Shera D, Berkowitz R, Fisler R, Sax G. Fluoxetine in posttraumatic stress disorder. J Clin Psychiatry 199; 55:517–522.
126. Robert R, Villarreal C, Blakeney P, Meyer W. An approach to timely treatment of acute stress disorder. J Burn Care Rehab 1999; 20:250–258.
127. Robert R, Blakeney P, Villarreal C, Rosenberg L, Meyer W. Imipramine treatment in pediatric burn patients with symptoms of acute stress disorder: A pilot study. J Am Acad Child Adolesc Psychiatry 199; 38:873–882.
128. Seed S, Stein D, Ziervogel C, Middleton T, Kaminer D, Emsley R, Rosouw W. Comparison of response to a selective serotonin reuptake inhibitor in children, adolescents, and adults with posttraumatic stress disorder. J Child Adolesc Psychopharmcol 2002; 12:37–46.
129. Brady K, Pearlstein T, Asnis G, Baker D, Rothbaum B, Cikes C, Farfel G. Efficacy and safety of sertraline treatment of posttraumatic stress disorder. JAMA 2000; 283:1837–1844.
130. Donnelly C, Amaya-Jackson L, March J. Psychopharmacology of pediatric posttraumatic stress disorder. J Child Adolesc Psychopharmcol 1999; 9:203–220.
131. Meyers-Paal R, Blakeney P, Murphy L, Robert R, Chinkes D, Meyer W, Desai M, Herndon D. Physical and psychological rehabilitation outcomes for pediatric patients who suffer > 80% total body surface area burn and > 70% 3rd degree burns. J Burn Care Rehab 2000; 43–49(1, Pt. 1).
132. Bandura A. Social Cognitive Theory. In Vasta R, Ed Annals of Child Development, Jai Press. 1989; 6:1–60.
133. Mannarino AP. The development of children's friendships. In Foot HC, Chapman AJ, Smith JR, Eds, Friendships and social relations in children. John Wiley & Sons. 1980:45–63.
134. Vaughan V, Litt I. Child and Adolescent Development, WB Saunders. 1990.
135. Bowden L, Feller I, Tholen D, Davidson T, James M. Self-esteem of severely burned patients. Arch of Phys Med Rehab 1980; 61:449–452.
136. Love B, Byrne C, Roberts J, Browne G, Brown B. Adult psychological adjustment following childhood injury: the effect of disfigurement. J Burn Care Rehab 1987; 8:280–285.

137. Cain LP, Cahners S. The Psychosocial impact of childhood burns: The adult's perspective. Proc Am Burn Assoc 28: abstract #131.

138. Sheridan R, Hinson M, Liang M, Nackel A, Schoenfeld DA, Ryan C, Mulligan J, Tompkins R. Long-term outcome of children surviving massive burns. JAMA 2000; 283:69–73.

139. Andriaenssen P, Boeck W, Gilles B, Meertens S, Nijs P, Pyck K. Impact of facial burns on the family. Scand J Plastic Reconstr Surg 1987; 21:303–305.

140. Knudson-Cooper M, Leuchtag A. The stress of a family move as a precipitating factor in children's burn accidents. J Human Stress 1982; 8:32–38.

141. LeDoux J, Blakeney P, Meyer W, Herndon D. Relationships between parental emotional states, family environment and behavioral adjustment of pediatric burn survivors. Burns 1998; 24:425–432.

142. Sawyer M, Minde K, Zuker R. The burned child — scarred for life? A study of psychosocial impact of burn injury at different developmental stages. Burns 1982; 9:205–213.

143. Meyer W, Blakeney P, Moore P, Murphy L, Robson M, Herndon D. Parental well-being; and behavioral adjustment of pediatric burn patients. J Burn Care Rehab 1994; 15:62–68.

144. Blakeney P, Moore P, Broemeling L, Hunt R, Herndon D, Desai M, Robson M. Parental stress as a cause and effect of pediatric burn injuries. J Burn Care Rehab 1993c; 14:73–79.

145. Moore P, Blakeney P, Broemeling L, Portman S, Herndon D, Robson M. Psychologic adjustment after childhood burn injuries as predicted by personality traits. J Burn Care Rehab 1993; 14:80–82.

146. LeDoux J, Meyer W, Blakeney P, Herndon D. Positive self-regard as a coping mechanism for pediatric burn survivors. J Burn Care Rehab 1996; 17:472–476.

147. Robert R, Blakeney P, Meyer W. Impact of disfiguring burn scars on adolescent sexual development. J Burn Care Rehab 1998; 19:430–435.

148. Robert R, Meyer W, Bishop S, Rosenberg L, Murphy L, Blakeney P. Disfiguring burn scars and adolescent self-esteem. Burns 1999; 25:581–585.

149. Faber E, Egeland B. Invulnerability among abused and neglected children. In Anthony EJ , Cohler BJ, Eds The Vulnerable Child, Guilford Press. 1987:253–288.

150. Holaday M, Blakeney P. A comparison of psychologic functioning in children and adolescents with severe burns on the Rorshach and the Child Behavior Checklist. J Burn Care Rehab 1994; 15:412–415.

151. Luthar S, Zigler E. Vulnerability and competence: a review of research on resilience in childhood. Am J Orthopsychiatry 1991; 61:6–22.

152. Achenbach TM. Manual for the Young Adult Self-Report and Young Adult Behavior Checklist, University of Vermont Dept of Psychiatry. 1997.

153. Cull JG, Gill WS. Suicide Probability Scale. Los Angeles. CA: Western Psychological Services, 1988.

154. Robert R, Berniger F, Thomas C, Blakeney P, Holzer C, Meyer W. Suicide probability in young adult survivors of pediatric burn injury. ISBI abstract, August 2002.

155. Luthar S, Zigler E. Vulernability and competence : a review of research on resilence in childhood. Am J Orthopsychiatry 1991; 61:6–22.

156. Baker C, Meyer W. Self-care skills of young adults burned as children. ISBI Abstract, August 2002.
157. Baker C, Mossberg K, Meyer W, Brown J, Ehlig A, Spencer H. Perceived health status of young adults burned as children. ISBI Abstract, August 2002.
158. Rosenberg M, Berniger F, Robert R, Thomas C, Holzer C, Blakeney P, Meyer W. Quality of life of eighty-five young adults having survived pediatric burn injury. Abstract, 9th Congress of the European Burn Assoc Lyon, France, 2001.
159. Evans DR, Cope WE. Manual for the Quality of Life Questionnaire. North Tonawanda. NY: Multi-Health Systems, Inc, 1989.
160. Doctor M, Meyer W, McShan S, Murphy L, Blakeney P. Burn camp: impact of psychosocial adjustment. 29th Annual meeting of the American Burn Association, New York City, 1997.
161. Rimmer R, Fornaciari GM, Caruso DM, Foster KN, Bay RC, Critt JT. The impact of a pediatric residential burn camp experience on burn survivor's perceptions toward self and attitudes regarding the camp community. Abstract, 9th Congress of the European Burns Assoc Lyon, France, 2001.
162. Gaskell SL. The impact of a burn camp on children's psychological well-being: a quantitative evaluation. Abstract. Lyon. France: European Burns Association, 2001.
163. Robinson E, Rumsey N, Partridge J. An evaluation of the impact of social interaction skills training for facially disfigured people. Br J Plast Surg 1996; 49:281–289.

Index

Note: Page numbers followed by f indicate figures; page numbers followed by p indicate pictures; and page numbers followed by t indicate tables.